WHAT YOU MUST KNOW ABOUT
VITAMINS, MINERALS, HERBS & MORE

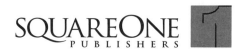

PAMELA WARTIAN SMITH, MD, MPH

SQUAREONE
PUBLISHERS

EDITOR: Ariel Colletti
COVER DESIGNER: Jeannie Tudor
TYPESETTER: Gary A. Rosenberg

The information and advice contained in this book are based upon the research and the personal and professional experiences of the author. They are not intended as a substitute for consulting with a health care professional. The publisher and author are not responsible for any adverse effects or consequences resulting from the use of any of the suggestions, preparations, or procedures discussed in this book. All matters pertaining to your physical health should be supervised by a health care professional. It is a sign of wisdom, not cowardice, to seek a second or third opinion.

Square One Publishers
115 Herricks Road
Garden City Park, NY 11040
(516) 535-2010 • (877) 900-BOOK
www.squareonepublishers.com

Library of Congress Cataloging-in-Publication Data

Smith, Pamela Wartian.
    What you must know about vitamins, minerals, herbs, and more /
Pamela Wartian Smith.
        p. cm.
    ISBN-13: 978-0-7570-0233-5 (quality pbk.)
    ISBN-10: 0-7570-0233-1 (quality pbk.)
    1. Naturopathy. 2. Dietary supplements. 3. Herbs—Therapeutic use.
4. Vitamins. 5. Nutrition. 6. Self-care, Health. I. Title.

    RZ440.S58   2008
    613—dc22

                                                    2007035197

Printed in Canada

10   9   8   7   6   5   4   3   2

Contents

Part 2 Health Conditions

Part 3   Maintaining Health

In memory of my father, Charles Wartian,
who taught me to never give up on my dreams.

Acknowledgments

The wisdom of so many fine people has led me to this book. I cannot hope to name them all. In thanking a few, I extend my thanks to all.

To Roger Williams and Linus Pauling, who were the forerunners in the field of orthomolecular/functional medicine.

To my contemporaries, Billie Sahley, David Perlmutter, Robert Crayhon, Steven Sinatra, Alan Gaby, Johnathan Wright, Ronald Klatz, Robert Goldman, Leo Galland, Michael Schmidt, Shari Lieberman, Mark Houston, Patrick Quillin, and Eric Braverman, who have taught me so much.

To Rudy Shur, Ariel Colletti, Joanne Abrams, and Marie Caratozzolo at Square One Publishers, for their hard work and dedication to this project.

To Jeffrey Bland, whose brilliance not only has instructed me but has rekindled my love for medicine.

To my husband, Christopher Smith, for his enduring patience and support.

To God, for always lighting my path.

Introduction

D o you need to take vitamins and other nutrients? In what amounts should you take them? Which supplements are the most effective? What should you take for a specific illness or chronic problem? Answering these questions is a fundamental aspect of good health and longevity—but there are so many countering viewpoints regarding nutrients and nutrient supplementation that it can be hard to know what to do. This book will provide you with the critical information necessary to find the answers that are right for you.

Various health committees have attempted to provide nutritional guidelines. The Food and Nutrition Board of the National Academy of Science, for example, developed its recommended daily allowance (RDA) and its reference daily intake (RDI). However, these dietary suggestions, which are often strictly adhered to by well-meaning individuals, are designed to prevent disease. They are not designed to help people achieve optimal wellness—which should be the goal.

Furthermore, the RDA and RDI were developed without considering that each person requires a different amount of vitamins, minerals, and other nutrients. To fully promote your body's health, your nutritional intake must reflect such factors as medications, vitamin interactions, soil depletion, need for more antioxidants, stress, age, lifestyle, and genetics. Therefore, you cannot trust that your healthy friend's nutritional plan will necessarily work for you. Dr. Linus Pauling first described this phenomenon in 1968.

Proper determination of what your body needs is imperative. Almost 75 percent of your health and life expectancy is based on lifestyle, environment, and nutrition. Just as importantly, these factors also greatly influence the number of years you spend healthy. This has been proven by studies which show that "not only do persons with better health habits

1

survive longer, but in such persons, disability is postponed and compressed into fewer years at the end of life." An article in the *New England Journal of Medicine* illustrated this point. After examining diet, lifestyle, and the risk of type 2 diabetes mellitus in women, the author concluded that the majority of type 2 diabetes cases are preventable with the adoption of a healthy lifestyle.

Similarly, researchers in the *Journal of the American Medical Association* stated, "Suboptimal vitamin states are associated with many chronic diseases including cardiovascular disease, cancer, and osteoporosis. It is important for physicians to identify patients with poor nutrition or other reasons for increased vitamin needs." They suggested that, "Most people do not consume an optimal amount of all vitamins by diet alone...it appears prudent for all adults to take vitamin supplements."

What You Must Know About Vitamins, Minerals, Herbs, and More provides the information you need to know about nutrients—including signs of deficiencies, how to treat various diseases and disorders, and the dangers of certain interactions. It will allow you to make informed decisions, optimize your health, and live your life well.

The Purpose
of this Book

Many people claim that good health is their top priority. They may eat healthy foods, exercise vigorously, and visit their doctor on a regular basis. Unfortunately, in today's society, these good habits aren't enough to maintain optimal health. As you read on page 1, vitamins and minerals have a direct effect on both life span and quality of life—and modern-day food does not contain all the essential nutrients.

There are several reasons why you can't get all the nutrients you need from food. Most soil is now depleted of many important minerals, including zinc and magnesium. Selenium, a trace mineral that contributes to good health in small amounts but can be toxic in large amounts, is depleted in some areas while in overabundance in others. If the soil in which fruits and vegetables are grown is not rich in the proper minerals, then these foods will not contain an adequate supply of nutrients.

Also, fruits and vegetables begin to lose their nutritional value immediately after they are picked. Cold storage continues this destruction of nutrients. Stored grapes, for example, lose up to 30 percent of their B vitamins by the time they arrive in most grocery stores. When tangerines are stored for eight weeks, they lose almost half of their vitamin C. Storing asparagus for one week can cause it to lose up to 90 percent of its vitamin C. The best and most effective time to eat fruits and vegetables is immediately after they are picked. Unfortunately, most of us are not in a position to do so.

Cold storage is usually not good for maintaining the nutritive value of food, but neither is cooking. In fact, the longer you cook fruits and vegetables, the less nutrients remain. Therefore, you should try to eat these foods raw or lightly steamed, and, if possible, soon after they are picked.

Along with cooking, most of the other processes by which food today is prepared destroys any nutritional value it may have retained after being

3

picked. Foods are processed, blanched, sterilized, canned, and frozen. These processes all decrease nutritional value. The milling of grains, for example, removes twenty-six essential nutrients and much of their fiber.

Because so much of the food we eat is deprived of essential vitamins and minerals, we must look elsewhere for these nutrients. In today's society, the consumption of supplements has become fundamental for good health. *What You Must Know About Vitamins, Minerals, Herbs, and More* will assist you in choosing the nutrients to keep you and your family healthy. It will also help you discover other nutrient-rich foods.

Unfortunately, however, even eating a nutrient-rich food does not guarantee that you are receiving the nutrients you need. The nutrients may not be in a form that is *bioavailable*—able to absorbed and utilized by the body. Despite the healthy perception of orange juice, for example, 40 percent of its vitamin C is biologically inactive. Yet most nutritional listings do not differentiate between nutrients that are biologically available and those that are biologically unavailable, leaving many health-conscious consumers in the dark.

There are also processes within your body that necessitate the constant refueling of nutrients. *Free radicals* are molecules created in the body by reactions that occur to produce energy and other substances. These molecules lack electrons. They search the body for healthy cells and steal their electrons, modifying or killing the cells as a result. This process, called *oxidation,* causes *oxidative stress,* which can lead to tissue damage, disease, and aging. Today, free radical production requires more nutrients to avoid this harmful oxidative stress than in previous generations—further increasing the importance of good nutrition.

Yet free radicals also occur in the environment. In fact, they now occur in the environment more than ever before. Causes of free radical production outside the body include television screens; cell phones; computer screens; airplane trips; hair dryers; fluorescent lights; microwaves; toxic exposure to chemicals in food, water, and air; and excessive sunlight.

This exposure to free radicals in the environment causes an extra load of oxidation that the body cannot handle. Oxidation in your body is like rust on your car. If extra free radicals are bombarding your body all day long, your system can "rust" on the inside. There may be physical results, such as cataract formation or sunburns. To stop the oxidative process, you can take *antioxidants,* which donate an electron to the free radical and help stop the destructive course.

There are different antioxidants that can be consumed to diminish oxidation. It is paramount that they be balanced. In certain conditions, too much of one antioxidant may hinder the protective effects of other antioxidants. Examples of antioxidants are vitamin A, vitamin C, vitamin E, selenium, coenzyme Q_{10}, alpha-lipoic acid, melatonin, garlic, and glutathione. I will describe these important antioxidants in further detail later in this book.

As you age, your body makes less vitamin D, alpha-lipoic acid, and coenzyme Q_{10}. Your body needs to find these nutrients elsewhere. As you will discover in later chapters, you can help your body age more comfortably by providing these nutrients in abundance. You will also read suggestions on which ones to consume.

The American Diet

According to most top nutritionists, the American diet is a serious cause for concern. As children develop, it is very important that they both receive necessary nutrients and learn healthy eating habits. Unfortunately, this is not the case for most American children. The following is an eye-opening list of the top three vegetables eaten by American children and teens.

- French fries—which account for 25 percent of all the vegetables they consume.
- Iceberg lettuce—which is 99-percent water with no nutritional value.
- Ketchup—which is one-half sugar.

Adults do not fare much better. The Second National Health and Nutrition Examination (NHANES II) conducted a survey which revealed the following.

- Less than 10 percent of Americans consume five servings of fruits and vegetables each day.
- 40 percent of Americans do not consume daily fruit or fruit juice.
- 50 percent of Americans do not consume daily garden vegetables.
- 70 percent of Americans do not consume daily fruit or vegetables rich in vitamin C.
- 80 percent of Americans do not consume daily fruit or vegetables rich in carotenoids.

Lifestyle is yet another factor that influences your need for vitamins. Stress, for example, depletes the body of certain vitamins and minerals, while drinking alcohol depletes the body of biotin, copper, zinc, and vitamins B_1, B_6, B_{12}, and C. Our eating habits can also cause major nutritional problems. As Dr. Michael Colgan states in his book *The New Nutrition*, "[T]he American diet is a major cause of disease." The American diet is examined in the inset on page 5.

Diet and nutrition play a major role in influencing how your genes express themselves. As Dr. Leo Galland pointed out, "It depends as much upon the milieu in which a gene functions as it does upon the DNA sequence of the genome." Therefore, even if you have inherited a gene for a particular illness such as Alzheimer's disease, whether the disease manifests itself depends on your environment, the food you eat, the toxins you are around, your stress level, and the nutrients your body receives. Dr. Roger Williams discusses this situation in his book *Biochemical Individuality: The Basis for the Genotropic Concept.* He states, "Nutrition applied with due concern for individual genetic variations, which may be large, offers the solution to many baffling health problems." Let's again compare your body to a car. If you feed it good fuel (nutritious food), it will run well, need little repair, and last a long time. If you put low octane fuel in your premium car (your body), it will not run well (develop disease and shorten life expectancy).

Some physicians say there is a lack of peer review studies or scientific evidence to show that vitamin and nutritional therapies work. Yet, every year, there are thousands of studies on vitamins published, and thousands more on antioxidants. In fact, more research has been published on nutrients than on medications!

The therapeutic techniques described throughout this book are supported by hundreds of literary references from respected, peer-reviewed scientific and medical publications. These references only scratch the surface of the voluminous amount of literature available. David Perlmutter, MD, a respected neurologist and author of BrainRecovery.com, said on his website, "It has been said that knowledge is power, but clearly in this context, knowledge is health." This knowledge is now available to you.

This book will begin by looking at vitamins, minerals, fatty acids, amino acids, and other nutrients that help maintain health and aid in reducing disease. The suggested dosages are for people twelve years old or older and at least one hundred pounds. They are given in either milligrams or international units (a unit of measurement used in phar-macology) unless otherwise stated. These can be consumed in supple-ments or from food sources, so you will also read suggestions on choosing supplements and lists of foods that contain high amounts of each nutrient. It is important to note that the numbered lists are in order: The closer to the beginning of the list a food item is found, the more of the nutrient the food contains. Lists that are not numbered are in alphabetical order.

The next section of the book describes different nutritional programs for various disorders and diseases. Then, you will read about suggested and selected therapies that myself and other healthcare practitioners have used to prevent disease, maintain optimal health, and treat certain disease processes.

As you read this book, keep in mind that, along with proper nutri-tional intake, choosing the proper healthcare provider is important to overall health. I strongly suggest finding a specialist fellowship-trained in anti-aging, regenerative, and functional medicine.

Anti-aging and regenerative medicine is a clinical/medical specialty and field of scientific research aimed at the early detection, prevention, treatment, and reversal of age-related decline. It is well documented by peer-reviewed medical and scientific journals and employs evidence-based methodologies to conduct patient assessments. The American Academy of Anti-Aging Medicine was established in 1997 as a profes-sional physician certification and review board. It offers physician recog-nition in the form of a specialty-based examination in anti-aging and regenerative medicine. Paraprofessionals may also now receive certifica-tion in this field. Anti-aging medicine is the newest and fastest growing medical specialty, and represents over 14,000 physicians, scientists, and other health professionals, as well as much of the health-minded public, from seventy-three countries worldwide.

Functional medicine is an integrative, science-based healthcare approach that treats illness and promotes wellness by focusing on the bio-chemically unique aspects of each patient, and then individually tailoring interventions to restore physiological, psychological, and structural bal-ance. Functional medicine focuses on understanding the fundamental physiological processes, the environmental inputs, and the genetic pre-dispositions that influence health and disease so that interventions are focused on treating the cause of the problem, rather than masking the symptoms.

Many essential vitamins and minerals are no longer available in the foods that we eat, yet they are essential to our health and longevity. At the same time, you may find it ncessary to look beyond your family doctor for the most beneficial nutritional advice. *What You Must Know About Vitamins, Minerals, Herbs, and More* will provide you with the proper education to promote and maintain optimal health in yourself and your family.

Mixing Supplements, Drugs, and Food

The importance of consuming vitamins, minerals, and other nutrients cannot be understated. At the same time, it is a process that must be monitored. The interaction of certain supplements, drugs, and food can be detrimental to your health rather than beneficial. Before starting any supplement regiment, therefore, you must be aware of possible side effects or contraindications. The following are examples of problems that can occur from some fairly common interactions. Other precautions can be found in the appropriate sections throughout this book.

COMBINING VITAMINS WITH MEDICATION

Some medications can deplete your body of specific vitamins and minerals. Similarly, some vitamins can increase or decrease your body's absorption of some medications. The following list provides common examples of both possibilities. If you are on any of the medications named here, you must discuss any nutritional changes with your doctor or healthcare professional. He will make sure your vitamins and medications do not interact, as well as aid you in replacing any depleted nutrients.

- Long-term use of antacids can lead to decreased folic acid absorption.

- Regular use of aspirin decreases folate levels.

- Birth control pills and other forms of estrogen replacement deplete the body of B vitamins.

- Too much vitamin B_6 can decrease the effectiveness of levodopa (an effective treatment for Parkinson's disease).

- Antiarrhythmic medications, such as Disopyramide (including Norpace) and Quinidine sulfate, can cause magnesium deficiency.

- Colchicine reduces the absorption of beta-carotene. It may also reduce the absorption of magnesium, potassium, and vitamin B_{12}.

- Methotrexate, used to treat cancer and autoimmune disorders, can decrease beta-carotene, folic acid, and vitamin B_{12}.

- Estrogen replacement increases calcium absorption.

- Anticonvulsants (seizure medication) can deplete the body of carnitine.

- Histamine-2 receptor antagonists (H2-blockers), such as cimetidine, can prevent or block the production of stomach acid and decrease vitamin D activity.

- HMG-CoA reductase inhibitors (statin drugs), used to lower cholesterol, stop your body from making coenzyme Q_{10}.

- Medications to lower blood sugar, such as glyburide (including Diabeta), acetohexamide (including Dymelor), and tolazamide (including Tolinase), can lead to coenzyme Q_{10} deficiency.

- Digoxin (a medication usually prescribed for heart-related problems) can increase the rate of calcium excretion from the body.

- Fiber can decrease the absorption of digoxin.

- Diuretics (water pills) decrease magnesium, potassium, sodium, and zinc levels.

- Potassium-sparing diuretics deplete your body of folic acid, calcium, and zinc.

- Calcium can decrease the absorption of beta blockers.

COMBINING FOOD WITH MEDICATION

The food you eat can affect the medication you are taking. You should be aware, for example, that grapefruit can increase the risk of side effects from a wide variety of drugs. The side effects described below can occur from eating grapefruit while on the specified medications.

- Grapefruit can cause flushing, headaches, and increased heart rate if eaten while taking calcium-channel blockers (such as nifedipine, amlodipine, verapamil, and felodipine), which help decrease blood pressure.

- Grapefruit increases quinidine levels.

- Grapefruit can cause irregular heart rhythms if eaten while taking the antihistamine terfenadine.

- Grapefruit can increase levels of benzodiazepines (sedatives that include alprazolam, diazepam, midazolam, and triazolam).

- Grapefruit can cause kidney and liver toxicity if eaten while taking cyclosporine.

- Grapefruit increases caffeine levels and can cause nervousness and insomnia.

- Grapefruit can decrease the absorption of macrolide antibiotics such as clarithromycin.

- Grapefruit can decrease the absorption of the antihistamine fexofenadine (such as Allegra).

- Grapefruit can increase the medication level of HMG-CoA reductase inhibitors (statin drugs).

- Grapefruit can increase the level of warfarin, a medication that affects blood clotting.

- Grapefruit can delay the absorption of Viagra, a male impotence medication.

- Grapefruit can cause hives if taken with the pain reliever naprosyn.

- Grapefruit can increase certain levels, which may lead to nausea, tremors, drowsiness, dizziness, or agitation, if eaten while taking carbamazepine (such as Tegretol).

- Grapefruit may elevate blood levels and cause nausea, drowsiness, tremors, or agitation if eaten while taking amiodarone.

- Grapefruit can increase estrogen levels in both men and women. No interaction with medication is necessary for this to occur.

COMBINING VITAMINS AND MINERALS

Vitamins and minerals can interact with each other, as well as with other nutrients. These relationships and interrelationships can have various effects. The following examples show how certain vitamins and minerals interact.

- A certain amount of vitamin C is necessary for your body to use selenium effectively.

- Vitamin C can enhance the availability of vitamin A.

- Too much zinc can decrease calcium absorption.

- Vitamin D increases the absorption of calcium and magnesium.

- Vitamin D helps your body use zinc effectively.

- Too much copper can decrease the uptake of manganese in your system.

- A vitamin A deficiency can decrease iron utilization.

- Too much iron can lower your manganese and copper levels.

- Too much vitamin B_2 (riboflavin) can cause a magnesium deficiency.

- Vitamin B_6 can cause a decrease in copper absorption.

- A vitamin E deficiency can decrease absorption of vitamin A.

- A vitamin B_6 (pyridoxine) deficiency can lead to a decreased use of selenium.

- Adequate phosphorus intake is needed to maintain vitamin D.

PART 1

Nutrients

1

Vitamins

itamins are substances that occur naturally in both plants and animals. They are divided into two categories: fat-soluble vitamins and water-soluble vitamins. *Fat-soluble vitamins* are stored in the fat cells of your body, and include vitamins A, D, E, and K. *Water-soluble vitamins,* such as vitamins B and C, are eliminated from your body the same day they are ingested. In this chapter, you will first read about fat-soluble vitamins. Then, you will turn your attention to water-soluble vitamins.

Although it has long been the topic of much debate, we now know that the type of vitamins you consume *does* make a difference. Whether or not the substance will work for you depends on factors including its form, purity, bioavailability, and third-party verification. (Bioavailability is discussed on page 16.) Vitamin supplements are divided into four grades, or quality categories that take these factors into account. See the inset "Categories of Vitamin Supplements" on page 16 for further information.

The chemical forms of minerals are not the elemental forms. For example, a 1,200-milligram tablet of calcium gluconate is only 9-percent elemental: It only contains 108 milligrams of calcium. You would, therefore, need to take eleven tablets a day to consume the recommended amount.

Also, whether the nutrients are in natural or synthetic form makes a difference with certain vitamins. Natural vitamin E, for example, is better absorbed and more active than the synthetic version.

Your herbal supplements should have an *adulteration screen,* which tests their purity. This examination will tell you if they contain any toxic metals, such as arsenic, lead, mercury, or cadmium. Supplements should also be screened for other contaminants, including other pharmaceuticals, and analyzed for pesticides, fungicides, insecticides, and other toxic ingredients. Unfortunately, there are no home tests available. To test a vitamin's contents and bioavailability, you have to take the vitamin to a laboratory for analyzation.

Categories of Vitamin Supplements

Vitamin supplements are divided into the following four quality categories. To fall into one of the better grades, a supplement must be tested by an outside source who can verify its quality. You should only buy supplements of pharmaceutical grade. See page 376 for a list of pharmaceutical grade companies.

- Pharmaceutical grade: Supplements of this grade meet the highest regulatory requirements for purity, dissolution (ability to be dissolved), and absorption.

- Medical grade: These supplements are of a high grade. Prenatal vitamins are usually in this category.

- Cosmetic, nutritional grade: These supplements are often not tested for purity, dissolution, or absorption. They may not have a high concentration of their listed active ingredient.

- Feed or agricultural grade: Supplements of this grade are used for veterinary purposes. Do not take supplements of this grade.

Many forms of nutrients are not *bioavailable*—they pass through the body without being absorbed into the bloodstream. For example, magnesium oxide is only one-tenth as bioavailable as magnesium aspartate, and therefore only one-tenth as useful. Despite this, manufacturers will frequently use the oxide form, because the aspartate form is more expensive and takes up a lot of room in the capsule. Using the magnesium oxide is, therefore, more cost effective.

Be sure to give careful consideration to the side effects and contraindications as you become familiar with each vitamin. As you read in "Mixing Supplements, Drugs, and Food," there are various reactions that can occur when different substances are taken together. Similarly, taking too much of a certain vitamin can result in either the deficit of another vitamin or health problems. Yet, as you will see, nutritional deficiencies can result in equally serious problems. Visit your healthcare professional if you have any questions as you develop your optimal vitamin regiment.

Every year, over 75 percent of your body is reconstructed from the nutrients you eat and take. This includes the DNA in your cells. The quality of vitamins and nutrients you consume determines the quality of your cells, how well they function, and their ability to prevent disease.

Vitamins are best stored in a refrigerator, and always taken with a full glass of water. You read on page 15 about water-soluble and fat-soluble vitamins. Fat-soluble vitamins should be taken once a day. Water-soluble vitamins, on the other hand, leave the body more quickly, so they should be taken twice daily. Therefore, if the daily dose of a water-soluble vitamin is 100 milligrams, you should take 50 milligrams twice a day. There will be more specific instructions on taking each type of vitamin as you read through this chapter.

VITAMIN A

Vitamin A is a fat-soluble vitamin that can be divided into two groups: retinoids (or aldehydes) and carotenoids. Retinoids come from animals and can also be called preformed or active vitamin A because they are already in a form that is usable by the body. Retinal and retinoic acid, which are both found in fish, are included in this grouping. Carotenoids, on the other hand, are found in plants, and are called *provitamins*, which means they are stored in the liver and converted into the usable vitamin as needed. These include beta-carotene, alpha-carotene, and gama-carotene. Beta-carotene is the most popular and thoroughly studied of the carotenoid varieties. After carotenoids are converted into vitamin A, they react as preformed vitamin A does in the body.

Functions of Active Vitamin A in Your Body

- Assists immune function (improves white blood cells, natural killer cells, macrophages, and T and B lymphocytes)
- Needed for the growth and support of the skin
- Needed to detoxify polychlorinated biphenyl (PCB; any of a group of highly toxic compounds often found in industrial waste) and dioxin
- Reduces risk for cancer (esophageal, bladder, stomach, and skin, as well as leukemia and lymphoma)
- Required for vision
- Responsible for healthy mucous membranes
- Strengthens bones during development

■ Symptoms of Vitamin A Deficiency

☐ Decreased steroid synthesis

☐ Dry eyes

☐ Fatigue

☐ Hypothyroidism (low thyroid production)

☐ Increased susceptibility to infections

☐ Increased susceptibility to vaginal yeast infections

☐ Night blindness

☐ Poor tooth and bone function

☐ Poor wound healing

☐ Rough, scaly skin

■ Causes of Vitamin A Deficiency

● Antibiotics

● Cholesterol-lowering medications

● Diabetes

● Laxatives

● Malabsorption

● Malnutrition

● Medication/products that decrease fat absorption

■ Substances that Increase Vitamin A Levels

● Birth control pills

■ Symptoms of Vitamin A Toxicity

☐ Appetite loss

☐ Bone pain

☐ Dry skin

☐ Fatigue

☐ Hair loss

☐ Headache

☐ Irritability

☐ Joint pain

☐ Weight loss

■ Recommended Dosage

5,000 to 10,000 international units daily

■ Side Effects and Contraindications

Excess vitamin A consumption can cause liver damage and even death. If you are taking a high dose, you need to have your doctor measure your calcium and liver enzymes on a regular basis. If you have liver disease, are a smoker, are exposed to asbestos, or are pregnant, you should not consume high doses of vitamin A. Also, a recent study suggested that a daily intake of even 5,000 international units of vitamin A from dietary sources for more than twenty years may increase hip fractures in women.

Food Sources of Vitamin A

The following foods are numbered so that the foods that contain the most vitamin A are at the beginning of the list. As the list proceeds, the foods contain progressively less vitamin A.

1. Lamb liver	19. Butternut squash	37. Whipped cream
2. Beef liver	20. Watercress	38. Peaches
3. Calf liver	21. Mangos	39. Acorn squash
4. Red chili peppers	22. Sweet red peppers	40. Eggs
5. Dandelion greens	23. Hubbard squash	41. Chicken
6. Chicken liver	24. Cantaloupe	42. Sour red cherries
7. Carrots	25. Butter	43. Butterhead lettuce
8. Dried apricots	26. Endive	44. Asparagus
9. Collard greens	27. Apricots	45. Tomatoes
10. Kale	28. Broccoli spears	46. Green chili peppers
11. Sweet potatoes	29. Whitefish	47. Green peas
12. Parsley	30. Green onions	48. Elderberries
13. Spinach	31. Romaine lettuce	49. Watermelon
14. Turnip greens	32. Papayas	50. Rutabagas
15. Mustard greens	33. Nectarines	51. Brussels sprouts
16. Swiss chard	34. Prunes	52. Okra
17. Beet greens	35. Pumpkin	53. Yellow cornmeal
18. Chives	36. Swordfish	54. Yellow squash

THE CAROTENOIDS

There are over 700 carotenoids on earth; only 60 are found in food. The typical American diet includes only six of them: alpha-carotene, beta-carotene, cryptoxanthin, lycopene, lutein, and zeaxanthin. Alpha-carotene, beta-carotene, and cryptoxanthin are converted into vitamin A inside your body, at which point they act like active vitamin A, described on page 17. Be aware, however, that if you have hypothyroidism, your body may be unable to convert beta-carotene into vitamin A. The other three common carotenoids will have the following effects.

LYCOPENE

The carotenoid lycopene is an antioxidant that may lower the risk of some types of cancers. It is best absorbed when cooked with fat. Pizza, therefore, which contains tomatoes that have been cooked with oil and cheese, is a good source of lycopene. Fresh tomatoes, on the other hand, are not a good source.

■ Functions of Lycopene in Your Body

- Decreases LDL (bad) cholesterol
- Helps prevent prostate cancer
- Lowers blood pressure

■ Recommended Dosage

5 to 20 milligrams daily

■ Side Effects and Contraindications

Carotenoids have to be taken carefully. Pharmacologic doses of a single carotenoid may result in inhibiting other carotenoids at your cell receptor sites. Also, a study called the Beta-Carotene and Retinol Efficacy Trial (CARET) has shown that smokers who take carotenoids may have a higher risk of developing lung cancer. However, high doses of carotenoids are non-toxic, unlike high doses of vitamin A, because excess carotenoids are stored in the liver until needed by the body.

Food Sources of Lycopene

- Dark green leafy vegetables
- Guavas
- Pink grapefruit
- Tomatoes
- Watermelon

LUTEIN AND ZEAXANTHIN

Lutein and zeaxanthin are carotenoids that are contained within the retina of the eye. They help the eye absorb light while also protecting it from various free radicals. (Free radicals were discussed on page 4.)

■ Functions of Lutein and Zeaxanthin in Your Body

- Help prevent cataracts
- Protect against macular degeneration

■ Recommended Dosage

6 to 12 milligrams daily

■ Side Effects and Contraindications

Carotenoids have to be taken carefully. Pharmacologic doses of a single carotenoid may result in inhibiting the other carotenoids at your cell receptor sites. Also, a study called the Beta-Carotene and Retinol Efficacy Trial (CARET) has shown that smokers who take carotenoids may have a higher risk of developing lung cancer. However, high doses of carotenoids are non-toxic, unlike high doses of vitamin A, because excess carotenoids are stored in the liver until needed by the body.

Food Sources of Lutein and Zeaxanthin

Of the following foods, egg yolks contain the most bioavailable forms of lutein and zeaxanthin.

- Collard greens
- Corn
- Egg yolks
- Green leafy vegetables
- Kale
- Spinach

CRYPTOXANTHIN

There has been less research with cryptoxanthin than with the carotenoids mentioned previously. However, there is significant evidence that it may effectively reduce the risk of cancer.

Food Sources of Cryptoxanthin

- Butter
- Egg yolk
- Oranges
- Papayas
- Peaches

■ Functions of Cryptoxanthin in Your Body

- May prevent cataracts and protect against macular degeneration
- May protect against various types of cancer, particularly cervical cancer

■ Recommended Dosage

4 milligrams daily

■ Side Effects and Contraindications

Carotenoids have to be taken carefully. Pharmacologic doses of a single carotenoid may result in inhibiting the other carotenoids at your cell receptor sites. Also, a study called the Beta-Carotene and Retinol Efficacy Trial (CARET) has shown that smokers who take carotenoids may have a higher risk of developing lung cancer. However, high doses of carotenoids are non-toxic, unlike high doses of vitamin A, because excess carotenoids are stored in the liver until needed by the body.

VITAMIN D

The fat-soluble vitamin D is actually not a vitamin (which must be consumed through diet) but a hormone (which is produced in the body). The active form is called 1,25 dihydroxycholecalciferol. Your body produces it after absorbing the sun's rays. I recommend getting sun exposure for ten to fifteen minutes, at least three times a week, if you are depending on the sun for your vitamin D. You can also get vitamin D from food, albeit in smaller doses. Vitamin D_3 comes from red meat and fish; vitamin D_2 comes from plants. In these forms, vitamin D must be metabolized in the body in order to be used by the body, and boron may be needed for the conversion. Vitamin-D receptors are located in your bones, pancreas, intestine, kidneys, brain, spinal cord, reproductive organs, thymus, adrenal glands, pituitary gland, and thyroid gland.

■ Functions of Vitamin D in Your Body

- Aids in the absorption of calcium from the intestinal tract
- Helps the body assimilate phosphorus
- Helps the pancreas release insulin
- Necessary for blood clotting
- Necessary for growth and development of bones and teeth
- Necessary for thyroid function
- Stimulates bone cell mineralization

■ Symptoms of Vitamin D Deficiency

- ☐ Bone disorders (rickets in children or osteomalacia in adults)
- ☐ Decreased calcium levels
- ☐ Decreased phosphate levels
- ☐ Increased risk of osteoporosis
- ☐ Muscle spasms

■ Causes of Vitamin D Deficiency

- Aging (which causes your body to make less vitamin D from the sun)
- Decreased fat absorption (as a result of short bowel syndrome, sprue, or certain medications)
- Fat-blocking medications and over-the-counter fat blockers used for weight loss
- Medications (such as phenytoin)
- Prednisone (a steroid that treats cancer and interferes with the conversion of vitamin D to its active form)
- Sunscreen (which prevents vitamin D absorption)

■ Diseases/Disorders that Can Be Treated with Vitamin D

- Autoimmune diseases
- Cancer prevention and treatment
- Cardiovascular disease
- Depression
- Diabetes
- Epilepsy
- Hypertension (high blood pressure)
- Inflammatory conditions
- Migraine headaches
- Multiple sclerosis
- Musculoskeletal pain
- Osteoarthritis
- Osteoporosis
- Polycystic ovary syndrome

Food Sources of Vitamin D

The following foods are numbered so that the foods that contain the most vitamin D are at the top of the list. As the list proceeds, the foods contain progressively less vitamin D.

1. Canned sardines
2. Salmon
3. Tuna
4. Shrimp
5. Butter
6. Sunflower seeds
7. Liver
8. Eggs
9. Fortified milk
10. Mushrooms
11. Natural cheese

■ Recommended Dosage

Consult your medical practitioner, who will conduct lab tests before deciding how much vitamin D you should consume. To get enough vitamin D from the sun's rays, you should expose your face and arms for ten to fifteen minutes, at least three times a week without sunscreen.

The use of sunscreen significantly decreases the absorption of vitamin D into the skin. If you are very fair and need to wear sunscreen, then you may need to intake more vitamin D. The preferred form of vitamin D with which to supplement is D_3.

■ Side Effects and Contraindications

Vitamin D is stored in the body and can become toxic for some people. At the same time, other people need much higher dosages. Consequently, for dosages above 1,000 international units a day, it is best to consult with your healthcare practitioner. It is necessary to take calcium when taking vitamin D.

VITAMIN E

Vitamin E, an antioxidant, is a group of eight fat-soluble compounds—alpha-tocopherol, beta-tocopherol, gamma-tocopherol, delta-tocopherol, alpha-tocotrienol, beta-tocotrienol, gamma-tocotrienol, and delta-tocotrienol. These compounds come in natural and synthetic forms. Natural vitamin E is called d-alpha (or d-beta, d-gamma, or d-delta) and synthetic vitamin E is noted as dl-alpha (or dl-beta, dl-gamma, or dl-delta). In its natural form, vitamin E is better absorbed by your body and better metabolized by your liver.

TOCOPHEROLS

Of the vitamin E compounds, alpha-tocopherol is the most biologically active, followed by beta-tocopherol, gamma-tocopherol, and delta-tocopherol.

Functions of Tocopherols in Your Body

- Can act as an estrogen substitute and relieve hot flashes
- Can stop cholesterol-like substances from damaging your blood vessels, which can cause heart disease or strokes
- Help prevent Alzheimer's disease
- Help prevent lung, esophageal, and colorectal cancer
- Help relieve atrophic vaginitis
- Improve the action of insulin
- Increase your immune system
- Inhibit platelet adhesion
- Needed by ovaries to function properly
- Protect vitamin A and increase its storage

Causes of Tocopherols Deficiency

- Alcohol
- Pectin (a natural substance added to thicken jams and jellies)
- Smoking
- Vitamin A
- Wheat bran

Recommended Dosage

100 to 400 international units daily

Side Effects and Contraindications

Ferrous sulfate, a common iron compound, destroys vitamin E and should not be taken with it. Other forms of iron, such as ferrous gluconate or ferrous fumarate, do not have this negative effect. Vitamin E is a blood

Food Sources of Tocopherols

The following foods are numbered so that the foods that contain the most tocopherols are at the beginning of the list. As the list proceeds, the foods contain progressively less tocopherols.

1. Wheat germ
2. Sunflower seeds
3. Sunflower seed oil
4. Safflower oil
5. Almonds
6. Sesame oil
7. Peanut oil
8. Corn oil
9. Wheat germ
10. Peanuts
11. Olive oil
12. Soybean oil
13. Roasted peanuts
14. Peanut butter
15. Butter
16. Spinach
17. Oatmeal
18. Bran
19. Asparagus
20. Salmon
21. Brown rice
22. Whole rye bread
23. Dark rye bread
24. Pecans
25. Wheat germ
26. Rye and wheat crackers
27. Whole wheat bread
28. Carrots
29. Peas
30. Walnuts
31. Bananas
32. Eggs
33. Tomatoes
34. Lamb

thinner, so if you are taking an anticoagulant (blood thinner), consult your physician as to the amount of vitamin E that is right for you. No toxicity is seen up to 3,200 international units.

■ Diseases/Disorders that Can Be Treated with Tocopherols

- Claudication (leg pain that occurs during exercise)
- Fibrocystic breast disease
- Heart disease
- Hepatitis
- Hot flashes
- Osteoporosis
- Painful menstrual cycles
- Premenstrual syndrome (PMS)
- Restless leg syndrome
- Scleroderma and other autoimmune diseases

TOCOTRIENOLS

Alpha-tocotrienol, beta-tocotrienol, gamma-tocotrienol, and delta-tocotrienol are active forms of vitamin E. Despite being less active than the tocopherols, tocotrienols perform important functions in your body.

■ Functions of Tocotrienols In Your Body

- Fight inflammation
- Lower cholesterol
- Reduce risk of cancer
- Reverse plaque build-up

■ Recommended Dosage

100 to 400 international units of mixed tocotrienols daily. They should be taken with other antioxidants since they have a *synergistic effect*—a result that is greater as a mixture than the sum of the results if the substances had worked alone. I recommend UltraTrienols, made by Designs for Health. (See Resources for availability.)

VITAMIN K

The fat-soluble vitamin K comes in two forms: K_1 and K_2. K_1 is found in green leafy vegetables. K_2 can be derived from K_1. It is also made in the gastrointestinal tract by friendly bacteria and found in egg yolk, butter, and fermented soy foods.

■ Functions of Vitamin K in Your Body

- Adequate bone mineralization
- Decreases calcifications, which lowers risk of heart disease
- Decreases the loss of calcium
- Helps your blood clot
- Needed for the synthesis of osteocalcin, which is involved in building bones
- Stimulates new bone growth

Food Sources of Vitamin K

The following foods are numbered so that the foods that contain the most vitamin K are at the beginning of the list. As the list proceeds, the foods contain progressively less vitamin K.

1. Turnip greens	10. Butter	18. Corn oil
2. Broccoli	11. Pork liver	19. Peaches
3. Lettuce	12. Oats	20. Beef
4. Cabbage	13. Green peas	21. Chicken liver
5. Beef liver	14. Whole wheat	22. Raisins
6. Spinach	15. Green beans	23. Tomato
7. Watercress	16. Pork	24. Milk
8. Asparagus	17. Eggs	25. Potato
9. Cheese		

■ Symptoms of Vitamin K Deficiency

☐ Decrease in amount of skin collagen (which makes skin look thinner)

☐ Increased breakdown of skin collagen

☐ Increased risk of coronary artery calcification

☐ Increased risk of osteoporosis

☐ Vitamin C levels, decrease in

■ Causes of Vitamin K Deficiency

- Antibiotic use
- Certain anticoagulants such as warfarin
- Cholesterol-lowering drugs
- Decreased consumption of green leafy vegetables
- Excess vitamins A and E
- Gallstones
- Hydrogenated food
- Liver disease
- Medication/products that decrease fat absorption
- Synthetic estrogen use
- Unhealthy intestinal tract

■ Recommended Dosage

100 to 500 micrograms daily

■ Side Effects and Contraindications

Synthetic vitamin K may cause toxicity. Also, the amount of vitamin K in your body can alter the effectiveness of any anticoagulants (drugs used to prevent clot formation or clots from enlarging, such as Coumadin) you may be taking. Discuss your vitamin-K intake with your doctor if you are prescribed an anticoagulant.

VITAMIN B COMPLEX

There are eleven vitamins in the vitamin B complex. The entire complex works together to help you achieve optimal health. The different vitamins, which are listed below and described on the following pages, are found in many of the same foods.

They are water soluble, which means they are eliminated from your body the same day they are ingested. Yet it is important to have an adequate amount of B vitamins in your body, so you should consume them at least twice a day. If you are on estrogen replacement therapy or birth control pills, you should take extra B vitamins since hormonal therapy leads to a deficiency. Also, high dose supplementation of a single B vitamin can cause imbalances of other B vitamins. Therefore, you should take a multi-vitamin that contains these vitamins rather than take each B vitamin individually.

■ Members of the Vitamin B Complex

These vitamins, except for vitamin B_{10}, are all described in detail in the following sections. However, there is no section for vitamin B_{10} (para-aminobenzoic acid) because there is not much known about it.

- B_1 (Thiamine)
- B_2 (Riboflavin)
- B_3 (Niacin and Niacinamide)
- B_5 (Pantothenic acid)
- B_6 (Pyridoxine)
- B_7 (Biotin)
- B_9 (Folic acid)
- B_{10} (Para-aminobenzoic acid)
- B_{12} (Cobalamin)
- Choline
- Inositol

■ Functions of B Vitamins in Your Body

- Help liver detoxify estrogen
- Help relieve leg cramps
- Metabolize glucose
- Stabilize brain chemistry
- Used in thyroid function

■ Symptoms of B-Vitamin Deficiency

- ☐ Change in appetite
- ☐ Impaired metabolism of medications
- ☐ Insomnia
- ☐ Irritability
- ☐ Poor scores in personality testing
- ☐ Reduced immune system
- ☐ Sugar cravings

■ Causes of B-Vitamin Deficiency

- Birth control pills
- Estrogen replacement therapy

B_1 (THIAMINE)

The first B vitamin discovered was thiamine (or thiamin). Thiamine is involved with many of the body's reactions, including the burning of carbohydrates for energy. You can find thiamine in individual supplements as well as supplements that contain all the B vitamins.

■ Functions of B_1 in Your Body

- Helps the body adapt to stress and avoid adrenal burnout
- Needed for proper metabolism of thyroid hormones
- Needed for synthesis of nucleic acids and certain coenzymes
- Needed for the making of aldosterone, a steroid hormone
- Required for energy production (Krebs cycle)
- Required for proper nerve function
- Used for activation of enzymes in the adrenal glands
- Used in the synthesis of acetylcholine

■ Symptoms of B₁ Deficiency

- ☐ Confusion
- ☐ Fatigue
- ☐ Forgetfulness
- ☐ Gastrointestinal disturbances
- ☐ General weakness
- ☐ Headache
- ☐ Irritability
- ☐ Loss of appetite
- ☐ Mild depression
- ☐ Nervousness
- ☐ Poor memory
- ☐ Racing heart
- ☐ Sleep disturbance
- ☐ Vision problems

■ Causes of B₁ Deficiency

- Alcohol
- Antibiotics
- Blueberries
- Brussels sprouts
- Coffee
- Diuretics
- Horseradish
- Oral contraceptives
- Pickled foods
- Red beet root
- Seafood such as fish, shrimp, clams, and mussels
- Sugar
- Sulfa drugs
- Sulfites (a food additive)
- Theophylline (an asthma medication)
- Tea

■ Recommended Dosage

10 to 100 milligrams daily. B vitamins are water soluble and leave the body quickly, so they should be taken twice a day. Therefore, you should take 5 to 50 milligrams of B₁ twice a day.

■ Side Effects and Contraindications

High doses of B₁ may deplete your body of vitamin B₆ or magnesium.

■ Diseases/Disorders that Can Be Treated with B₁

- Alcoholism
- Confusion
- Dementia
- Depression
- Fatigue
- Memory loss
- Neuropathy
- Pain

Food Sources of Vitamin B_1

The following foods are numbered so that the foods that contain the most vitamin B_1 are at the beginning of the list. As the list proceeds, the foods contain progressively less vitamin B_1. Note that grains lose up to 100 percent of their thiamine content when processed. Also, marinating your meat in wine, soy sauce, or vinegar depletes its level of thiamine by 50 to 75 percent.

1. Brewer's yeast
2. Wheat germ
3. Sunflower seeds
4. Rice polishings
5. Pine nuts
6. Peanuts (with skins)
7. Brazil nuts
8. Pork
9. Pecans
10. Soybean flour
11. Pinto and red beans
12. Split peas
13. Millet
14. Wheat bran
15. Pistachio nuts
16. Navy beans
17. Buckwheat
18. Oatmeal
19. Whole wheat flour
20. Whole wheat grain
21. Dry lima beans
22. Hazelnuts
23. Heart, lamb
24. Wild rice
25. Whole grain rye
26. Cashews
27. Lamb liver
28. Mung beans
29. Whole-ground cornmeal
30. Lentils
31. Beef kidneys
32. Green peas
33. Macadamia nuts
34. Brown rice
35. Walnuts
36. Garbanzo beans
37. Garlic cloves
38. Beef liver
39. Almonds
40. Fresh lima beans
41. Pumpkin and squash seeds
42. Fresh chestnuts
43. Soybean sprouts
44. Red chili peppers
45. Hulled sesame seeds

B_2 (RIBOFLAVIN)

Vitamin B_2, or riboflavin, is very much involved with your body's energy processes, as well as many other processes. It is vital, for example, for healthy eyes, the production of antibodies, and proper tissue repair.

■ Functions of B$_2$ in Your Body

- Catalyzes several reactions that process carbohydrates, fats, and proteins
- Crucial to the cytochrome P450 system, which metabolizes medications and xenobiotics (environmental toxins)
- Involved in the metabolism of vitamin K
- Needed for energy metabolism
- Needed in the regeneration of glutathione (the strongest antioxidant produced by your body)
- Needed to convert vitamin B$_6$, folic acid, vitamin A, and niacin into their active forms

---

Food Sources of Vitamin B$_2$

The following foods are numbered so that the foods that contain the most vitamin B$_2$ are at the beginning of the list. As the list proceeds, the foods contain progressively less vitamin B$_2$. Processing food decreases its riboflavin content by up to 80 percent.

1. Brewer's yeast	16. Soy flour	31. Pine nuts
2. Lamb liver	17. Wheat bran	32. Sunflower seeds
3. Beef liver	18. Mackerel	33. Pork
4. Calf liver	19. Collards	34. Navy beans
5. Beef kidneys	20. Dry soybeans	35. Beet and mustard greens
6. Chicken liver	21. Eggs	36. Lentils
7. Lamb kidneys	22. Split peas	37. Prunes
8. Chicken giblets	23. Beef tongue	38. Rye
9. Almonds	24. Kale	39. Whole grain
10. Wheat germ	25. Parsley	40. Mung beans
11. Wild rice	26. Cashews	41. Pinto and red beans
12. Mushrooms	27. Rice bran	42. Black-eyed peas
13. Egg yolks	28. Veal	43. Okra
14. Millet	29. Salmon	
15. Hot red peppers	30. Broccoli	

- Required for proper thyroid function
- Used in lipid metabolism
- Used in the formation of aldosterone (a steroid hormone that balances blood) by the adrenal glands

■ Symptoms of B_2 in Deficiency

☐ Depression ☐ Dry, cracking skin ☐ Light sensitivity

■ Substances that Reduce the Bioavailability of B_2

- Adriamycin
- Alcohol
- Amitriptyline
- Antacids
- Caffeine
- Copper
- Imipramine
- Phenothiazines
- Phenytoin
- Saccharin
- Theophylline
- Tryptophan
- Vitamin B_3
- Vitamin C
- Zinc

■ Recommended Dosage

10 to 100 milligrams daily. You need more B_2 during illness or athletic training. B vitamins are water soluble and leave the body quickly, so they should be taken twice a day. Therefore, you should take 5 to 50 milligrams of B_2 twice a day.

■ Side Effects and Contraindications

None. However, high dose supplementation of a single B vitamin can cause imbalances of other B vitamins.

■ Diseases/Disorders that Can Be Treated with B_2

- Acne
- Alcoholism
- Arthritis
- Athlete's foot
- Baldness
- Cataracts
- Depression
- Diabetes mellitus
- Diarrhea
- Failure to detoxify effectively
- Hysteria
- Indigestion
- Light sensitivity
- Migraines
- Nerve damage
- Reddening of eyes
- Scrotal skin changes
- Seborrhic dermatitis
- Skin changes around the mouth
- Stress
- Visual changes

B₃ (NIACIN AND NIACINAMIDE)

Vitamin B₃ includes both niacin (or nicotinic acid) and its derivative niacinamide. The lists below, however, refer to niacin, a vitamin made from tryptophan, B₆, B₂, and iron. It is used in at least forty chemical reactions in your body. Niacin has shown to have positive effects on cholesterol levels, particularly when used in conjunction with a statin drug. As stated in "Side Effects and Contraindications" (on pages 36 to 37), however, taking niacin by itself may result in increased homocysteine levels.

◼ Functions of Niacin in Your Body

- Can decrease lipoprotein A (high amounts of which are related to heart disease)
- Can lower LDL (bad) cholesterol and raise HDL (good) cholesterol
- Decreases fibrinogen (high amounts of which are related to heart disease)
- Involved in energy production
- Lowers triglycerides
- May improve the health of people with diabetes
- Needed for the proper function of the adrenal glands
- Provides energy needed to convert cholesterol to pregnenolone (a hormone that, among other things, is involved with memory)
- Used in the metabolism of carbohydrates, proteins, and fats
- Used in the metabolism of tryptophan and serotonin

◼ Symptoms of Niacin Deficiency

☐ Anorexia	☐ Headaches	☐ Mouth ulcers
☐ Confusion	☐ Inability to detoxify	☐ Muscle weakness
☐ Depression	☐ Indigestion	☐ Nausea
☐ Dermatitis	☐ Insomnia	☐ Skin changes around the mouth
☐ Fatigue	☐ Irritability	

◼ Recommended Dosage

50 to 3,000 milligrams daily. However, see your doctor if you want to consume doses greater than 100 milligrams. If you find yourself needing

Food Sources of Niacin

The following foods are numbered so that the foods that contain the most niacin are at the beginning of the list. As the list proceeds, the foods contain progressively less niacin.

1. Brewer's yeast	16. Mackerel	31. Beef
2. Rice bran	17. Fresh chicken	32. Pork
3. Rice polishings	18. Fresh swordfish	33. Brown rice
4. Wheat bran	19. Fresh turkey	34. Pine nuts
5. Peanuts with skin	20. Fresh goose	35. Whole-grain buckwheat
6. Lamb liver	21. Beef heart	36. Red chili peppers
7. Pork liver	22. Salmon	37. Whole wheat grain
8. Peanuts without skin	23. Veal	38. Whole wheat flour
9. Beef liver	24. Beef kidneys	39. Wheat germ
10. Calf liver	25. Wild rice	40. Barley
11. Turkey, light meat	26. Chicken giblets	41. Herring
12. Chicken liver	27. Lamb	42. Almonds
13. Chicken, light meat	28. Chicken flesh and skin	43. Shrimp
14. Trout	29. Sesame seeds	44. Split peas
15. Halibut	30. Sunflower seeds	45. Haddock

more niacin, try taking NADH, a reduced form of the vitamin that is also more active. B vitamins are water soluble and leave the body quickly, so they should be taken twice a day. Therefore, you should take 25 to 1,500 milligrams of niacin twice a day.

■ Side Effects and Contraindications

When you are first beginning niacin treatment, it is fairly common to experience skin flushing, sensations of heat, stomach problems, or dry skin. However, these reactions typically subside within several weeks. Also, taking an aspirin 30 minutes before supplementing with niacin can help prevent skin flushing. High doses of niacin or extended-release niacin can cause liver damage, peptic ulcers, high uric acid levels, or glucose intolerance. Do not take niacin without taking the other vitamins in the B complex because doing so can cause your homocysteine levels to elevate, increasing your risk of heart disease and memory loss. If statin drugs (which lower cholesterol) and niacin are taken together, rhabdomyolysis (a potentially fatal breakdown of skeletal muscle) may occur. Therefore, niacin should only be taken under the supervision of a doctor.

■ Diseases/Disorders that Can Be Treated with Niacin

- Acne
- Depression
- Diabetes mellitus
- High cholesterol
- High lipoprotein(a)
- High triglycerides
- Intermittent claudication (leg pains due to circulation changes)

- Low HDL (good) cholesterol
- Memory loss
- Osteoarthritis
- Painful menstrual cycles
- Parkinson's disease
- Rheumatoid arthritis

B_5 (PANTOTHENIC ACID)

Like the other elements of the vitamin B complex, B_5—pantothenic acid—is involved in the body's metabolism of carbohydrates, fats, and proteins. It is named "pantothenic," which is derived from a Greek word that means "everywhere," because this vitamin can be found, albeit in small quantities, in many, many different foods.

■ Functions of B_5 in Your Body

- Aids in the formation of antibodies
- Aids in wound healing
- Helps convert food into energy
- Helps with fatty acid transport
- Helps your body use other vitamins
- Needed for synthesis of coenzyme A
- Needed to make fatty acids
- Stimulates adrenal gland
- Used in red cell production

- Used in the synthesis of several amino acids
- Used to make vitamin D

■ Symptoms of B$_5$ Deficiency

- ☐ Adrenal exhaustion
- ☐ Allergies
- ☐ Arthritis
- ☐ Burning sensation in your feet
- ☐ Constipation
- ☐ Decreased antibody formation
- ☐ Decreased production of hydrochloric acid in stomach
- ☐ Depression
- ☐ Duodenal ulcers
- ☐ Eczema
- ☐ Enlarged, chunky, furrowed tongue
- ☐ Fatigue

- ☐ Gout
- ☐ Graying hair
- ☐ Headache
- ☐ High blood pressure
- ☐ Insomnia
- ☐ Intestinal inflammation
- ☐ Muscle cramps
- ☐ Nerve degeneration
- ☐ Restlessness
- ☐ Upper respiratory tract infections
- ☐ Vomiting

■ Causes of B$_5$ Deficiency

- Caffeine
- Estrogen supplementation
- Sleeping pills

■ Recommended Dosage

50 to 250 milligrams daily. B vitamins are water soluble and leave the body quickly, so they should be taken twice a day. Therefore, you should take 5 to 125 milligrams of B$_5$ twice a day.

■ Side Effects and Contraindications

None. However, high dose supplementation of a single B vitamin can cause imbalances of other B vitamins.

Food Sources of Vitamin B₅

The following foods are numbered so that the foods that contain the most vitamin B₅ are at the top of the list. As the list proceeds, the foods contain progressively less vitamin B₅.

1. Brewer's yeast	14. Eggs	27. Hazelnuts
2. Calf liver	15. Lobster	28. Turkey, dark meat
3. Chicken liver	16. Oatmeal, dry	29. Brown rice
4. Beef kidneys	17. Buckwheat flour	30. Whole wheat flour
5. Peanuts	18. Sunflower seeds	31. Sardines
6. Mushrooms	19. Lentils	32. Red chili peppers
7. Soybean flour	20. Rye flour, whole	33. Avocados
8. Split peas	21. Cashews	34. Veal
9. Beef tongue	22. Fresh salmon	35. Dry black-eyed peas
10. Perch	23. Camembert cheese	36. Wild rice
11. Blue cheese	24. Garbanzo beans	37. Cauliflower
12. Pecans	25. Wheat germ, toasted	38. Chicken, dark meat
13. Soybeans	26. Broccoli	39. Kale

■ Diseases/Disorders that Can be Treated with B₅

- Acne
- Adrenal dysfunction
- Allergies
- Cold sores
- Detoxification
- Elevated triglycerides
- Genital herpes
- Fatigue
- Infection
- Osteoarthritis
- Rheumatoid arthritis
- Shingles
- Ulcerative colitis

B₆ (PYRIDOXINE)

Pyridoxine acts as a partner for more than one hundred different enzymes. As you get older, the efficiency with which you utilize B₆ decreases, so it may be necessary to increase your intake of B₆ as you age.

■ Functions of B$_6$ in Your Body

- Detoxifies chemicals
- Involved in strengthening connective tissue

Food Sources of Vitamin B$_6$

The following foods are numbered so that the foods that contain the most B$_6$ are at the beginning of the list. As the list proceeds, the foods contain progressively less B$_6$.

1. Brewer's yeast
2. Sunflower seeds
3. Toasted wheat germ
4. Fresh tuna
5. Beef liver
6. Dry soybeans
7. Chicken liver
8. Walnuts
9. Fresh salmon
10. Fresh trout
11. Calf liver
12. Fresh mackerel
13. Pork liver
14. Soybean flour
15. Dry lentils
16. Dry lima beans
17. Buckwheat flour
18. Dry black-eyed peas
19. Navy beans, dry
20. Brown rice
21. Hazelnuts
22. Garbanzo beans, dry
23. Dry pinto beans
24. Bananas
25. Pork
26. Fresh albacore
27. Fresh halibut
28. Beef kidneys
29. Avocados
30. Veal kidneys
31. Whole wheat flour
32. Fresh chestnuts
33. Egg yolks
34. Kale
35. Rye flour
36. Spinach
37. Turnip greens
38. Sweet peppers
39. Potatoes
40. Prunes
41. Raisins
42. Sardines
43. Brussels sprouts
44. Elderberries
45. Fresh perch
46. Fresh cod
47. Barley
48. Camembert cheese
49. Sweet potatoes
50. Cauliflower
51. Popped popcorn
52. Red cabbage
53. Leeks

- Key to the synthesis of several neurotransmitters, including the metabolism of tryptophan to serotonin
- Needed for REM sleep
- Needed for the absorption of fats and proteins
- Needed for the immune system
- Needed for the production of hydrocholoric acid
- Needed for the transfer of amino groups
- Used in the metabolism of amino acids
- Used in the methylation process, which lowers homocysteine levels (high levels of which can be a risk factor for heart disease and memory loss)

■ Symptoms of B₆ Deficiency

☐ Depression

☐ Fatigue

☐ Hyperactivity

☐ Insomnia

☐ Irritability

☐ Mental confusion

☐ Mouth ulcers

☐ Nervousness

☐ Numbness

☐ Skin lesions around the mouth

☐ Weakness

■ Causes of B₆ Deficiency

- Aminoglycosides
- Amphetamines
- Antidepressants
- Bumetanide
- Cephalosporins
- Chlortetracycline
- Cigarette smoking
- Cortisone
- Demeclocycline
- Diethylstilbestrol
- Dopamine
- Doxycycline
- Estrogen supplementation
- Ethacrynic acid
- Excessive exercise
- Fluoroquinolones
- Food additives (FDC yellow #5)
- Hydralazine
- Hydrochlorothiazide
- Isoniazid
- Macrolides
- Minocycline
- Oral contraceptives
- Oxytetracycline
- Penicillamine
- Penicillins
- Pesticides
- Phenelzine
- Quinestrol
- Raloxifene
- Sulfonamides
- Tetracyclines
- Theophylline
- Torsemide
- Trimethoprim

■ Recommended Dosage

30 to 500 milligrams daily. B vitamins are water soluble and leave the body quickly, so they should be taken twice a day. Therefore, you should take 15 to 250 milligrams of B_6 twice a day.

■ Side Effects and Contraindications

At too high a dose (more than 500 milligrams a day), pyridoxine can cause a neuropathy (nerve disorder). If you are taking levodopa for Parkinson's disease, do not take B_6 without first consulting your doctor. Also, high dose supplementation of a single B vitamin can cause imbalances of other B vitamins.

■ Diseases/Disorders that Can Be Treated with B_6

- Asthma
- Atherosclerosis
- Autism
- Carpal tunnel syndrome
- Constipation
- Depression
- Diabetes mellitus
- Eczema
- Epilepsy
- Infertility
- Irritability
- Monosodium glutamate (MSG) sensitivity or intolerance
- Nausea and vomiting related to pregnancy
- Nervous system dysfunction
- Osteoporosis
- Premenstrual syndrome (PMS)
- Prevention of calcium oxalate kidney stones
- Schizophrenia
- Seborrheic dermatitis
- Sickle cell disease

B_7 (BIOTIN)

Biotin is a B vitamin made by the flora of your gastrointestinal tract. It is involved in the metabolism of fats and proteins. Excessive amounts of biotin synthesize with bacteria and kill it. If you take antibiotics all of the time, the bacteria that synthesizes biotin are killed off and you will not make enough.

■ Functions of B₇ in Your Body

- Increases insulin sensitivity
- Needed for fatty acid synthesis
- Strengthens nails
- Used in energy metabolism

■ Symptoms of B₇ Deficiency

- ☐ Cradle cap (in newborns)
- ☐ Dandruff
- ☐ Depression
- ☐ Hair loss
- ☐ Hallucinations
- ☐ Localized numbness and tingling
- ☐ Muscle pain
- ☐ Nausea
- ☐ Reduced appetite
- ☐ Scaly dermatitis

■ Causes of B₇ Deficiency

- Alcohol excess
- Anticonvulsants (phenytoin, carbamazepine, primidone, phenobarbital)
- Raw egg whites

Food Sources of Vitamin B₇

The following foods are numbered so that the foods that contain the most vitamin B₇ are at the beginning of the list. As the list proceeds, the foods contain progressively less vitamin B₇.

1. Brewer's yeast
2. Lamb liver
3. Pork liver
4. Beef liver
5. Soy flour
6. Soybeans
7. Rice bran
8. Rice germ
9. Rice polishings
10. Egg yolk
11. Peanut butter
12. Walnuts
13. Roasted peanuts
14. Barley
15. Pecans
16. Oatmeal
17. Canned sardines
18. Whole eggs
19. Black-eyed peas
20. Split peas
21. Almonds
22. Cauliflower
23. Mushrooms
24. Whole wheat cereal
25. Canned salmon
26. Textured vegetable protein
27. Bran
28. Lentils
29. Brown rice

■ Ways to Increase B₇ Level

• Vegetarian diet

■ Recommended Dosage

300 to 600 micrograms daily. B vitamins are water soluble and leave the body quickly, so they should be taken twice a day. Therefore, you should take 150 to 300 micrograms of B₇ twice a day.

■ Side Effects and Contraindications

None. However, high dose supplementation of a single B vitamin can cause imbalances of other B vitamins.

■ Diseases/Disorders that Can Be Treated with B₇

• Brittle nails

• Diabetes mellitus

• Diabetic neuropathy

• Seborrheic dermatitis

B₉ (FOLIC ACID)

Vitamin B₉ has many functions in the body but is especially important for energy production and the immune system. Part of the B₉ you need is made in your intestine, while the rest can be found in food or supplements. The synthetic form of B₉ is folic acid; the natural form found in food is called folate.

■ Functions of B₉ in Your Body

• Detoxifies hormones (such as estrogen)

• Detoxifies phenols (by-products of manufacturing) from the environment

• Essential for central nervous system function

• Essential for DNA synthesis

- Involved in methylation (which decreases homocysteine)
- Metabolic conversion of dopamine, a neurotransmitter
- Needed for proper health of all tissues, especially mucous membrane tissues of the digestive tract, vagina, and cervix
- Needed for the synthesis of hemoglobin
- Produces complex phospholipids for neurological function
- Produces S-adenosylmethionine (SAMe), an important compound found in all living cells
- Protects baby from neural tube defects, such as spina bifida

■ Symptoms of B₉ Deficiency

- ☐ Birth defects affecting the neural tube
- ☐ Decreased resistance to infection
- ☐ Depression
- ☐ Diarrhea
- ☐ Drowsiness
- ☐ Graying hair
- ☐ Indigestion
- ☐ Inflamed and sore tongue with smooth and shiny appearance
- ☐ Insomnia
- ☐ Irritability
- ☐ Mental illness
- ☐ Numbness or tingling in hands and feet
- ☐ Slow, weakened pulse
- ☐ Toxemia
- ☐ Weakness
- ☐ Wound healing, impaired

■ Problems Associated with B₉ Deficiency

- ☐ Adrenal dysfunction
- ☐ Anemia
- ☐ Depression
- ☐ Impaired synthesis of estrogen and progesterone by the ovaries
- ☐ Increased number of ovarian cysts
- ☐ Increased risk of cervical cancer
- ☐ Increased risk of heart disease and memory loss due to high homocysteine levels
- ☐ Low vitamin C levels

Food Sources of Vitamin B$_9$

1. Brewer's yeast
2. Black-eyed peas
3. Rice germ
4. Soy flour
5. Wheat germ
6. Beef liver
7. Lamb liver
8. Soy beans
9. Pork liver
10. Bran
11. Kidney beans
12. Mung beans
13. Lima beans
14. Navy beans
15. Garbanzo beans
16. Asparagus
17. Lentils
18. Walnuts
19. Fresh spinach
20. Kale
21. Hazelnuts
22. Beet and mustard greens
23. Textured vegetable protein
24. Peanuts, roasted
25. Peanut butter
26. Broccoli
27. Barley
28. Split peas
29. Whole wheat cereal
30. Brussels sprouts
31. Almonds
32. Whole wheat flour
33. Oatmeal
34. Cabbage
35. Dried figs
36. Avocados
37. Green beans
38. Corn
39. Fresh coconut
40. Pecans
41. Mushrooms
42. Dates
43. Blackberries
44. Ground beef
45. Oranges

◼ Causes of B$_9$ Deficiency

- Alcohol
- Aspirin
- Barbituates
- Birth control pills
- Carbamazepine
- Celecoxib
- Cholestyramine
- Cimetidine
- Colestipol
- Corticosteroids
- Ethosuximide
- Famotidine
- Fosphenytoin
- Hydrochlorothiazide
- Indomethacin
- Methotrexate
- Methsuximide
- Non-steroidal anti-inflammatory drugs (NSAIDs)
- Phenobarbital
- Phenytoin
- Primidone
- Ranitidine
- Salsalate
- Sulfasalazine
- Tobacco
- Triamterene
- Trimethoprim
- Valproic acid

■ Recommended Dosage

Up to 400 micrograms daily. B vitamins are water soluble and leave the body quickly, so they should be taken twice a day. Therefore, you should take up to 200 micrograms of B_9 twice a day. Higher doses should only be taken under the direction of a physician. After taking digestive enzymes, wait at least two hours before taking folic acid or your absorption of the vitamin may be effected.

■ Side Effects and Contraindications

Dosages should not exceed 400 micrograms per day since folic acid supplementation may mask the symptoms of B_{12} deficiency. Large doses can cause insomnia, irritability, and gastrointestinal problems. If you are taking phenytoin (an anticonvulsant), do not take high doses of folic acid. Folic acid also interferes with seizure medications such as valproic acid, carbamazepine, and primidone, so consult your doctor before taking this vitamin if you are on any of these medications.

■ Diseases/Disorders that Can Be Treated by B_9

- Birth defects such as neural tube and cleft palate (prevention)
- Cancer prevention
- Cervical dysplasia
- Depression
- Gingivitis
- Gout
- Lower homocysteine
- Psoriasis
- Restless leg syndrome

B_{12} (COBALAMIN)

Vitamin B_{12} is called either cobalamin or cyanocobalamin, and is synthesized by bacteria. It performs many important functions in the body, and exists in most animal foods. Vegetarians and vegans should take B_{12} supplements or eat fortified breakfast cereals, which are a valuable source of this vitamin. Hydrochloric acid releases B_{12} from food, at which point the vitamin can be absorbed by the body.

■ Functions of B_{12} in Your Body

- Essential for DNA synthesis

- Facilitates the metabolism of folic acid
- Functions as a methyl donor, which lowers homocysteine levels (high levels of which can be a risk factor for heart disease and memory loss)
- Helps synthesize proteins
- Involved in the production of neurotransmitters
- Needed for carnitine metabolism (which breaks down fat to provide energy)
- Needed for nervous system function
- Needed for red blood cell metabolism
- Required for proper digestion

■ Symptoms of B_{12} Deficiency

- ☐ Confusion
- ☐ Constipation
- ☐ Decreased estrogen in women
- ☐ Decreased progesterone in women
- ☐ Depression
- ☐ Diarrhea
- ☐ Dizziness
- ☐ Drowsiness
- ☐ Elevated levels of homocysteine
- ☐ Fatigue
- ☐ Hallucinations

- ☐ Increased cortisol levels
- ☐ Insomnia
- ☐ Irritability
- ☐ Memory loss
- ☐ Moodiness
- ☐ Numbness and tingling of extremities
- ☐ Poor appetite
- ☐ Ringing in ears
- ☐ Sore tongue
- ☐ Stiffness
- ☐ Weakness

■ Causes of B_{12} Deficiency

- Antacids (which can decrease absorption from food but not from supplementation)
- Colchicine (gout medication)
- Digestive disorders
- Nitrous oxide
- Potassium citrate and chloride
- Some oral hypoglycemic agents (which lower blood sugar)

Food Sources of Vitamin B$_{12}$

1. Lamb liver
2. Clams
3. Beef liver
4. Lamb kidneys
5. Calf liver
6. Beef kidneys
7. Chicken liver
8. Oysters
9. Sardines
10. Beef heart
11. Egg yolks
12. Lamb heart
13. Trout
14. Fresh salmon
15. Fresh tuna
16. Lamb
17. Thymus sweetbreads
18. Eggs
19. Dried whey
20. Beef
21. Edam cheese
22. Swiss cheese
23. Brie cheese
24. Gruyere cheese
25. Blue cheese
26. Fresh haddock
27. Fresh flounder
28. Scallops
29. Cheddar cheese
30. Cottage cheese
31. Mozzarella cheese
32. Halibut
33. Perch fillets
34. Fresh swordfish

Drugs that Deplete B$_{12}$ from Your Body

- Aminoglycosides
- Cephalosporins
- Certain cholesterol-lowering medications
- Chlorotetracycline
- Cholestyramine
- Cimetidine
- Co-trimoxazole
- Doxycycline
- Famotidine
- Fluoroquinolones
- Histamine blockers
- Lansoprazole
- Macrolides
- Metformin
- Minocycline
- Neomycin
- Nizatidine
- Omeprazole
- Oral contraceptives
- Oxytetracycline
- Penicillins
- Phenytoin
- Ranitidine
- Sulfonamides
- Tetracyclines
- Trimethoprim
- Zidovudine and other HIV/AIDS medications

Recommended Dosage

400 to 5,000 micrograms daily. B vitamins are water soluble and leave the body quickly, so they should be taken twice a day. Therefore, you should take 200 to 2,500 micrograms of B$_{12}$ twice a day.

■ Side Effects and Contraindications

None. However, high dose supplementation of a single B vitamin can cause imbalances of other B vitamins.

■ Diseases/Disorders that Can Be Treated with B$_{12}$

- AIDS
- Anemia
- Anxiety
- Asthma
- Ataxia
- Bell's palsy
- Dementia
- Depression
- Epilepsy

- Fatigue
- Hepatitis
- Infertility
- Insomnia
- Irritability
- Leg cramps at night
- Multiple sclerosis
- Neuropathy
- Numbness

- Psychosis
- Retinopathy
- Sciatica
- Seborrheic dermatitis
- Tingling
- Tinnitus
- Trigeminal neuralgia
- Vitiligo
- Xanthelasma

CHOLINE

Choline is an important nutrient that plays a role in almost every bodily system. The important compounds acetylcholine and lecithin are derived from this B vitamin. Acetylcholine is believed to protect against certain types of age-related dementia.

■ Functions of Choline in Your Body

- Aids in metabolism of fats
- Allows movement and coordination
- Component of every cell membrane

Food Sources of Choline

- Beef
- Brewer's yeast
- Chicken

- Egg yolks
- Iceberg lettuce
- Nuts

- Oats
- Peanut butter
- Soy

- Lowers LDL (bad) cholesterol
- Precursor to acetylcholine (the main neurotransmitter involved with memory)
- Required for normal brain function

■ Symptoms of Choline Deficiency

- ☐ High blood pressure
- ☐ High cholesterol levels
- ☐ Nervous system disorders

■ Causes of Choline Deficiency

- Alcohol
- Folic acid deficiency
- High sugar intake
- Nicotine

■ Recommended Dosage

400 to 500 milligrams daily. Do not take more than 3 grams a day. Also, B vitamins are water soluble and leave the body quickly, so they should be taken twice a day. Therefore, you should take 200 to 250 milligrams of choline twice a day.

■ Diseases/Disorders that Can Be Treated with Choline

- Alzheimer's disease
- Hepatitis
- High cholesterol
- Liver disease
- Manic depression (bipolar disease)

INOSITOL

Inositol is part of the vitamin B complex. It helps synthesize phospho-lipids, which are essential to the digestion, absorption, and transportation of fats in the body. Sufficient amounts of inositol are vital for good health—both mental and physical.

■ Functions of Inositol in Your Body

- Can reduce LDL (bad) cholesterol
- Has a calming effect

- Helps form lecithin, an important antioxidant
- Helps keep arteries from hardening
- Improves quality of sleep
- Involved in augmenting effects of neurotransmitter release
- Involved with metabolizing fats and cholesterol in the arteries and liver
- Supports the metabolism of estrogen and progesterone
- Used to treat depression and panic disorders

■ Symptoms of Inositol Deficiency

☐ Anxiety

☐ Depression

☐ Difficulty falling asleep

☐ Fibroid tumors

☐ Premenstrual syndrome (PMS) symptoms

■ Causes of Inositol Deficiency

- Caffeine

■ Recommended Dosage

200 milligrams to 12 grams daily. However, dosages larger than 200 milligrams should only be taken under physician supervision. Also, B vitamins are water soluble and leave the body quickly, so they should be taken twice a day. Therefore, you should take around 100 milligrams of inositol twice a day.

Food Sources of Inositol

- Beans
- Brewer's yeast
- Fruits
- Grains
- Meat
- Milk
- Nuts
- Raisins

■ Side Effects and Contraindications

Do not take inositol if you have kidney failure.

■ Diseases/Disorders that Can Be Treated with Inositol

- Depression
- Fibroids
- Liver disease
- Neuropathy
- Panic attacks
- Premenstrual syndrome (PMS)

VITAMIN C

Vitamin C must be consumed in food or supplements because it cannot be made by our bodies. This water-soluble vitamin is essential for many of your body's systems to function properly. The immune system, in particular, relies on vitamin C. Rutin, a bioflavonoid, inhibits the oxidation of this vitamin, making it more useful to the body.

If you are diabetic, you need to take vitamin C. This is because vitamin C and glucose enter your cells through the same pathways. Consequently, vitamin C will be competing with glucose to enter your cells—and glucose will win, leaving the cells deficient in vitamin C.

■ Functions of Vitamin C in Your Body

- Aids in the healing of wounds
- Aids in the synthesis of collagen
- Benefits immune system by increasing number of white blood cells and interferons (proteins that can fight viruses and cancer)
- Decreases adrenal steroid production
- Decreases production of leukotrienes (which contribute to symptoms of allergic reactions)
- Decreases rate of gum disease
- Decreases rate of stomach cancer
- Decreases risk of heart disease
- Helps carnitine synthesis (which breaks down fatty acids and releases energy)
- Helps in the metabolism of tyrosine (an amino acid that synthesizes proteins)
- Helps regenerate vitamin E, glutathione, and uric acid
- Increases fertility

- Increases HDL (good) cholesterol
- Increases nitric oxide
- Inhances the body's absorption of iron
- Involved in catecholamine synthesis (which prepares the body for activity or to handle stress)
- Involved in production of serotonin (a neurotransmitter involved in many important brain functions, including mood and appetite)
- Is a diuretic
- Is a powerful antioxidant
- Lowers blood pressure
- Lowers incidence of cataracts
- Lowers sorbitol levels, which can prevent cataracts
- Lowers triglycerides
- Needed for progesterone production
- Needed to maintain glutathione levels (which are very important for good health)
- Prevents formation of nitrosamines (compounds which can cause cancer)
- Prevents free radical damage of LDL (bad) cholesterol
- Prevents some forms of lung disease
- Reduces bruising
- Reduces damage (such as diabetes or stiffening tissues) due to glycation
- Reserves the energy-producing capacity of the mitochondria

■ Symptoms of Vitamin C Deficiency

☐ Bleeding gums	☐ Impaired wound healing
☐ Cardiovascular disease	☐ Joint pain
☐ Easy bruising	☐ Loose teeth
☐ Fatigue	☐ Scurvy
☐ Frequent infections	☐ Weight loss

Food Sources of Vitamin C

The following foods are numbered so that the foods that contain the most vitamin C are at the beginning of the list. As the list proceeds, the foods contain progressively less vitamin C.

The vitamin C content of foods is easily destroyed by light, heat, and chemicals. Fresh-cut lettuce, for example, loses half of its vitamin C in forty-eight hours unless it is stored in a dark refrigerator.

1. Red chili peppers
2. Guavas
3. Red sweet peppers
4. Kale leaves
5. Parsley
6. Collard leaves
7. Turnip greens
8. Green sweet peppers
9. Broccoli
10. Brussels sprouts
11. Mustard greens
12. Watercress
13. Cauliflower
14. Persimmons
15. Red cabbage
16. Strawberries
17. Papayas
18. Spinach
19. Oranges
20. Orange juice
21. Cabbage
22. Lemon juice
23. Grapefruit
24. Grapefruit juice
25. Elderberries
26. Calf liver
27. Turnips
28. Mangos
29. Asparagus
30. Cantaloupes
31. Swiss chard
32. Green onions
33. Beef liver
34. Okra
35. Tangerines
36. New Zealand spinach
37. Oysters
38. Young lima beans
39. Black-eyed peas
40. Soybeans
41. Green peas
42. Radishes
43. Raspberries
44. Chinese cabbage
45. Yellow summer squash
46. Loganberries
47. Honeydew melon
48. Tomatoes

◼ Causes of Vitamin C Deficiency

- Aging
- Antibiotics
- Aspirin
- Birth control pills
- Cortisone
- Diabetes mellitus
- High blood pressure
- High fever
- Painkillers
- Smoking
- Stress
- Sulfa drugs

■ Symptoms of Toxicity

Doses of vitamin C higher than 5,000 milligrams can be ingested, but may cause diarrhea. Mineral ascorbates and Ester-C are buffered forms of vitamin C that cause less diarrhea.

■ Recommended Dosage

1,000 to 5,000 milligrams daily. Vitamin C is water soluble and leaves the body quickly, so it should be taken twice a day. Therefore, you should take 500 to 2,500 milligrams of C twice a day.

■ Side Effects and Contraindications

Hemochromatosis occurs when the body accumulates excess iron. Vitamin C can increase this accumulation, so people with hemochromatosis should avoid taking extra vitamin C. If you have a glucose-6-phosphate dehydrogenase (G6PD) deficiency, do not have vitamin C given to you intravenously.

2

Minerals

Many important bodily functions require certain minerals in order to operate correctly. Yet minerals, unlike vitamins, cannot be produced by our bodies. Therefore, adequate consumption of minerals is very important for your health.

At the same time, you cannot simply load up on these nutrients. Every mineral is required by your body in a specific amount. This precise amount depends on many factors including diet, mineral content of the soil in which your food is grown, medications, health, and the interaction of the mineral with other substances. (See page 9 for more on nutritional interactions.)

Minerals are divided into two groups: macro (or major) and micro (or minor). *Macrominerals* are required by your body in relatively high quantities. Generally, people need more than 200 milligrams of these nutrients a day. Calcium, chloride, magnesium, phosphorus, potassium, and sodium are all macrominerals.

Microminerals, on the other hand, are required by your body in trace amounts. Generally, people need less than 200 milligrams of these nutrients a day. Arsenic, boron, chromium, cobalt, copper, fluoride, iodine, iron, manganese, molybdenum, nickel, selenium, silicon, tin, vanadium, and zinc are microminerals.

In this chapter, macrominerals are discussed first, while the second half of the chapter describes microminerals. The nutrients are arranged alphabetically within these two sections. You will read important information about each mineral, including its functions, food sources, and recommended dosage. All dosages include what is consumed in both food and supplements. You will also read about the symptoms that can occur if your body's storage of that mineral becomes deficient. This will allow you to plan your daily mineral intake and promote your optimal health.

The microminerals arsenic, cobalt, fluoride, nickel, and tin are not elaborated on because these minerals are sufficiently consumed through diet. There is, however, the possibility of ingesting too much of these nutrients. A toxic metal screen test can determine whether you are ingesting too much of these minerals. See Resources for the names and contact information of several laboratories that perform this test.

CALCIUM

Calcium is the most abundant mineral in your body, and an essential component of a healthy diet. It is important that everyone, regardless of age, consumes proper amounts of calcium, but most doctors advise people to increase their intake as they get older. However, your body can only

---

Acid-Creating Foods

The average American diet includes many foods that, once eaten, create acid in your body. If you eat a majority of acidic foods and not enough alkaline foods, your body has to find alkalizing minerals elsewhere to neutralize its pH levels. It often has to resort to using the calcium and protein in your bones. As a result, your bones can become weakened, possibly irrevocably, and your bodily systems can age at an accelerated pace, resulting in a slew of related problems. The following foods create particularly high acidity levels in your body.

- Chocolate
- Dairy products, such as butter, cheese, ice cream, milk, and yogurt
- Drinks, such as beer, black tea, coffee, and soft drinks
- Fish, such as haddock
- Fruit, such as blueberries, cranberries, and dried fruit
- Grains, such as barley, oats, rice, wheat, and white bread
- Honey
- Meat products, such as beef, chicken, ham, turkey, and veal
- Nuts, such as peanuts and walnuts
- Processed soybeans
- Sugar
- Vegetables, such as corn
- White vinegar

---

absorb about 500 milligrams of calcium at a time, so your daily intake should be divided into separate doses.

■ Functions of Calcium in Your Body

- Activates numerous enzymes
- Helps cholesterol make sex hormones
- Needed for the absorption of vitamin B_{12}
- Plays a crucial role in nerve impulse transmission
- Regulates ion transport in your cells
- Required (along with vitamin K) for blood to clot
- Used by muscles in energy production
- Vital for development of bones and teeth

■ Symptoms of Calcium Deficiency (Hypocalcemia)

- ☐ Hypertension (high blood pressure)
- ☐ Muscle spasms and twitching
- ☐ Osteoporosis (bone loss)

■ Causes of Calcium Deficiency (Hypocalcemia)

- Acidic foods (see inset on page 58)
- Alcohol
- Aspartame
- Aspirin
- Caffeine
- Chocolate
- Cholestyramine
- Excess protein in your diet
- Excessive thyroid replacement
- Fiber*
- Heavy exercise
- Heparin (an anticoagulant)
- High phosphorus-containing foods (such as soft drinks and white flour)
- Increased fat in diet
- Increased zinc consumption
- Methotrexate (treatment for cancer and autoimmune diseases)
- Oxalic acid-containing foods (such as chocolate, cocoa, kale, rhubarb, and spinach)
- Phenobarbital
- Steroids
- Sugar
- Tetracyclines
- Whole wheat

*After eating fiber, wait two hours before taking calcium supplements.

■ Substances that Increase Calcium Absorption

- Ascorbic acid
- Citric acid
- Glycine
- Hydrochloric acid
- Lysine

■ Symptoms of Calcium Toxicity (Hypercalcemia)

Since the body is limited in its ability to absorb calcium, there are few short-term effects (namely, constipation and kidney stones) of ingesting too much. However, long-term consumption of too much calcium can result in *hypercalcemia*—high levels of calcium in the blood. Additionally, combining excess calcium with excess vitamin D, which helps the body absorb calcium, can be very dangerous. There are also several diseases, such as certain cancers, that can cause calcium toxicity.

- ☐ Blocked uptake of manganese (see page 91)
- ☐ Clogged arteries (which can predispose you to heart disease)
- ☐ Constipation
- ☐ Decreased iron absorption
- ☐ Decreased magnesium absorption
- ☐ Decreased vitamin K production
- ☐ Decreased zinc absorption
- ☐ Kidney stones
- ☐ Problems with your thyroid hormones

■ Recommended Dosage

As you read on pages 58 to 59, your body can only absorb 500 milligrams of calcium at a time. Therefore, to fully utilize your ingestion of calcium, the following suggestions for daily calcium consumption should be split into dosages. These amounts refer to your entire calcium intake, including what you eat *and* the supplements you take.

- Adults: 800 milligrams daily
- Menopausal women: 1,600 milligrams daily
- Perimenopausal women: 1,000 milligrams daily
- Pregnant or lactating women: 1,200 milligrams daily

Food Sources of Calcium

The following list is reprinted with permission from Jeffrey Bland's *Clinical Nutrition: A Functional Approach*. Foods that contain the most calcium are listed first, followed by foods that contain progressively less calcium. The number to the left of each food describes how many milligrams of calcium are in 100 grams (3.5 ounces) of that food.

1093	Kelp	99	English walnut	32	Sweet potato
925	Swiss cheese	94	Cottage cheese	32	Brown rice
750	Cheddar cheese	93	Spinach	29	Garlic
352	Carob flour	73	Cooked soybeans	28	Summer squash
296	Dulse	73	Pecans	27	Onion
250	Collard leaves	72	Wheat germ	26	Lemon
246	Turnip greens	69	Peanuts	26	Fresh green peas
245	Barbados molasses	68	Miso	25	Cauliflower
		68	Romaine lettuce	25	Cooked lentils
234	Almonds	67	Dried apricots	22	Sweet cherry
210	Brewer's yeast	66	Rutabaga	22	Asparagus
203	Parsley	62	Raisins	22	Winter squash
200	Corn tortillas with lime	60	Black currant	21	Strawberries
		59	Dates	20	Millet
187	Dandelion greens	56	Green snap beans	19	Mung bean sprouts
186	Brazil nuts	51	Globe artichoke		
151	Watercress	51	Dried prunes	17	Pineapple
129	Goat's milk	51	Pumpkin and squash seeds	16	Grapes
128	Tofu			16	Beets
126	Dried figs	50	Cooked dry beans	14	Cantaloupe
121	Buttermilk	49	Common cabbage	14	Jerusalem artichoke
120	Yogurt	48	Soybean sprouts		
119	Beet greens	46	Hard winter wheat	13	Tomato
119	Wheat bran			12	Eggplant
118	Whole milk	41	Orange	12	Chicken
114	Buckwheat, raw	39	Celery	11	Orange juice
110	Hulled sesame seeds	38	Cashews	10	Beef
		38	Rye grain	8	Banana
106	Ripe olives	37	Carrot	7	Apple
103	Broccoli	34	Barley	3	Sweet corn

■ Diseases/Disorders that Can Be Treated with Calcium

- Colon cancer
- Elevated triglycerides
- High blood pressure
- Increased cholesterol

- Leg cramps
- Osteoporosis
- Preeclampsia
- Premenstrual syndrome (PMS)

■ Side Effects and Contraindications

- Decreases absorption of ciprofloxacin and most fluoroquinolone antibiotics
- Decreases aluminum absorption
- Increases the toxicity of digoxin
- Inhibits absorption of tetracycline
- Interferes with the absorption of thyroid medication
- May interfere with the absorption of magnesium, zinc, iron, manganese, and phosphorus

■ Other Important Factors

- Always use only pharmaceutical-grade supplements. Lower-grade products may be contaminated with lead, mercury, arsenic, aluminum, or cadmium. (See page 376 for a list of pharmaceutical grade companies.)
- Calcium carbonate is not a good form of calcium because most of its calcium is not bioavailable.
- Calcium citrate and hydroxyapatite are both good sources of calcium. Bioavailability of calcium citrate is 2.5 times that of calcium carbonate.
- Milk is not the best source of calcium because pasteurization destroys up to 32 percent of its available calcium.
- Tums (antacids) are not a good source of calcium because the calcium they contain is poorly absorbed by the body.
- Vitamin C increases calcium absorption by 100 percent.

CHLORIDE

Electrolytes are molecules in your plasma—the liquid portion of your blood—that maintain either a positive or negative charge. These charges allow them to respond to messages from your nervous system by conducting electrical currents through your body, enabling and regulating many bodily functions and systems. Chloride is one of your body's most important electrolytes. It is located in the extracellular fluid compartments—area outside the cells. Your body's chloride levels are directly related to its sodium levels.

■ Functions of Chloride in Your Body

- Balances the fluid inside and outside cells along with sodium and potassium
- Component of stomach acid
- Generates and conducts electrical signals that play roles in many bodily functions
- Maintains pH balance

■ Electrolyte Imbalance

It is very important that your body's electrolytes—such as chloride, sodium, and potassium—remain at their proper levels. *Electrolyte imbalance* (which is also called electrolyte disturbance) can occur if any of these substances has a sudden, abnormal change. The change can be elevation or depletion of the electrolyte, and may be due to renal failure or water loss, such as from long-time laxative abuse or excessive vomiting, diarrhea, or sweating. Therefore, sufferers of anorexia and bulimia are at particularly high risk. Electrolyte imbalance is usually the result of an underlying problem, such as dehydration or dysfunction of the endocrine system or kidneys, and is usually corrected by treating the initial problem. If an electrolyte imbalance is left untreated, it can cause heart-related issues, organ failure, problems with the nervous system, or death.

Chloride Deficiency (Hypochloremia)

Chloride can exit the body through urine, sweat, or vomit, or from kidney or adrenal gland disease. *Hypochloremia* occurs when too much chloride exits the body, resulting in a deficiency. Although there are often no symptoms, some people experience headaches, nausea, or cardiac arrest. Others experience water loss and dehydration.

Chloride Elevation (Hyperchloremia)

Although there are often no symptoms, some people with elevated levels

Food Sources of Chloride

Most people get a majority of their chloride from table salt or sea salt. (Salt also contains potassium and sodium.) Chloride can also be found in the following foods.

- Celery
- Lettuce
- Olives
- Tomatoes

of chloride—*hyperchloremia*—also experience dehydration, diarrhea, muscle tension, or kidney disease. Diabetics with elevated chloride levels have a very difficult time maintaining healthy blood sugar levels. There is usually an underlying cause of this disorder, and treatment should involve pinpointing and treating this problem.

■ Recommended Dosage

Because salt is so common in most of our diets, it is usually not necessary to take supplements or eat more salt-containing foods. However, some people do need to add salt to their diets. People with adrenal failure, for example, need to increase their salt intake. Your healthcare provider can help determine whether or not you need more or less salt in your diet.

■ Possible Side Effects of Excess Chloride Consumption

Any excess of chloride is usually removed from the body in urine. However, be cautious about consuming too much salt, which also contains sodium and potassium, and may contribute to muscle cramps, heartburn, dizziness, high blood pressure, or even electrolyte disturbances in people who are susceptible to this condition.

MAGNESIUM

Magnesium is a *cofactor*—a molecule that binds to and stimulates an enzyme—that is involved in the activation of over 300 enzymes in your body. It is involved in the production of adenosine triphosphate (ATP), one of the body's main energy sources. Half of your body's magnesium is found in your bones and prevents bone loss.

■ Functions of Magnesium in Your Body

- Acts as a natural anticonvulsant
- Acts as a natural tranquilizer
- Assists with nerve function
- Assists with skeletal muscle function
- Can help induce sleep
- Decreases blood vessel constriction
- Decreases risk of tooth decay
- Enhances the function of various brain antioxidants
- Essential to the life of all cells
- Helps heal wounds
- Helps prevent labor complications
- Helps synthesize and oxidize fatty acids
- Important for functions of immune system
- Improves glucose uptake by insulin
- Improves muscle strength and endurance
- Increases HDL (good) cholesterol
- Maintains the normal rhythm of your heart
- Maximizes heart health
- May reduce risk of arrhythmias (irregular heart rhythm) after bypass surgery
- Metabolizes fats and carbohydrates for energy production
- Necessary for bone formation
- Necessary for steroid hormone production
- Necessary for teeth formation
- Necessary for protein synthesis
- Prevents production of inflammation-increasing chemicals
- Relaxes electrical impulses and encourages calmness
- Relaxes muscles
- Removes excess ammonia

▪ Symptoms of Magnesium Deficiency

☐ Anxiety

☐ Back pain or spasm

☐ Chest tightness

☐ Confusion

☐ Decreased appetite

☐ Depression

☐ Fatigue

☐ Hyperexcitability

☐ Hyperventilation

☐ Insomnia

☐ Irritability

☐ Memory loss

☐ Muscle cramps, soreness, or twitches

☐ Neck pain or spasm

☐ TMJ (joint between the jaw and skull) pain

☐ Weakness

▪ Causes of Magnesium Deficiency

• Alcoholism

• Antibiotics (such as amphotericin B, carbenicillin, and gentamicin)

• Asthma medications (such as beta-agonists and epinephrine)

• Caffeine intake

• Cyclosporine

• Diarrhea

• Digoxin use

• Diuretics (water pills), except those that are potassium sparing

• Drugs for chemotherapy (such as cisplatinum, bleomycin, and vinblastine)

• Excessive sugar intake

• Extreme athletic competition

• Fiber excess

• Foods high in oxalic acid (such as almonds, cocoa, spinach, and tea)

• Laxatives

• Phosphates in soft drinks

• Steroids

• Stress

• Surgery

• Trans fatty acids

• Trauma

■ Disease States Associated with Magnesium Deficiency

- Abnormal calcium deposits
- Aggressive behavior
- Agoraphobia (fear of large crowds, open spaces, and/or being someplace from which there is no escape)
- Alcoholism
- Anxiety
- Attention deficit disorder (ADD)
- Autism
- Carbohydrate craving
- Cardiovascular disease
- Cold hands and feet
- Constipation
- Delirium
- Dementia (mental deterioration)
- Depression
- Diabetes
- Difficulty swallowing
- Endometriosis
- Excitability
- Fatigue
- Heart attack
- Heart arrhythmia (irregular heart rate)
- Hypertension
- Hypoglycemia (low blood sugar)
- Insomnia
- Learning disabilities
- Loud noise sensitivity
- Lupus
- Mental confusion
- Migraine headaches
- Mitral valve prolapse (a common heart problem that is usually not life threatening)
- Numbness
- Osteoporosis
- Palpitations
- Photophobia (extreme sensitivity to light)
- Poor wound healing
- Premenstrual syndrome (PMS)
- Problem pregnancy
- Psychosis
- Salt craving
- Schizophrenia
- Seizures
- Stress
- Tingling
- Tremors
- Urinary spasms

■ Symptoms of Magnesium Toxicity

Diarrhea may occur if more than 600 milligrams of magnesium are ingested in a day. Symptoms of more severe toxicity include drowsiness, lethargy, and weakness.

Food Sources of Magnesium

The following list is reprinted with permission from *Clinical Nutrition: A Functional Approach* by Jeffrey Bland. Foods that contain the most magnesium are listed first, followed by foods that contain progressively less magnesium. The number to the left of each food describes how many milligrams of magnesium are in 100 grams (3.5 ounces) of that food.

760	Kelp	71	Dried figs	30	Blackberry
490	Wheat bran	65	Swiss chard	25	Beets
336	Wheat germ	62	Dried apricots	24	Cauliflower
270	Almonds	58	Dates	23	Carrot
267	Cashews	57	Collard leaves	22	Celery
258	Blackstrap molasses	51	Shrimp	21	Beef
		48	Sweet corn	20	Asparagus
231	Brewer's yeast	45	Avocado	19	Chicken
229	Buckwheat	45	Cheddar cheese	18	Green pepper
225	Brazil nut	41	Parsley	17	Winter squash
220	Dulse	40	Dried prunes	16	Cantaloupe
184	Hazelnuts	38	Sunflower seeds	16	Eggplant
175	Peanuts	37	Cooked common beans	14	Tomato
162	Millet			13	Cabbage
160	Wheat grain	37	Barley	13	Grapes
142	Pecan	36	Dandelion greens	13	Milk
131	English walnut	36	Garlic	13	Mushroom
115	Tofu	35	Raisins	12	Onion
106	Beet greens	35	Fresh green peas	11	Orange
90	Dry coconut meat	34	Potato with skin	11	Iceberg lettuce
88	Cooked soybeans	34	Crab	9	Plum
88	Spinach	33	Banana	8	Apple
88	Brown rice	31	Sweet potato		

■ Recommended Dosage

400 to 800 milligrams daily. Some people will have diarrhea if over 600 milligrams a day are taken, and should take less than this amount. Magnesium citrate, magnesium glycinate, magnesium gluconate, and magnesium lactate are more easily absorbed than magnesium oxide.

■ Diseases/Disorders that Can Be Treated with Magnesium

- Angina
- Asthma
- Calcium-oxalate kidney stones
- Cardiac arrhythmias (irregular heart rhythm)
- Cardiomyopathy (enlarged heart)
- Chronic fatigue syndrome
- Chronic obstructive pulmonary disease (COPD)
- Claudication (pain in legs due to decreased circulation)
- Congestive heart failure
- Diabetes mellitus
- Fibromyalgia
- Heart attack
- High blood pressure
- Hypoglycemia (low blood sugar)
- Low HDL (good) cholesterol
- Migraine
- Mitral valve prolapse (a common heart problem that is usually not life threatening)
- Muscle spasms
- Osteoporosis
- Pregnancy complications
- Premenstrual syndrome (PMS)
- Restless leg syndrome
- Sickle cell anemia
- Urinary problems

PHOSPHORUS

Phosphorus is essential to many important life processes in all living organisms. The second-most abundant mineral in your body, phosphorus is mainly stored in your bones. There are also phosphate-containing molecules called phospholipids, which are located in your cell membranes and lipoprotein particles, and have many responsibilities on the cellular level.

■ Functions of Phosphorus in Your Body

- Assists with growth and healing of bones and teeth

- Develops and repairs body tissue
- Helps regulate enzymes
- Involved in many biochemical reactions
- Major component of bones and teeth
- Necessary for lipid metabolism
- Needed for energy production
- Used in buffering system (which maintains acid-alkaline balance)

■ Symptoms of Phosphorus Deficiency (Hypophosphatemia)

☐ Anorexia   ☐ Joint stiffness

☐ Fragile bones   ☐ Weakness

■ Causes of Phosphorus Deficiency (Hypophosphatemia)

Most Americans are not deficient in phosphorus because it is found in most foods, including soft drinks and fast foods. The following actions, however, can lower your phosphorus levels, sometimes dangerously.

- Alcoholism
- Excess calcium intake
- Overconsumption of antacids
- Overconsumption of calcium

supplements (which can be avoided by taking a supplement that contains both calcium and phosphorus)
- Vitamin D deficiency

■ Symptoms of Phosphorus Toxicity (Hyperphosphatemia)

There are not many side effects of having high phosphorus levels, or *hyperphosphatemia*. The most common problem when experiencing phosphorus toxicity is diarrhea. However, it can also result in decreased calcium levels, or *hypocalcemia*.

■ Recommended Dosage

People with severe kidney disease or problems regulating their calcium levels should consult their medical practitioner before beginning a regiment of phosphorus supplements. Although most people in the United States are not deficient in phosphorus (particularly because soft drinks contain the mineral), it is suggested that everyone ingest the following amounts.

Food Sources of Phosphorus

The following list is reprinted with permission from Jeffrey Bland's *Clinical Nutrition: A Functional Approach.* Foods that contain the most phosphorus are listed first, followed by foods that contain progressively less phosphorus. The number to the left of each food describes how many milligrams of phosphorus are in 100 grams (3.5 ounces) of that food.

1753	Brewer's yeast	202	Garlic	51	Spinach
1276	Wheat bran	175	Crab	44	Green beans
1144	Pumpkin and squash seeds	152	Cottage cheese	44	Pumpkin
		150	Beef	42	Avocado
1118	Wheat germ	150	Lamb	40	Beet greens
837	Sunflower seeds	119	Cooked lentils	39	Swiss chard
693	Brazil nuts	116	Mushrooms	38	Winter squash
592	Hulled sesame seeds	116	Fresh peas	36	Carrot
		111	Sweet corn	36	Onions
554	Dried soybeans	101	Raisins	35	Red cabbage
504	Almonds	93	Whole milk	33	Beets
478	Cheddar cheese	88	Globe artichoke	31	Radish
457	Dried pinto beans	87	Yogurt	29	Summer squash
		80	Brussels sprouts	28	Celery
409	Peanuts	79	Prunes, dried	27	Cucumber
400	Wheat	78	Broccoli	27	Tomato
380	English walnuts	77	Dried figs	26	Banana
376	Rye grain	69	Yams	26	Persimmon
373	Cashews	67	Soybean sprouts	26	Eggplant
353	Beef liver	64	Mung bean sprouts	26	Lettuce
338	Scallops			24	Nectarine
311	Millet	63	Dates	22	Raspberries
290	Pearled barley	63	Parsley	20	Grapes
289	Pecans	62	Asparagus	20	Orange
267	Dulse	59	Bamboo shoots	17	Olives
240	Kelp	56	Cauliflower	16	Cantaloupe
239	Chicken	53	Potato with skin	10	Apple
221	Brown rice	51	Okra	8	Pineapple
205	Eggs				

- Adults aged 19 to 24 years: 2,400 milligrams daily
- Adults aged 25 years and older: 800 milligrams daily
- Pregnant women: 1,200 milligrams daily

POTASSIUM

Electrolytes are molecules that serve to conduct electricity through your body. Every electrolyte has either a positive or negative charge that reacts to messages sent through your body by your nervous system. They react to these messages by conducting electric currents, which regulate many functions and systems in your body. Potassium is an electrolyte that remains within your body's cells (intracellular), while electrolytes sodium and chloride remain outside the cells (extracellular). Together, these three macrominerals maintain balance between the intra- and extracellular compartments in order to regulate many functions, including nerve transmission and muscle contractions.

◼ Functions of Potassium in Your Body

- Aids in maintaining cellular integrity (keeps the cell together)
- Needed for muscle contraction
- Preserves the acid-base balance
- Regulates fluid balance
- Transmits electrical signals between cells and nerves
- Used in glucose and glycogen metabolism

◼ Electrolyte Imbalance

It is very important that your body's electrolytes—such as chloride, sodium, and potassium—remain at their proper levels. Electrolyte imbalance can occur if any of these has a sudden, abnormal change. It is usually the result of an underlying problem, and can often be corrected by treating this initial problem. The change, which can be elevation or depletion of the electrolyte, may be due to dysfunction of the endocrine or hormone systems, renal failure, or dehydration. If electrolyte imbalance is left untreated, it can cause heart-related issues, organ failure, problems with the nervous system, or death.

Symptoms of Potassium Deficiency (Hypokalemia)

☐ Arrhythmia (irregular heartbeat)
☐ Cardiac weakness
☐ Central nervous system changes
☐ Death
☐ Fragile bones
☐ Muscle weakness or pain
☐ Slow heart rate

Causes of Potassium Deficiency (Hypokalemia)

- Aging
- Burns
- Diarrhea
- Excessive water loss
- Kidney disease
- Low levels of magnesium (because magnesium is necessary for the body to process potassium)
- Low-potassium diet
- Medications (such as diuretics or water pills)
- Starvation
- Vomiting

Symptoms of Potassium Elevation (Hyperkalemia)

☐ Arrhythmia (irregular heartbeat)
☐ Chest pain
☐ Diarrhea
☐ General malaise
☐ Increased urination
☐ Muscle pain
☐ Paralysis

Causes of Potassium Elevation (Hyperkalemia)

- Breakdown of cell function
- Certain anti-inflammatory drugs
- Congestive heart failure
- Endocrine problems
- Hormone problems
- Ineffective elimination from body
- Kidney disease
- Laxative abuse
- Problems with adrenal gland
- Severe dehydration

■ Recommended Dosage

500 milligrams daily. Potassium supplements should be taken with water because they can damage the esophagus if they get caught in the throat.

■ Side Effects and Contraindications

Do not take potassium if you have kidney failure.

Food Sources of Potassium

The following list is reprinted with permission from Jeffrey Bland's *Clinical Nutrition: A Functional Approach.* Foods that contain the most potassium are listed first, followed by foods that contain progressively less potassium. The number to the left of each food describes how many milligrams of potassuim are in 100 grams (3.5 ounces) of that food.

8060	Dulse	416	Beans, cooked	234	Papaya
5273	Kelp	414	Mushrooms	214	Eggplant
920	Sunflower seeds	407	Potato with skin	213	Green pepper
827	Wheat germ			208	Beets
773	Almonds	382	Broccoli	202	Summer squash
763	Raisins	370	Banana	200	Orange
727	Parsley	370	Meats	199	Raspberries
715	Brazil nuts	369	Winter squash	191	Cherries
674	Peanuts	366	Chicken	164	Strawberry
648	Dates	341	Carrots	162	Grapefruit juice
640	Dried figs	341	Celery	158	Grapes
604	Avocado	322	Radishes	157	Onions
603	Pecans	295	Cauliflower	146	Pineapple
600	Yams	282	Watercress	144	Whole milk
550	Swiss chard	278	Asparagus	141	Lemon juice
540	Cooked soybeans	268	Red cabbage	130	Pear
529	Garlic	264	Lettuce	129	Eggs
470	Spinach	251	Cantaloupe	110	Apple
450	English walnuts	249	Cooked lentils	100	Watermelon
430	Millet	244	Tomato	70	Cooked brown rice
		243	Sweet potato		

■ Potassium Supplementation

There are certain drugs which treat hypertension and congestive heart failure that can be very effective, but can also cause potassium levels to drop dangerously. Potassium-sparing medications (such as ACE inhibitors or spironolactone), when taken with these drugs, counter this effect by holding potassium in the body. However, if you are taking these medications, do not take potassium supplements because the excess potassium could cause your levels to become toxic.

If you have been taking potassium supplements and are not showing signs of improvement, the underlying problem may be a magnesium deficiency, which is known as hypomagnesemia. Magnesium is needed for the body to properly process potassium. Therefore, taking potassium supplements when your magnesium levels are low will be ineffective because your body will be unable to process the potassium.

■ Diseases/Disorders that Can Be Treated with Potassium

- Diabetes mellitus
- Fatigue
- High blood pressure

- Postural low blood pressure (lightheadedness or dizziness from sitting or standing up)
- Stroke prevention

SODIUM

Electrolytes are molecules that serve to conduct electricity through your body. Every electrolyte has either a positive or negative charge that reacts to messages sent through your body by your nervous system. They react to these messages by conducting electric currents, which regulate many functions and systems in your body. Sodium, chloride, and potassium are important electrolytes. Along with chloride, sodium remains outside of your body's cells, while potassium remains on the inside. These three electrolytes regulate many of your body's systems.

■ Functions of Sodium in Your Body

- Generates and conducts electricity, which is involved with many bodily functions
- Helps transport carbon dioxide
- Needed for muscle contraction
- Required for amino acid transport

- Required for proper function of nervous system
- Responsible for nerve transmission

■ Electrolyte Imbalance

It is very important that your body's electrolytes—such as chloride, sodium, and potassium—all remain at their proper levels. Electrolyte imbalance can occur if any of these has a sudden, abnormal elevation or depletion. Electrolyte imbalance is usually the result of an underlying problem, such as dehydration or dysfunction of the endocrine, kidney, or hormone systems, and is usually corrected by treating this initial problem. If electrolyte imbalance is left untreated, it can cause heart-related issues, organ failure, problems with the nervous system, or death.

Symptoms of Sodium Deficiency (Hyponatremia)

Hyponatremia, or sodium deficiency, is the most common electrolyte disorder. It is usually caused by drinking an excessive amount of water. Sometimes it occurs as a side effect to other disorders or diseases, such as severe diarrhea, hyperglycemia, or malaria. Taking certain diuretics in conjunction with one of these problems or a low-sodium diet can also result in hyponatremia. Doctors can usually treat hyponatremia fairly easily, but the underlying cause may be more difficult to cure.

☐ Change in body's acid-base balance

☐ Confusion

☐ Decreased elasticity of subcutaneous tissue (the layer of skin under the cutis)

☐ Diminished reflexes

☐ Fall in blood pressure

☐ Fall in cardiac output

☐ General malaise

☐ Headache

☐ Impaired adrenal function

☐ Increased hematocrit (portion of blood that contains red blood cells)

☐ Neurological disorders

☐ Tiredness

☐ Vomiting

Symptoms of Sodium Elevation (Hypernatremia)

Hypernatremia, or elevated levels of sodium in the body, is usually caused by dehydration. Whenever a body is losing more water than it is consuming for an extended period of time, there is a risk for hypernatremia.

Food Sources of Sodium

The following list is reprinted with permission from Jeffrey Bland's *Clinical Nutrition: A Functional Approach.* Foods that contain the most sodium are listed first, followed by foods that contain progressively less sodium. The number to the left of each food describes how many milligrams of sodium are in 100 grams (3.5 ounces) of that food, unless another measurement is given.

3007	Kelp	122	Eggs	30	Dried lentils
2400	Green olives	110	Cod	30	Sunflower seeds
2132	One teaspoon of salt	71	Spinach	27	Raisins
		70	Lamb	26	Red cabbage
1428	Dill pickles	65	Pork	19	Garlic
1319	Soy sauce, one tablespoon of	64	Chicken	19	White beans
		60	Beef	15	Broccoli
828	Ripe olives	60	Beets	15	Mushrooms
747	Sauerkraut	60	Sesame seeds	13	Cauliflower
700	Cheddar cheese	52	Watercress	10	Onion
265	Scallops	50	Whole cow's milk	10	Sweet potato
229	Cottage cheese	49	Turnip	9	Lettuce
210	Lobster	47	Carrot	6	Cucumber
147	Swiss chard	47	Yogurt	5	Peanuts
130	Beet greens	45	Parsley	4	Avocado
130	Buttermilk	43	Artichoke	3	Tomato
126	Celery	34	Dried figs	2	Eggplant

It may, for example, occur during a long marathon, or to a patient in a coma who is not receiving water infusions. Occasionally it is caused by excessive salt consumption, but this is fairly unusual.

☐ High blood pressure   ☐ Kidney problems   ☐ Seizures

☐ Irritability   ☐ Neurological damage   ☐ Weakness

BORON

Boron, a micromineral, is required by the body in trace amounts. As an *activating agent*, it is responsible for triggering many important bodily functions, including helping the body respond to various hormone activities. It also manages the balance of other essential minerals. Because it is involved in so many processes in your body, a boron deficiency can be quite serious and result in a number of problems.

■ Functions of Boron in Your Body

- Aids vitamin D in increasing mineral content of your bones
- Decreases inflammation
- Enhances cartilage formation
- Fights tooth decay
- Helps maintain memory and improve other brain functions
- Increases absorption and regulates levels of calcium, magnesium, and phosphorus
- Increases estrogen production in women
- Reduces risk of prostate cancer
- Regulates hormone production in both men and women

■ Symptoms of Boron Deficiency

☐ Arthritis	☐ Muscle pain or weakness
☐ Carpal tunnel syndrome	☐ Osteoporosis
☐ Depression	☐ Receding gum lines
☐ Hormonal imbalance	☐ Tooth decay
☐ Memory problems	☐ Weak or brittle bones

■ Symptoms of Boron Toxicity

☐ Dermatitis	☐ Inability to properly metabolize riboflavin
☐ Diarrhea	
☐ Hormonal imbalance	☐ Lethargy
☐ Inability to properly metabolize phosphorus	☐ Nausea
	☐ Vomiting

Food Sources of Boron

- Apples
- Broccoli
- Cauliflower
- Grapes
- Green leafy vegetables, such as kale
- Legumes
- Nuts
- Peaches
- Pears
- Prunes
- Tomatoes

■ Recommended Dosage

1,000 micrograms daily

CHROMIUM

The micronutrient chromium is essential to your health, but your body has a difficult time absorbing it when it is by itself. Combining it with another substance, such as the protein picolinate, allows it to enter the blood stream more easily. Picolinate also increases the absorption of zinc, copper, and iron.

■ Functions of Chromium in Your Body

- Aids in fat loss

- Burns calories

- Decreases total cholesterol and LDL (bad) cholesterol

- Helps decrease sugar cravings

- Helps hold onto calcium and prevent osteoporosis

- Helps increase the hormone dehydroepiandrosterone (DHEA), which has many roles as a steroid hormone but is also believed to be effective against several diseases

- Helps regulate blood sugar by making insulin work more effectively

- Increases antibodies

- Increases HDL (good) cholesterol

- Increases physical endurance
- Lowers excess cortisol
- Reduces bone loss
- Stimulates muscle development

■ Symptoms of Chromium Deficiency

- ☐ Anxiety
- ☐ Atherosclerosis
- ☐ Decreased insulin binding and receptor number, which infringes upon the cells' ability to perform properly
- ☐ Elevated insulin levels
- ☐ Fatigue
- ☐ Heart disease

- ☐ High blood sugar, and possibly hyperglycemia or impaired glucose tolerance (IGT)
- ☐ Increased cholesterol and triglyceride levels
- ☐ Low blood sugar, and possibly hypoglycemia
- ☐ Neuropathy (disorders involving nerves)

■ Causes of Chromium Deficiency

- Age
- Antacid use
- Exercise

- High carbohydrate diet
- High intake of refined sugar
- Soil in which food is grown may be low in chromium

■ Factors that Increase Chromium Levels

- Amino acids
- Physical trauma
- Vitamin C

■ Symptoms of Chromium Toxicity

- ☐ Lightheadedness
- ☐ Rashes

■ Recommended Dosage

50 to 200 micrograms daily. Higher dosages may be used to treat a specific disease process, such as those listed on page 81. See your doctor about increasing your chromium intake.

Food Sources of Chromium

Chromium can be found in the following foods. However, up to 90 percent of the chromium content of food is lost in food processing. If eaten for their chromium content, the following foods should be eaten unprocessed and, most likely, along with chromium supplementation.

This list is reprinted with permission from *Clinical Nutrition: A Functional Approach* by Jeffrey Bland. Foods that contain the most chromium are listed first, followed by foods that contain progressively less chromium. The number to the left of each food describes how many milligrams of chromium are in 100 grams (3.5 ounces) of that food.

112	Brewer's yeast	15	Chicken	8	Dry navy beans
57	Round beef	14	Apple	7	Shrimp
55	Calf's liver	13	Butter	7	Lettuce
42	Whole wheat bread	13	Parsnips	5	Orange
		12	Cornmeal	5	Lobster tail
38	Wheat bran	12	Lamb chops	5	Blueberries
30	Rye bread	11	Scallops	4	Green beans
30	Fresh chili	11	Swiss cheese	4	Cabbage
26	Oysters	10	Banana	4	Mushrooms
24	Potatoes	10	Spinach	3	Beer
23	Wheat germ	10	Pork chops	3	Strawberries
19	Green pepper	9	Carrots	1	Milk
16	Eggs				

■ Diseases/Disorders that Can Be Treated with Chromium

- Diabetes/insulin resistance
- High cholesterol levels
- High triglyceride levels
- Hypothyroidism
- Osteoporosis
- Sarcopenia (muscle wasting)
- Weight gain
- Yeast overgrowth

COPPER

The essential micromineral copper travels through your body in your bloodstream. The highest concentrations of copper can be found in your kidneys, liver, brain, heart, and bones. This mineral is in our food, air, and water, usually in negligible amounts. However, people in certain situations or environments may be overexposed to copper. Short-term exposure causes "metal fever," which passes after a couple of days; long-term exposure, however, can be extremely bad for your health. (See page 83 for more information on copper overexposure.)

▓ Functions of Copper in Your Body

- Aids in energy production
- Antioxidant protection
- Assists thyroid function (converts certain hormones into their more active forms)
- Decreases inflammation
- Helps wound healing
- Metabolizes catecholamine (important chemical compounds in the brain)
- Metabolizes cholesterol
- Metabolizes protein
- Necessary for heart health
- Necessary for skeletal mineralization (when cartilage becomes bone)
- Needed for the production of adrenal and ovarian hormones
- Oxidative phosphorylation (cellular process that releases energy)
- Promotes healthy nerve function
- Red blood cells formation
- Regulates body temperature
- Regulates glucose metabolism
- Strengthens immune system
- Synthesizes connective tissue, including collagen

- Synthesizes melanin pigment (which provides color in skin, pupils, and hair)
- Synthesizes myelin (which facilitates proper functioning of the nervous system)
- White blood cells formation

■ Symptoms of Copper Deficiency

- Anemia
- Bone abnormalities
- Broken blood vessels
- Decreased hair and skin pigmentation
- Fatigue

- Hypochromic microcytic anemia (small and unhealthy red blood cells)
- Limb edema (swelling)
- Loss of muscle tone
- Low white blood cell count

■ Causes of Copper Deficiency

- Antacid use
- Excess calcium
- Excess iron
- Excess molybdenum (a micromineral described in detail on page 94)
- Excess vitamin C
- Excess zinc

- Fiber
- Non-steroidal anti-inflammatory drugs, such as aspirin and ibuprofen
- Penicillamine (such as Cuprimine and Depen)
- Poor digestion
- Vegetarian diet

■ Symptoms of Copper Toxicity

- Abdominal pain
- Brain damage

- Diarrhea
- Headaches

- Kidney damage
- Liver damage

■ Causes of Copper Overexposure

- Environmental exposure to copper water pipes, cookware, birth control pills, and dental materials
- Estrogen (which can increase the body's copper levels)

Food Sources of Copper

The following list is reprinted with permission from Jeffrey Bland's *Clinical Nutrition: A Functional Approach.* Foods that contain the most copper are listed first, followed by foods that contain progressively less copper. The number to the left of each food describes how many milligrams of copper are in 100 grams (3.5 ounces) of that food.

13.7	Oysters	0.7	Lamb chops	0.3	Garlic
2.3	Brazil nuts	0.5	Sunflower oil	0.2	Millet
2.1	Soy lecithin	0.4	Butter	0.2	Whole wheat
1.4	Almonds	0.4	Rye grain	0.2	Chicken
1.3	Hazelnuts	0.4	Pork loin	0.2	Eggs
1.3	Walnuts	0.4	Barley	0.2	Corn oil
1.3	Pecans	0.4	Gelatin	0.2	Ginger root
1.2	Split peas, dry	0.3	Shrimp	0.2	Molasses
1.1	Beef liver	0.3	Olive oil	0.2	Turnips
0.8	Buckwheat	0.3	Clams	0.1	Green peas
0.8	Peanuts	0.3	Carrots	0.1	Papaya
0.7	Cod liver oil	0.3	Coconut	0.1	Apple

■ Recommended Dosage

1.5 to 3 milligrams daily. It is very important that your body maintains a proper ratio of zinc to copper—between 10:1 and 15:1—so you may want to take a multi-vitamin that contains both minerals. Also, the bioavailability of cupric oxide is almost zero, so it should not be taken as a supplement. Instead, try copper sulfate, copper gluconate, cupric acetate, or alkaline copper carbonate.

■ Side Effects and Contraindications

Do not take copper supplements if you have Wilson's disease.

IODINE

Iodine is added to many table salts produced in the United States in order to prevent iodine deficiency, the effects of which can be incredibly devastating, particularly for children—and, according to the World Health Organization, up to 72 percent of the world's population is affected by an iodine deficiency disorder. These salts are called iodized salts. Sea salt, however, is *not* rich in iodine. The main function of iodine is to allow the thyroid gland to produce its hormones. Therefore, two-thirds of your body's iodine is stored in the thyroid.

■ Functions of Iodine in Your Body

- Fights bacteria

- Involved in energy production

- Involved in nerve function

- Maintains healthy breast tissue in women

- Needed for the development and functioning of the thyroid gland and hormones

- Promotes hair and skin growth

- Protects against toxic effects from radioactive material

- Relieves pain and soreness associated with fibrocystic breast disease

- Required for normal function of thyroid, breast, prostate, kidneys, spleen, liver, blood, salivary glands, and intestines

■ Symptoms of Iodine Deficiency

☐ Cold extremities	☐ Fatigue	☐ Insomnia
☐ Decreased mental capabilities	☐ Goiter (an enlarged thyroid)	☐ Neurological defects
☐ Depression	☐ Hypothyroidism	☐ Tenderness of sternum
☐ Dry eyes	☐ Impaired thyroid hormone synthesis	☐ Weight gain

■ Causes of Iodine Deficiency

- Asthma inhalers that contain fluoride or bromide
- Being born from an iodine-deficient mother
- Diet high in pasta and breads which contain bromide
- Diet without fish or sea vegetables (such as seaweed)
- Fluoride use (which inhibits iodine binding)
- Eating food from ground deplete of iodine
- Low-salt diet
- Sucralose (which contains chlorinated table sugar)
- Vegan and vegetarian diets

■ Foods that Interfere with Iodine in Your Body

If you eat large amounts of the following foods, you may develop a goiter (an enlarged thyroid) or any of the other problems listed under "Symptoms of Iodine Deficiency."

- Broccoli
- Cabbage
- Cauliflower
- Soybeans

■ Symptoms of Iodine Toxicity

- ☐ Acne-like skin lesions
- ☐ Goiter (an enlarged thyroid)

■ Diseases/Disorders that Can Be Treated with Iodine

- Dupuytren's contracture
- Excess mucous production
- Fatigue
- Fibrocystic breast disease
- Headaches including migraines
- Hemorrhoids
- Keloids
- Ovarian cysts
- Parotid duct stones
- Peyronie's disease
- Sebaceous cysts
- Thyroid disorders

■ Recommended Dosage

- Adults who are not pregnant: 150 micrograms daily
- Pregnant women: 220 micrograms daily

Food Sources of Iodine

The following list is reprinted with permission from Jeffrey Bland's *Clinical Nutrition: A Functional Approach*. Foods that contain the most iodine are listed first, followed by foods that contain progressively less iodine. The number to the left of each food describes how many milligrams of iodine are in 100 grams (3.5 ounces) of that food.

90 Clams	16 Canned tuna	9 Green peppers
65 Shrimp	14 Eggs	9 Butter
62 Haddock	11 Peanuts	7 Milk
50 Oysters	11 Whole wheat bread	6 Cream
50 Salmon		6 Cottage cheese
46 Halibut	11 Cheddar cheese	6 Beef
37 Canned sardines	10 Pork	3 Lamb
19 Beef liver	10 Lettuce	3 Raisins
16 Pineapple	9 Spinach	

Sea vegetables are also a good source of iodine.

IRON

The micromineral iron is key to good health because it is involved in many important functions in your body. Luckily, it is found in many food products, which are listed on page 90.

It is important to note that heme iron, which is found in red meat, fish, and poultry, is much more readily and efficiently absorbed by your body than nonheme iron, which is found in vegetables and other plant foods. Despite this, the iron used to enrich iron-fortified food is nonheme iron. The absorption of nonheme iron can be improved by the consumption of vitamin C and proteins found in meat.

Interestingly, the precise amount of iron absorbed from food is directly related to the amount of iron your body needs. Therefore, your body will absorb more iron from food consumed if you have an iron deficiency than it will if your iron levels are already normal. Yet iron toxicity is quite possible and can have devastating consequences. (See page 89 for details on iron toxicity.) Once in your body, iron is stored in *hemoglobin*—the part of red blood cells that carries oxygen from your lungs to your tissues.

Pregnant women may need to increase their iron intake to insure that their babies, if carried full-term, are born with a sufficient amount of iron to last several months. At that point, breast milk or iron-fortified formula provides the baby with a necessary amount of this mineral, so they should not be given supplements. (Ask the baby's healthcare provider for a recommendation if the baby was born premature.) Cow's milk, on the other hand, contains significantly less iron than breast milk. Cow's milk is also unhealthy for babies for other reasons, and should not be fed to children under one year of age.

■ Functions of Iron in Your Body

- Essential component of hemoglobin (oxygen-containing part of red blood cells)
- Involved in immune system efficiency
- Involved in oxygen transport
- Key element in many enzymatic reactions
- Necessary for collagen synthesis
- Needed for good cognition and behavior
- Regulates cell growth

■ Symptoms of Iron Deficiency

- ☐ Craving for ice
- ☐ Decreased cognitive functioning
- ☐ Decreased immune system
- ☐ Decreased memory
- ☐ Fatigue
- ☐ Hair loss
- ☐ Headache
- ☐ Hypochromic microcytic anemia (small and unhealthy red blood cells)
- ☐ Impaired ability to maintain body temperature
- ☐ Impaired growth
- ☐ Increased blood sugar
- ☐ Increased body tension
- ☐ Increased fearfulness
- ☐ Increased risk of jitteriness that can result from taking tricyclic antidepressants
- ☐ Inflammation of the tongue
- ☐ Pallor (lack of color in skin)
- ☐ Rapid heart rate
- ☐ Restless leg syndrome
- ☐ Short attention span
- ☐ Shortness of breath
- ☐ Spoon nails (soft, concave nails)
- ☐ Unhappiness
- ☐ Weakness

■ Causes of Iron Deficiency

- Black tea
- Bleeding from any part of the body
- Calcium
- Coffee
- Copper
- Green tea
- Manganese
- Menstrual cycles
- Oxalate
- Partially digested proteins
- Phytates (which are found in pita bread, matzoh, wheat germ, vanilla extract, cacao powder, oats, and nuts)
- Polyphenolic compounds (which are found in certain plant foods)
- Problems in the small intestine or gastrointestinal tract (which is where iron is absorbed)
- Red wine
- Soy products
- Vegetarian diet
- Zinc

■ Symptoms of Iron Toxicity

- ☐ Decreased absorption and utilization of vitamin E
- ☐ Diabetes
- ☐ Gut disturbances
- ☐ Hair loss
- ☐ Increase in free radical production (which can increase your risk of cancer, cause inflammation, or worsen arthritis symptoms; see page 4 for more information on free radicals)
- ☐ Liver disease
- ☐ Predisposition to heart disease

■ Substances that Increase Iron Absorption

- Cysteine
- Folic acid
- Meat
- Vitamin B$_6$
- Vitamin C
- Zinc

■ Recommended Dosage

Men over the age of fifty and menopausal women should consume no supplemental iron unless instructed by their doctor.

- Males: 10 milligrams daily
- Pregnant women: 30 milligrams daily
- Pre-menopausal women: 15 milligrams daily

Foods Sources of Iron

The following list is reprinted with permission from Jeffrey Bland's *Clinical Nutrition: A Functional Approach.* Foods that contain the most iron are listed first, followed by foods that contain progressively less iron. The listed number describes how many milligrams of iron are in 100 grams (3.5 ounces) of food.

Iron in meat is more bioavailable than iron found in vegetables. Additionally, your body will absorb more iron from vegetables if they are eaten *with* meat than if they were eaten alone.

100.0	Kelp	2.9	Pork	0.8	Red cabbage
17.3	Brewer's yeast	2.7	Cooked dry beans	0.8	Pumpkin
16.1	Blackstrap molasses	2.4	Hulled sesame seeds	0.8	Mushrooms
14.9	Wheat bran	2.4	Pecans	0.7	Banana
11.2	Pumpkin and squash seeds	2.3	Eggs	0.7	Beets
		2.1	Lentils	0.7	Carrot
9.4	Wheat germ	2.1	Peanuts	0.7	Eggplant
8.8	Beef liver	1.9	Lamb	0.7	Sweet potato
7.1	Sunflower seeds	1.9	Tofu	0.6	Avocado
6.8	Millet	1.8	Green peas	0.6	Figs
6.2	Parsley	1.6	Brown rice	0.6	Potato
6.1	Clams	1.6	Ripe olives	0.6	Corn
4.7	Almonds	1.5	Chicken	0.5	Pineapple
3.9	Dried prunes	1.3	Artichoke	0.5	Nectarine
3.8	Cashews	1.3	Mung bean sprouts	0.5	Watermelon
3.7	Lean beef			0.5	Winter squash
3.5	Raisins	1.2	Salmon	0.5	Cooked brown rice
3.4	Jerusalem artichoke	1.1	Broccoli		
		1.1	Currants	0.5	Tomato
3.4	Brazil nuts	1.1	Whole wheat bread	0.4	Orange
3.3	Beet greens			0.4	Cherries
3.2	Swiss chard	1.1	Cauliflower	0.4	Summer squash
3.1	Dandelion greens	1.0	Cheddar cheese	0.3	Papaya
		1.0	Strawberries	0.3	Celery
3.1	English walnut	1.0	Asparagus	0.3	Cottage cheese
3.0	Dates	0.9	Blackberries	0.3	Apple

■ Iron Supplementation

There are two different kinds of iron supplements: ferrous (such as ferrous sulfate, ferrous fumarate, and ferrous gluconate) and ferric (such as ferric citrate). Ferrous supplements are much more easily absorbed by your body than ferric supplements. Ferrous sulfate, the most popular iron supplement, can cause intestinal problems—such as constipation or nausea—in some users. If you experience a problem like this, you can switch to a different form of ferrous supplement, with which you will most likely have a different reaction, or you can switch to another form of iron. Ask your doctor for advice.

■ Medications that have Decreased Absorption when Taken with Iron

- Blood thinners
- Captopril
- Ciprofloxacin
- Levothyroxine
- Norfloxacin
- Penicillamine

MANGANESE

Consuming enough manganese is very important for good health. Most Americans eat enough manganese-containing foods each day and do not need to take supplements. Manganese is a component of some metals and is sometimes inhaled. However, inhaled manganese is not treated by the body the same way ingested manganese is treated. While consumption of manganese has many health benefits, inhaling manganese can cause mental and emotion problems and even brain damage. However, it usually takes months or years of exposure for this to occur.

■ Functions of Manganese in Your Body

- Aids in protein digestion and synthesis
- Essential for a healthy nervous system
- Essential for the utilization of vitamins B and C in adrenal health
- Helps with carbohydrate metabolism
- Is a cofactor for enzymes involved in energy production
- Needed for a good immune system

- Needed for brain health
- Needed for the synthesis of cartilage, collagen, and other connective tissue
- Part of the antioxidant defense mechanism
- Required for fatty acid synthesis
- Required for the production of estrogen and progesterone
- Used for bone growth and maintenance
- Used in blood formation

▓ Symptoms of Manganese Deficiency

☐ Decreased hair and nail growth

☐ Decreased HDL (good) cholesterol

☐ Decreased lipid metabolism

☐ Impaired carbohydrate metabolism

☐ Impaired coordination

☐ Impaired growth

☐ Loss of hair color

☐ Skeletal problems

☐ Skin rash

▓ Substances that Lower Your Manganese Levels

- Aluminum
- Iron

- Phytates in bread and grains (which bind to manganese and prevent it from being bioavailable)

▓ Symptoms of Manganese Toxicity (Manganism)

Like many of the other microminerals, manganese is needed by your body in trace amounts but can be toxic in large quantities. The following list includes the most common symptoms of manganese toxicity.

☐ Anxiety

☐ Delusions

☐ Disorientation

☐ Emotional problems

☐ Hallucinations

☐ Memory loss

☐ Neurological problems

☐ Permanent brain damage

☐ Slurred speech

☐ Tremors

▓ Recommended Dosage

2.5 to 5 milligrams daily

Food Sources of Manganese

The following list is reprinted with permission from Jeffrey Bland's *Clinical Nutrition: A Functional Approach*. Foods that contain the most manganese are listed first, followed by foods that contain progressively less manganese. The number to the left of each food describes how many milligrams of manganese are in 100 grams (3.5 ounces) of that food. Besides the foods listed below, cloves, ginger, thyme, bay leaves, and tea also contain manganese.

3.5	Pecans	0.3	Oatmeal	0.05	Eggs
2.8	Brazil nuts	0.2	Cornmeal	0.04	Beets
2.5	Almonds	0.2	Millet	0.04	Coconut
1.8	Barley	0.19	Gorgonzola cheese	0.03	Apple
1.3	Rye			0.03	Orange
1.3	Buckwheat	0.16	Carrots	0.03	Pear
1.3	Split peas, dry	0.15	Broccoli	0.03	Lamb chops
1.1	Whole wheat	0.14	Brown rice	0.03	Cantaloupe
0.8	Walnuts	0.14	Whole wheat bread	0.03	Tomato
0.8	Fresh spinach			0.02	Whole milk
0.7	Peanuts	0.13	Swiss cheese	0.02	Chicken breasts
0.6	Oats	0.13	Corn	0.02	Green beans
0.5	Raisins	0.11	Cabbage	0.02	Apricot
0.5	Turnip greens	0.10	Peach	0.01	Beef liver
0.5	Rhubarb	0.09	Butter	0.01	Scallops
0.4	Beet greens	0.06	Tangerine	0.01	Halibut
0.3	Brussels sprouts	0.06	Peas	0.01	Cucumber

■ Diseases/Disorders that Can Be Treated with Manganese

In addition to the disorders listed on page 94, manganese may be helpful in treating diabetes and epilepsy. However, this has not been proven conclusively.

- Arrhythmias (irregular heart rhythm)
- Arthritic pains
- Back pain
- Myasthenia gravis
- Premenstrual syndrome (PMS)

■ Side Effects and Contraindications

You must be extra cautious consuming manganese if you have gallbladder or liver disease. If you have either of these chronic problems, manganese may be toxic to you. Consult your doctor if you wish to start a manganese regiment but have gallbladder or liver problems.

MOLYBDENUM

Molybdenum is an essential micromineral. A component of three major enzymes, molybdenum is involved in several of your body's metabolism and oxidation processes. It is found in your liver, kidneys, and adrenal glands.

■ Functions of Molybdenum in Your Body

- Acts as a coenzyme in uric acid formation
- Acts as an electron transport agent in oxidation/reduction reactions
- Antagonist to copper
- Coenzyme in alcohol detoxification
- Helps body utilize stored iron
- Used to detoxify sulfites

■ Symptoms of Molybdenum Deficiency

- ☐ Decreased uric acid in urine
- ☐ Disorientation
- ☐ Headache
- ☐ Irritability
- ☐ Mental disturbance
- ☐ Tachycardia (fast heart rate)
- ☐ Visual problems

■ Symptoms of Molybdenum Toxicity

- ☐ Copper deficiency
- ☐ Gout
- ☐ Increased uric acid production
- ☐ Kidney problems

Food Sources of Molybdenum

The following list is reprinted with permission from Jeffrey Bland's *Clinical Nutrition: A Functional Approach*. Foods that contain the most molybdenum are listed first, followed by foods that contain progressively less molybdenum. The number to the left of each food describes how many milligrams of molybdenum are in 100 grams (3.5 ounces) of that food.

155	Lentils	50	Rye bread	24	Lamb
135	Beef liver	45	Corn	21	Green beans
130	Split peas	42	Barley	19	Crab
120	Cauliflower	40	Fish	19	Molasses
110	Green peas	36	Whole wheat	16	Cantaloupe
109	Brewer's yeast	32	Whole wheat bread	14	Apricots
100	Wheat germ	32	Chicken	10	Raisins
100	Spinach	31	Cottage cheese	10	Butter
77	Beef kidney	30	Beef	7	Strawberries
75	Brown rice	30	Potatoes	5	Carrots
70	Garlic	25	Onions	5	Cabbage
60	Oats	25	Coconut	3	Whole milk
53	Eggs	25	Pork	1	Goat milk

■ Recommended Dosage

75 to 250 micrograms daily

SELENIUM

Selenium is an essential micromineral that is important for growth and reproduction, as well as several organs including the heart and liver. However, as an essential micromineral, it can be toxic in large dosages. Brazil nuts are the best food source of selenium.

Each food's content of selenium depends on the soil in which it is grown. In the United States, the selenium-deficient states are Connecticut, Delaware, Illinois, Indiana, Massachusetts, New York, Ohio, Oregon, Pennsylvania, and Rhode Island. Selenium levels are also low in the District of Columbia. Although selenium supplements have not been proven effective for the prevention of heart disease, a study at the Cleveland Clinic in Ohio suggested that people who lived in states with low selenium content in their soil were three times more likely to die of heart disease than people who lived in states with adequate selenium content in their soil.

◼ Functions of Selenium in Your Body

- Helps prevent cancer (due to its role in DNA repair)
- Involved in thyroid function
- May prevent heart disease
- Needed for immune system
- Reduces heavy metal toxicity
- Works with vitamin E as an antioxidant

◼ Symptoms of Selenium Deficiency

☐ Cataracts   ☐ Recurrent infections

☐ Inflammatory disease   ☐ Skeletal muscle problems

☐ Loss of pigment in skin and hair   ☐ Thyroid enlargement

☐ Low sperm count   ☐ Weakness

◼ Causes of Selenium Deficiency

- AIDS   • Infertility (in males)
- Autoimmune disease   • Inflammatory bowel disease
- Cancer   • Thyroid disease

◼ Symptoms of Selenium Toxicity

☐ Bad breath   ☐ Hair loss

☐ Dry hair   ☐ Irritability

☐ Fatigue   ☐ Nervous system problems

Food Sources of Selenium

The following list is reprinted with permission from Jeffrey Bland's *Clinical Nutrition: A Functional Approach*. Foods that contain the most selenium are listed first, followed by foods that contain progressively less selenium. The number to the left of each food describes how many milligrams of selenium are in 100 grams (3.5 ounces) of that food.

146	Butter	49	Oysters	12	Mushrooms
141	Smoked herring	48	Milk	12	Chicken
123	Smelt	43	Cod	10	Swiss cheese
111	Wheat germ	39	Brown rice	5	Cottage cheese
103	Brazil nuts	34	Top round steak	5	Wine
89	Apple cider vinegar	30	Lamb	4	Radishes
77	Scallops	27	Turnips	4	Grape juice
66	Barley	26	Molasses	3	Pecans
66	Whole wheat bread	25	Garlic	2	Hazelnuts
65	Lobster	24	Barley	2	Almonds
63	Bran	19	Orange juice	2	Green beans
59	Shrimp	19	Gelatin	2	Kidney beans
57	Red Swiss chard	19	Beer	2	Onion
56	Oats	18	Beef liver	2	Carrots
55	Clams	18	Lamb chops	2	Cabbage
51	King crab	18	Egg yolk	1	Orange

■ Recommended Dosage

200 micrograms once a day

■ Side Effects and Contraindications

Selenium may interfere with the absorption of medications such as proton-pump inhibitors (PPIs, used to treat reflux) and histamine blockers.

SILICON

Silicon is an essential micronutrient. Although it is found in many forms, the only form that is useful to humans is orthosilicic acid. Foods high in fiber usually contain silicon.

■ Functions of Silicon in Your Body

- Bone and cartilage development
- Responsible for elasticity of connective tissue
- Responsible for skin, hair, and nail health
- Supports and improves function of thymus gland

■ Symptoms of Silicon Deficiency

☐ Brittle bones   ☐ Irritability

☐ Cramps in muscles   ☐ Osteoporosis

☐ Insomnia   ☐ Poor bone development

■ Symptoms of Silicon Toxicity

As mentioned earlier, silicon is only useful to human health in the form of orthosilicic acid. However, as the second-most abundant element in the universe, it is in our environment in many other forms, including silicon dioxide, or silica. This crystallized element is toxic if inhaled in abundance. Located in rock, sandstone, concrete, and paint, silica is released when these materials are crushed, drilled, or otherwise broken. The inhalation of silica can cause *silicosis,* an irreversible and potentially fatal respiratory disease.

Food Sources of Silicon

• Apples	• Horsetail (an herb)	• Oranges
• Celery	• Legumes	• Rice bran
• Cherries	• Oats	• Root vegetables
• Endive	• Onions	• Unrefined grains

■ Recommended Dosage

1 to 2 milligrams daily

■ Diseases/Disorders that Can Be Treated with Silicon

- Acne
- Boils
- Eczema
- Psoriasis

VANADIUM

Vanadium is needed by the body in trace amounts, and is found in most soils. Therefore, most people consume enough vanadium in their regular daily diet and do not need to take supplements.

■ Function of Vanadium in Your Body

- Aids metabolism of glucose

Food Sources of Vanadium

The following list is reprinted with permission from Jeffrey Bland's *Clinical Nutrition: A Functional Approach.* Foods that contain the most vanadium are listed first, followed by foods that contain progressively less vanadium. The number to the left of each food describes how many milligrams of vanadium are in 100 grams (3.5 ounces) of that food.

100	Buckwheat	15	Corn	5	Onions
80	Parsley	14	Green beans	5	Whole wheat
70	Soybeans	11	Peanut oil	4	Lobster
64	Safflower oil	10	Carrots	4	Beets
42	Eggs	10	Cabbage	3	Apples
41	Sunflower seed oil	10	Garlic	2	Plums
35	Oats	6	Tomatoes	2	Lettuce
30	Olive oil	5	Radishes	2	Millet
15	Sunflower seeds				

- Improves insulin sensitivity
- Involved in metabolism of fats

■ Symptoms of Vanadium Toxicity

☐ Bipolar disorder

☐ Decreased coenzyme A

☐ Elevated blood pressure

☐ Increased triglyceride levels

☐ Interference with cellular energy production

☐ Lowered coenzyme Q_{10} levels

☐ May deplete body of chromium, lithium, or vitamin C

■ Recommended Dosage

10 to 50 milligrams daily. Do not take more than 50 milligrams a day without the supervision of a doctor because some of the side effects of vanadium toxicity—such as bipolar disorder—are very serious.

ZINC

Although zinc is a micromineral, and therefore needed by your body only in small quantities, it is very important for your overall physical and mental health. It is used in many enzymatic reactions in your body. Furthermore, there are one hundred enzymes that need zinc as a cofactor. (A cofactor is molecule to which another molecule must bind in order to activate or function.) A recent study revealed that zinc supplementation increases the production of insulin-like growth factor-1 (IGF-1)—which is associated with growth and healthier aging. The other functions of zinc are described below.

■ Functions of Zinc in Your Body

- Boosts immune defenses
- Breaks down and metabolizes proteins
- Contributes to a healthy prostate
- Decreases the body's requirement for insulin
- Enhances the biochemical actions of vitamin D
- Essential component of hormones

- Essential for cell division and replication of both DNA and RNA
- Essential for fertility and reproduction
- Has anti-inflammatory effects
- Helps absorption of vitamin A
- Helps assemble proteins inside the cell
- Helps balance blood sugar levels
- Helps stabilize cell membrane and structures within the cell
- Important component of superoxide dismutase, an essential antioxidant
- Improves taste and appetite
- Inhibits the enzyme that reduces levels of the male hormone dihydrotestosterone (DHT)
- Is an antioxidant
- Metabolizes carbohydrates
- Necessary for the proper maintenance of vitamin E
- Needed for the formation of bone and skin
- Promotes thyroid activity
- Related to sexual maturation
- Thyroid function (converts certain hormones into their more active forms)
- Transports vitamin A to retinas, thereby improving night vision

■ Diseases/Disorders that Cause a Predisposition to Zinc Deficiency

- AIDS
- Aging (zinc absorption decreases with age)
- Alcoholism
- Anorexia nervosa
- Celiac disease
- Chronic renal failure
- Cirrhosis
- Cystic fibrosis
- Hemolytic anemia
- Increased calcium ingestion
- Infection
- Inflammatory bowel disease
- Iron supplementation
- Nephrotic syndrome
- Pancreatic insufficiency
- Pancreatitis
- Rheumatoid arthritis
- Short bowel syndrome
- Smoking
- Some diuretics
- Surgery

Food Sources of Zinc

The following list is reprinted with permission from Jeffrey Bland's *Clinical Nutrition: A Functional Approach*. Foods that contain the most zinc are listed first, followed by foods that contain progressively less zinc. The number to the left of each food describes how many milligrams of zinc are in 100 grams (3.5 ounces) of that food. Black pepper, paprika, mustard, chili powder, thyme, and cinnamon are not included on the list but are also high in zinc.

148.7 Fresh oysters	3.1 Almonds	0.4 Black beans
6.8 Ginger root	3.0 Walnuts	0.4 Raw milk
5.6 Ground round steak	2.9 Sardines	0.4 Pork chops
	2.6 Chicken	0.4 Corn
5.3 Lamb chops	2.5 Buckwheat	0.3 Grape juice
4.5 Pecans	2.4 Hazel nuts	0.3 Olive oil
4.2 Dry split peas	1.9 Clams	0.3 Cauliflower
4.2 Brazil nuts	1.7 Anchovies	0.2 Spinach
3.9 Beef liver	1.7 Tuna	0.2 Cabbage
3.5 Nonfat dry milk	1.7 Haddock	0.2 Lentils
3.5 Egg yolk	1.6 Green peas	0.2 Butter
3.2 Whole wheat	1.5 Shrimp	0.2 Lettuce
3.2 Rye	1.2 Turnips	0.1 Cucumber
3.2 Oats	0.9 Parsley	0.1 Yams
3.2 Peanuts	0.9 Potatoes	0.1 Tangerine
3.1 Lima beans	0.6 Garlic	0.1 String beans
3.1 Soy lecithin	0.5 Whole wheat bread	

■ Symptoms of Zinc Deficiency

- ☐ Acne
- ☐ Anemia
- ☐ Anorexia
- ☐ Arthritis
- ☐ Behavioral disturbances (such as apathy, confusion, depression, hostility, or irritability)
- ☐ Brittle nails
- ☐ Craving for sugary foods
- ☐ Dandruff
- ☐ Decreased ability to taste
- ☐ Decreased desire for protein-rich foods
- ☐ Decreased sense of smell

- ☐ Decreased sexual function
- ☐ Delayed sexual maturation
- ☐ Diarrhea
- ☐ Eczema
- ☐ Enlargement of the spleen and liver
- ☐ Fatigue
- ☐ Frontal headaches
- ☐ Growth retardation
- ☐ Hair loss
- ☐ Immune deficiencies
- ☐ Impaired nerve conduction
- ☐ Impaired wound healing

- ☐ Impotence
- ☐ Infertility
- ☐ Low sperm count
- ☐ Memory impairment
- ☐ Negative nitrogen balance
- ☐ Nerve damage
- ☐ Night blindness
- ☐ Poor appetite
- ☐ Psoriasis
- ☐ Reduced salivation
- ☐ Sleep disturbances
- ☐ Stretch marks
- ☐ White spots on nails

■ Substances that Decrease Zinc Absorption

- Coffee and other caffeinated beverages
- Cortisone
- Diuretics
- Excess copper
- Foods rich in oxalic acid (such as spinach, sweet potatoes, and rhubarb)

- Foods rich in phytic acid (such as unleavened bread, raw beans, seeds, nuts, and grains)
- Teas containing tannin
- Tetracycline

■ Symptoms of Zinc Toxicity

☐ Alcohol intolerance

☐ Anemia

☐ Decreased immune system

☐ Dizziness

☐ Drowsiness

☐ Hallucinations

☐ Increased sweating

☐ Loss of muscular coordination

☐ Premature heartbeats (heartbeats that occur before the regular heartbeat)

■ Recommended Dosage

25 to 50 milligrams. Try to take zinc at a different time of day from calcium, copper, iron, and soy, because zinc can interfere with the absorption of these nutrients. When buying zinc supplements, look for zinc picolinate and zinc citrate. These are the two forms of zinc that are best absorbed by your body.

■ Side Effects and Contraindications

Zinc decreases the absorption of fluoroquinolones and tetracyclines, two groups of antibiotics.

■ Diseases/Disorders that Can Be Treated With Zinc

- Acne
- Anorexia nervosa
- Colds
- Diabetes mellitus
- Eczema
- Enlarged prostate
- Furuncles (bacteria-caused boils)
- Gastric ulcers
- Growth retardation
- Immune function
- Impaired taste sensation
- Infertility
- Macular degeneration (chronic deterioration of retina)
- Rheumatoid arthritis
- Tinnitus

3

Fatty Acids

Many people regard fat as an adversary to their good health. It *is* true that excessive intake of certain fats can result in serious medical problems. However, not all fats are the same. In fact, your body requires certain fatty acids—a major component of fats—to maintain health and prevent disease. Fats are also an important source of energy and help your body perform a variety of functions. Recognizing the difference between "good" and "bad" fats is crucial as you strive to achieve optimal health.

There are several different types of fats. *Saturated fats* are "bad" fats because they can raise cholesterol levels and cause unhealthy weight gain. They are primarily found in foods that come from animals, including fatty meats (such as beef and pork) and dairy products (such as whole milk and butter), and are usually solids at room temperature.

Unsaturated fats primarily come from vegetable foods and tend to be liquids at room temperature. They consist of polyunsaturated fats and monounsaturated fats, both of which are "good" fats. *Polyunsaturated fats,* which are found in corn, soybean, and safflower oils, can positively affect your body by lowering your LDL (bad) cholesterol. However, they can also lower your HDL (good) cholesterol. (For further discussion on cholesterol, see the inset on page 106.) *Monounsaturated fats,* on the other hand, lower LDL cholesterol but do not affect HDL cholesterol. Yet, the impact made on LDL cholesterol is usually minor. Monounsaturated fats are found in olive oil and canola oil.

Production of most fatty acids occurs within your body from the breakdown of fat molecules, but there are two important polyunsaturated fatty acids—omega-3 and omega-6—that cannot be manufactured in your body and must be provided through diet or taken as supplements. Therefore, although certain low-fat diets can be healthier than diets high in fat, a major shift in food consumption to a low-fat diet may deprive your body of these essential nutrients. These two "good" fats are termed *essential fatty acids* (EFAs). Starting on page 108, omega-3 and omega-6 fatty acids are described further.

Trans fatty acids are another type of unsaturated fat. In nature, they occur only in small dosages that don't have negative effects on your body. (See the inset on page 114 for an example of a naturally occurring trans fatty acid.) However, the food industry has started producing this type of fat to help food stay fresh longer. As you will see later in this chapter,

Cholesterol

Cholesterol is a soft, waxy substance that is found in your bloodstream and carried through your body in lipoprotein particles. It is both made by your body and consumed in animal foods. Although needed by your body, the intake of too much cholesterol can clog your arteries, resulting in your heart receiving less blood and oxygen. This can cause serious cardiovascular problems.

There are two types of cholesterol: high-density lipoprotein (HDL) and low-density lipoprotein (LDL). LDL is known as the "bad" (or "lousy") cholesterol because it can form as plaque along your arteries and increase your risk of heart disease. HDL, on the other hand, is the "good" (or "happy") cholesterol. Its main job is to collect, breakdown, and excrete the LDL that is already in your body.

Therefore, your goal for optimal health should include a low LDL count and a high HDL count. Your doctor will be able to test your cholesterol levels from a blood sample. Ideally, your total cholesterol (LDL plus HDL) should be under 200 milligrams per deciliter (mg/dL) and your HDL should be over 40 milligrams per deciliter (mg/dL). If it is not, your doctor may need to run further tests.

If your cholesterol is high or has a sudden increase, you may wish to change your dietary habits. Although a portion of your cholesterol levels is due to heredity, limiting your intake of "bad" cholesterol while increasing exercise to elevate "good" cholesterol are important steps you can take to lower your risk for heart disease. There are suggestions of vitamins and other nutrients that can help improve your cholesterol levels throughout this book.

manufactured trans fatty acids are *very* unhealthy "bad" fats. There are even mandates against their use in Europe—but in the United States, they can be found in baked goods, breads, candies, chocolate, frozen dinners, and processed meats.

It is also important to continue your intake of the vitamins and minerals discussed in Chapters 1 and 2. Your body requires vitamin A, the B vitamins, vitamin C, biotin, magnesium, niacin, zinc, and other nutrients to convert fatty acids into usable hormones. Protein is necessary as well. Proper intake of these nutrients as well as good fats will contribute to your good health.

However, alcohol, stress, and certain medications can cause your body to use these fatty acids incorrectly. At the same time, intake of fatty acids may change the amount of medication you need. For example, increased fatty acid intake may result in your needing less Prozac or insulin. Your healthcare provider can provide you with the knowledge you need to make this decision. Similarly, consult your doctor about your fatty acid consumption if you are taking a blood thinner. As you will read, some fatty acids have major effects on your blood's ability to clot.

Instead of the complete elimination of fat from your diet, you need to eat less "bad" fats while adding more "good" fats to your eating and nutrient supplementation programs. This chapter will explain which foods contain which fats, the effects each fat can have on your body, and how much of each you should consume.

SATURATED FATTY ACIDS

Saturated fats are "bad" fats because they have negative effects on your overall health. They are the main dietary source of high cholesterol levels and can cause unhealthy weight gain. Saturated fats are mainly found in animal products such as meat and dairy.

■ Types of Saturated Fats and their Food Sources

- Arachidic acid occurs in peanuts.
- Butyric acid occurs in butter and certain cheeses.

- Palmitic acid occurs in coconut, palm, and palm kernel oils.
- Stearic acid occurs in beef, butter, cocoa butter, mutton, and pork.

■ Diseases/Disorders that Can Be Caused by High Intake of Saturated Fats

- Atherosclerosis
- Coronary heart disease
- Decreased effectiveness of arteries

- Heart disease
- High cholesterol levels
- Stroke
- Weight gain

■ Recommended Intake

The amount of saturated fat in a food can be found on its label. Avoid or limit foods that are high in saturated fat, such as fatty meats and whole-milk dairy products. Instead, eat meats that are lean and high in protein.

ESSENTIAL FATTY ACIDS

Essential fatty acids (EFAs) are polyunsaturated fatty acids that are necessary for good health. They cannot be produced by the body, so they must be consumed in food or supplements. The two most important EFAs are omega-3 fatty acids and omega-6 fatty acids.

OMEGA-3 FATTY ACIDS

Omega-3 fatty acids can lower your cholesterol and reduce your risk of coronary heart disease (a build-up of plaque that can result in a heart attack). They must be consumed in food or supplements. If you rely on food for your omega-3, be sure to eat fish, lamb, nuts, or other foods that contains this fatty acid twice a week.

■ Types of Omega-3 Fatty Acids and their Food Sources

- Alpha-linolenic acid (ALA)
- Docosahexaenoic acid (DHA)

- Eicosapentaenoic acid (EPA)
- Stearidonic acid (also known as moroctic acid)

■ Functions of Omega-3 Fatty Acids

- Crucial for many brain functions

- Decrease arrhythmias (irregular heart rhythm)

- Decrease inflammation

- Diminish build-up of plaque in arteries

- Enhance insulin function

- Help convert nutrients from food into usable forms of energy

- Important component of brain structure and function

- Important for mitochondrial function (which is to produce energy for your cells)

- Improve immune function in infants

- Involved in cell-to-cell communication

- Lower blood pressure

- Lower triglycerides (a type of fat that may be directly related to cholesterol levels)

- Make blood less "sticky" and less likely to clot in dangerous places

- May decrease homocysteine levels (therefore decreasing risk of coronary heart disease)

- May protect against ischemic heart disease (which results in a damaged or inefficient heart and can be fatal)

- Necessary for normal development and function of your adrenal glands, brain, eyes, inner ear, and reproductive tract

- Needed to make certain prostaglandins (hormones which affect inflammation, decrease menstrual cramps, and increase immune function)

Food Sources of Omega-3 Fatty Acids

- Alpha-linolenic acid (ALA) occurs in canola oil, dark green leaves, flax, hemp seed, soy bean, and walnuts.

- Docosahexaenoic acid (DHA) occurs in fish (such as albacore tuna, mackerel, salmon, and sardines), lamb, and nuts.

- Eicosapentaenoic acid (EPA) occurs in fish (such as albacore tuna, mackerel, salmon, and sardines), lamb, and nuts.

- Stearidonic acid (also known as moroctic acid) occurs in black currant seeds.

- Provide structural support for the membranes (outer walls) of your body's cells
- Raise HDL (good) cholesterol
- Reduce premenstrual syndrome (PMS)
- Used to manufacture red blood cells

■ Symptoms of Omega-3 Deficiency

- ☐ Age-related memory decline
- ☐ Arthritis
- ☐ Asthma
- ☐ Behavioral changes
- ☐ Brittle nails
- ☐ Craving fatty foods
- ☐ Dandruff
- ☐ Depression
- ☐ Dry skin
- ☐ Excessive urination
- ☐ Fatty infiltration of the liver
- ☐ Growth retardation
- ☐ Hair loss
- ☐ Impaired immune response
- ☐ Impaired motor coordination
- ☐ Increase in allergies
- ☐ Increase in arthritis
- ☐ Inflammation
- ☐ Learning disorders
- ☐ Mental deterioration
- ☐ Mood swings
- ☐ Psychological disturbances
- ☐ Thirst
- ☐ Tingling feeling in arms or legs

■ Causes of Omega-3 Deficiency

- Alcoholism
- Carnitine deficiency
- Decreased intake of "good" fatty acids
- Decreased intake of nutrients needed as cofactors
- Excessive consumption of omega-6 fatty acids
- High intake of saturated fats
- Inability to absorb fatty acids
- Increased intake of sugar
- Increased intake of trans fatty acids
- Stress
- Type I diabetes

■ Recommended Dosage

It is important that your intake of omega-6 fatty acids and omega-3 fatty acids maintain a proper ratio—between 3:1 and 6:1—or you may become deficient in omega-3. This is because the two EFAs compete for use in the body. Unfortunately, the standard American diet is very high in omega-6 and very low in omega-3, so most Americans maintain a ratio of between 10:1 and 25:1. You should either eat foods (such as fish) that are high in omega-3 twice a week or take daily omega-3 supplements. Have your doctor measure your essential and metabolic fatty acids. This test is available through Genova Diagnostics and other laboratories. (See Resources for contact information.)

Take vitamin E when ingesting omega-3 fatty acids to prevent oxidation. (Oxidation is a chemical process that results in free radicals in your body. Page 4 explains more about free radicals.) You should also consume vitamin A, the B vitamins, vitamin C, biotin, magnesium, niacin, zinc, and protein to convert all fatty acids into usable hormones.

Omega-3s can become rancid if oxidized before eaten. This can be prevented through refrigeration. If you have trouble "burping them up," you can put them in the freezer. This does not destroy their effectiveness.

■ Diseases/Disorders that Can Be Treated with Omega-3

- ADD/ADHD
- Arthritis (rheumatoid and degenerative)
- Asthma
- Atherosclerosis
- Autism
- Autoimmune disorders
- Bipolar disorder
- Cancer of the breast, colon, lung, prostate, and skin (prevention)
- Cardiovascular disease
- Cerebral palsy
- Certain benign tumors (inhibits)

- Chronic fatigue syndrome
- Cognitive decline
- Crohn's disease
- Depression
- Diabetes (prevention and treatment)
- Down's syndrome
- Drug abuse
- Eczema
- High blood pressure
- High cholesterol
- High triglyceride levels
- Inflammation
- Irritable bowel syndrome

- Memory decline
- Menopausal symptoms
- Menstrual cramps
- Migraine headaches
- Multiple sclerosis
- Neuropathy (nerve disorder)
- Postpartum depression
- Psoriasis
- Schizophrenia
- Stroke (prevention, recovery)
- Type II diabetes
- Unwanted blood clots

OMEGA-6 FATTY ACIDS

Omega-6 fatty acids must be consumed in food or supplements. Like omega-3s, omega-6 fatty acids are crucial to good health. They help your body produce prostaglandins, which are important hormones, and they have many other bodily functions. However, most Americans consume significantly more omega-6 fatty acids than they need, which can lead to a number of health problems.

◼ Types of Omega-6 Fatty Acids

- Arachidonic acid (AA)
- Dihomogamma-linolenic acid (DGLA)
- Gamma-linolenic acid (GLA)
- Linoleic acid

◼ Functions of Omega-6 Fatty Acids

- Essential for normal development and function of your adrenal glands, brain, eyes, inner ear, and reproductive tract
- Help convert nutrients from food into usable forms of energy
- Involved in cell-to-cell communication
- Lower LDL (bad) cholesterol
- Make blood "sticky," which allows it to clot
- Necessary for brain development and function
- Needed to make certain prostaglandins (hormones)
- Nourishment of skin and hair
- Promote inflammation

Food Sources of Omega-6 Fatty Acids

- Arachidonic acid (AA) occurs in meats and other animal products.
- Dihomogamma-linolenic acid (DGLA) occurs in mother's milk.
- Gamma-linolenic acid (GLA) occurs in black current seed, borage oil, and evening primrose oil.
- Linoleic acid occurs in flax oil, hemp, pumpkin, safflower, sesame, soybean, sunflower, and walnut.

- Provide structural support for the membranes (outer walls) of the body's cells
- Reduce premenstrual syndrome (PMS)
- Used to manufacture red blood cells

■ Symptoms of Omega-6 Deficiency

☐ Behavioral changes   ☐ Dry eyes   ☐ Poor vision

☐ Cardiovascular   ☐ Dry skin   ☐ Reproductive
   abnormalities   ☐ Hair loss   problems

☐ Dehydration   ☐ Kidney problems   ☐ Stunted growth

■ Recommended Dosage

As you have read, omega-6 fatty acids have to be ingested in food or supplements because they cannot be produced in the body. Yet it is important that your intake of omega-6 fatty acids and omega-3 fatty acids maintain a proper ratio—between 3:1 and 6:1—or it can lead to chronic inflammation as well as many other health problems (listed on page 110). Unfortunately, the standard American diet is very high in omega-6 and low in omega-3, so that most Americans maintain a ratio of between 10:1 and 25:1. It is, therefore, to your advantage to decrease your intake of omega-6 while increasing your intake of omega-3. The average Mediterranean diet, on the other hand, contains many less omega-6 fatty acids and many more omega-3 fatty acids. Symptoms of omega-3 deficiency are listed on page 110.

TRANS FATTY ACIDS

Unsaturated fats have a tendency to become rancid (chemically altered) rather quickly. To combat this problem, manufacturers began to *hydrogenate*—stabilize by adding a hydrogen molecule to—these fats. This developed a new type of fatty acid, the *trans fatty acid*, that allows foods and cooking oils to be stored for much longer periods of time. These fats can also stay solid at room temperatures, which is unusual for unsaturated fats.

Unfortunately, these fats are "bad" fats. They increase your choles-

Food Sources of Trans Fatty Acids

Foods that contain trans fatty acids will read "hydrogenated" or "partially hydrogenated" on their labels.

- Baked goods
- Breads
- Candies
- Chocolates
- Corn chips
- Donuts

- French fries
- Fried foods
- Frozen dinners
- Margarine (particularly in stick form)

- Mayonnaise
- Pastries
- Potato chips
- Processed meats
- Processed oils
- Shortening

terol levels as well as your risk of heart disease. Trans fatty acids are so unhealthy that some countries have banned them completely, but they are still found in many manufactured foods in the United States. You can learn to avoid unhealthy amounts of trans fatty acids by becoming aware of which foods contain them.

However, there are some trans fatty acids that occur naturally, although usually in very small quantities. These trans fats are not "bad" fats, and some even have healthful functions. Conjugated linoleic acid (CLA), one

Conjugated Linoleic Acid

Conjugated linoleic acid (CLA) is a naturally occuring trans fatty acid. Unlike manufactured fatty acids, CLA can have positive effects on your overall health. It is currently being marketed as a dietary supplement because it has been shown to aid in weight loss. When used for this purpose, CLA should be consumed in quantities of 3,000 to 4,000 milligrams a day.

CLA is beneficial in many other ways, as well. It is an antioxidant, lowers cholesterol, fortifies the immune system, and improves insulin sensitivity. It is also believed to fight breast and colon cancer. For these preventative measures, 100 to 500 milligrams of CLA should be consumed daily.

CLA is found in low quantities in beef, kangaroo meat, and lamb. However, in order to ingest the suggested dosages, it is best to take CLA supplements.

such example, is described in the inset on page 114. The rest of this section will look at the more common trans fats: the ones that are manufactured by companies in order to preserve foods for longer shelf-life.

■ Diseases/Disorders that Can Be Caused by High Intake of Trans Fatty Acids

- Clogged arteries
- Decreased HDL (good) cholesterol
- Heart disease
- Increased LDL (bad) cholesterol
- Increased triglycerides
- Interference with your body's ability to make its own DHA (an omega-3 essential fatty acid)
- Leaking cell membranes, which can disrupt cellular metabolism and allow toxins to enter your cells
- Obesity
- "Stickier" blood, which can increase blood clots
- Type II diabetes

■ Recommended Intake of Trans Fatty Acids

If you live in the United States, you are surrounded by foods that contain trans fatty acids. Try to eliminate as many as possible from your diet. If you are healthy, do not have a personal history of heart disease, and do not have very high cholesterol, you can consume more fatty acids than you would be able to otherwise. However, regardless of your current health status, it is important for your future well-being that you limit your intake of non-natural trans fatty acids. Their potential effects on your health are all negative.

4

Amino Acids

There are 40,000 *proteins* in your body. They are a main source of energy, promote repair of damaged tissue, and function as the building blocks of muscle. They also perform a variety of other important functions.

Proteins consist of *amino acids* linked by *peptide bonds*. Although amino acids are the main components and the nutritional part of these complex compounds, most of the 40,000 proteins in your body are made from only twenty amino acids. These *standard amino acids* are included in the genetic code of every living being. After the proteins are constructed by your body, however, some of these amino acids become attached to other functional groups (such as phosphates or lipids), at which point they are structurally changed into different amino acids. These, too, are important for nutritional health.

All amino acids are divided into three categories. Some are *essential amino acids* because your system cannot manufacture them on its own. Others are *nonessential amino acids*—although important for your health, they are made in sufficient quantities by your body and do not need to be ingested. The last group is *conditionally essential amino acids*. These can be made by your body under normal conditions. However, you may need to ingest them in certain situations: factors such as fever, illness, diet, or chemotherapy may cause a person to be unable to manufacture these amino acids, or a process such as detoxification may be using all the amino acids the body has made. (Detoxification is further discussed on page 346.) Amino acids are divided into these three groups in Table 4.1.

This chapter focuses on some of the most important amino acids found in your body. For a more comprehensive text of this subject, read *Heal with Amino Acids and Nutrients* by Dr. Billie Sahley.

If you exhibit several of the symptoms from the list on page 119, it

TABLE 4.1. AMINO ACIDS

Essential Amino Acids	Conditionally Essential Amino Acids	Nonessential Amino Acids
Histidine	Cysteine	Alanine
Isoleucine	Cystine	Arginine
Leucine	Glutamine	Asparagine
Lysine	Taurine	Aspartic acid
Methionine	Tyrosine	Carnitine
Phenylalanine		5-HTP
Threonine		GABA
Tryptophan		Glutamate
Valine		Glycine
		Proline
		Serine

may indicate an amino acid deficiency. Your doctor can perform an amino acid analysis test to determine the dosages of amino acids you should take. If you are deficient in one or two amino acids, you can buy amino acid supplements from any of the pharmaceutical grade companies from which they are offered. If you are deficient in several amino acids, your doctor can contact a *compounding pharmacist,* who can formulate amino acids into a prescription specific for you. The Professional Compounding Centers of America (PCCA) can help you find a compounding pharmacist near you. (See Resources for contact information.)

When you are buying amino acids, be sure to buy only those of pharmaceutical grade. You should also attempt to buy *free amino acids,* which are amino acids that are in their purest form and do not need to be digested before being utilized. Instead, they are absorbed directly into the bloodstream and immediately put to use by your body.

You will see that most amino acids come in two forms: D- and L- (such as D-carnitine and L-carnitine). The D-amino acid is a mirror image of the L-amino acid. They are very similar, and both can be taken as supplements. However, the L- form is preferable because it is the exact image of the amino acid in its natural form as found in your body (while the D-form is backwards). For that reason, the L- form is considered more effective than the D- form for overall human health. (The amino acids glycine and taurine are each available in only one form, and are therefore not designated D- or L-.)

Your body needs vitamin B_6 (pyridoxine) to metabolize most amino acid supplements. (See page 39 for more information on this vitamin.) Also, consult a physician before taking any amino acid supplements if you have diabetes, hypertension, kidney disease, or liver disease.

■ Symptoms of an Amino Acid Deficiency

- ☐ ADD/ADHD
- ☐ Aggressive behavior
- ☐ Alcoholism
- ☐ Anxiety
- ☐ Arthritis
- ☐ Blood sugar disorders
- ☐ Chronic fatigue
- ☐ Craving carbo-hydrates and sugar
- ☐ Depression
- ☐ Fibromyalgia
- ☐ Food or chemical allergies
- ☐ Frequent colds
- ☐ Frequent headaches
- ☐ Hyperactivity
- ☐ Immune dysfunction
- ☐ Insomnia
- ☐ Mental or emotional problems
- ☐ Mood swings or disorders
- ☐ Neurological disorders
- ☐ Obsessive compulsive disorder (OCD)
- ☐ Panic attacks
- ☐ Premenstrual syndrome (PMS)
- ☐ Recurrent ear infections

ALANINE

The standard amino acid alanine is one of the simplest structured amino acids. It is also one of the most widely used amino acids in your body. Alanine is nonessential, and requires vitamin B_6 for metabolism.

■ Functions of Alanine in Your Body

- Converts into glucose when energy is needed or blood sugar levels decrease
- Helps break down glucose, which provides your body with energy
- Helps form neurotransmitters
- Involved in production of antibodies
- Is an inhibitory neurotransmitter in the brain
- Required for the metabolization of tryptophan

Food Sources of Alanine

- Beans
- Brewer's yeast
- Dairy products

- Duck
- Fish
- Nuts

- Sausage
- Turkey
- Wheat germ

■ Recommended Dosage

200 to 600 milligrams daily. Since alanine can be made in the body, most people do not need to take supplements. However, people with hypoglycemia tend to have low levels of alanine and may benefit from increased intake.

■ Side Effects and Contraindications

Check with your doctor before starting an amino acid regiment if you have kidney or liver disease.

ARGININE

Arginine is a standard amino acid that can be synthesized in your body from ornithine. (Arginine can also be synthesized *into* ornithine.) Some bodybuilders take arginine supplements because it increases muscle mass while decreasing body fat. However, it is also involved in a number of essential bodily functions, described below.

■ Functions of Arginine in Your Body

- Builds muscle
- Decreases platelet stickiness, lowering risk of unhealthy blood clots
- Enhances fat metabolism
- Enhances immune function
- Helps wounds heal
- Important for gut health
- Increases circulation
- Increases human growth hormone (HGH) production

- Increases immune function by increasing natural killer cell activity
- Increases sperm count
- Inhibits plaque accumulation in your arteries
- Needed for protein production
- Reduces pain from claudication (poor circulation)
- Used to produce nitric oxide
- Vital for secretion of glucagon and insulin

■ Symptoms of Arginine Deficiency

☐ Coma

☐ Constipation

☐ Fatty liver

☐ Hair loss and breakage

☐ Hepatic cirrhosis

☐ Poor wound healing

☐ Skin rash

■ Recommended Dosage

1,000 to 3,000 milligrams daily

■ Side Effects and Contraindications

- Diarrhea
- Increase in outbreaks of herpes simplex infections (cold sores or genital herpes. The addition of the amino acid lysine to your supplementation program can limit this effect.)
- Nausea
- Tightness in chest or throat

Food Sources of Arginine

- Asparagus
- Avocados
- Beans
- Brewer's yeast
- Broccoli
- Chocolate
- Corn
- Dairy products
- Eggs
- Fish
- Green peas
- Legumes
- Meat
- Nuts
- Oatmeal
- Onion
- Popcorn
- Potatoes
- Raisins
- Seafood
- Seeds
- Sesame seeds
- Soy
- Spinach
- Sunflower seeds
- Swiss chard
- Whey
- Whole grains

ASPARAGINE

Asparagine, a standard amino acid involved in making protein, is nonessential because it can be synthesized in your body. It is synthesized from aspartic acid and adenosine triphosphate. When necessary, your body can convert asparagine back into aspartic acid.

■ Functions of Asparagine in Your Body

- Forms part of DNA
- Helps ammonia detoxify
- Helps protect the liver
- Metabolizes carbohydrates via the Krebs cycle (which produces energy)
- Promotes mineral uptake in the intestinal tract
- Transport nitrogen

■ Symptoms of Asparagine Deficiency

☐ Allergies

☐ Fatigue

■ Recommended Dosage

Have your doctor perform an amino acid analysis test. From your results, he will be able to recommend a daily dosage.

Food Sources of Asparagine

- Asparagus
- Cheese
- Chicken
- Dairy products
- Pork
- Potatoes
- Sausage
- Turkey
- Wheat germ

ASPARTIC ACID

Aspartic acid is an amino acid as well as an excitatory neurotransmitter. It is made in the body from glutamic acid and requires the presence of B_6. Aspartic acid is a nonessential amino acid so it is not necessary to seek it out in supplements or diet. Instead, some people have elevated levels, which can lead to the problems listed below.

■ Functions of Aspartic Acid

- Forms parts of DNA
- Involved in metabolism of ammonia
- Involved in urea cycle
- May play a role in the immune system
- May encourage endurance
- Metabolizes carbohydrates via the Krebs cycle
- Necessary for brain health
- Necessary for the production of glucose

■ Symptoms of Aspartic Acid Toxicity

☐ Depression   ☐ Epilepsy   ☐ Stroke

Food Sources of Aspartic Acid

- Beef
- Chicken
- Cottage cheese
- Fish
- Pork
- Ricotta cheese
- Sausage
- Turkey
- Wheat germ

CARNITINE

Carnitine is made from lysine and methionine in your liver, kidneys, and brain. Therefore, your being deficient in carnitine implies that you may lack lysine and methionine. Iron, niacin, vitamin B_6, and vitamin C are also necessary to make carnitine.

■ Functions of Carnitine in Your Body

- Can be converted to acetyl choline in your body
- Energizes the heart
- Enhances short- and long-term memory
- Helps convert stored body fat into energy

- Improves mental focus and energy

- Increases oxygen availability and respiratory efficiency

- Lowers LDL (bad) cholesterol

- May slow the progression of Alzheimer's disease

- Needed for the transport of long-chain fatty acids into the cells

- Prevents DNA degeneration

- Promotes DNA repair from mutations that occur from free radical production

- Raises HDL (good) cholesterol

- Reduces the build-up of acids and metabolic waste

- Reduces triglycerides

■ Causes of Carnitine Deficiency

- Deficiency of folic acid

- Deficiency of S-adenosylmethionine (SAMe), an important compound found in all living cells

- Deficiency of vitamin B_6, B_{12}, or C

- Ipecac syrup (used to remove poisons before they can be absorbed)

- Iron deficiency

- Lysine deficiency

- Pivampicillin (an antibiotic)

- Pyrimethamine (antiparasitic and antimalaria drug)

- Sulfadiazine (used to treat infection)

- Valproic acid (an anticonvulsant)

- Vegetarian diet

■ Nutrients that Increase Carnitine Effectiveness

- Alpha-lipoic acid

- B vitamins

- Docosahexaenoic acid (DHA)

- Eicosapentaenoic acid (EPA)

- Phosphatidylcholine (a phospholipid)

- Phosphatidylserine (a phospholipid described on page 204)

■ Recommended Dosage

500 to 4,000 milligrams daily. Acetyl-L-carnitine (ALCAR) is the form of carnitine that can effectively help maintain memory and recover from a stroke.

■ Side Effects and Contraindications

Although side effects of carnitine supplementation are rare, they include agitation, headache, increased appetite, nausea, skin rash, and vomiting. Some people also experience body odor, which can be prevented by taking riboflavin. If you have kidney or liver disease, contact your physician before starting a carnitine regiment.

■ Diseases/Disorders that Can Be Treated with Carnitine

- Alzheimer's disease
- Angina pectoris
- Attention deficit disorder (ADD)
- Brain injuries
- Congestive heart failure
- Depression
- High cholesterol levels
- Immune enhancement
- Increased triglycerides
- Infertility
- Memory enhancement
- Mitral valve prolapse
- Nerve injury
- Parkinson's disease
- Recovery from heart attack or stroke
- Renal disease
- Senility
- Stroke
- Weight loss

CARNOSINE

Carnosine is an amino acid that is formed when a beta-alanine molecule and a histidine molecule join together. Stored in your brain, heart, and muscles, it protects your body from *glycation*—a process which results in free radicals in your body and causes signs of aging. Do not confuse this nutrient with the similar-sounding amino acid carnitine (page 123).

■ Functions of Carnosine in Your Body

- Binds metal ions that cause tissue damage
- Blocks the aging effects of glycation
- Helps maintain memory
- Is an antioxidant
- Protects muscle tissue from lactic acid
- Regulates levels of copper and zinc

Food Source of Carnosine

- Beef
- Chicken
- Pork

■ **Recommended Dosage**

1,000 to 2,000 milligrams daily

■ **Side Effects and Contraindications**

If you have kidney or liver disease, contact your doctor before taking carnosine. Also, be aware that taking too much carnosine can result in hyperactivity.

■ **Diseases/Disorders that Can Be Treated with Carnosine**

- Aging
- Alzheimer's disease
- Atherosclerosis
- Autism
- Brain injury
- Cataracts
- Diabetes mellitus
- Hypertension
- Stroke
- Wound healing

CYSTEINE

Cysteine is a nonessential amino acid that is made in your liver. N-acetyl cysteine (NAC) is the most frequently used form of cysteine. It has many important functions, including helping synthesize protein and aiding your body in making the strong antioxidant glutathione. The amino acid cystine is the stable form of cysteine. The conversion of cysteine into cystine occurs as your body requires it.

■ **Functions of Cysteine in your Body**

- Aids in cancer protection (by stimulating natural killer cells)
- Aids in healing after surgery
- Boosts your immune system
- Breaks down homocysteine

- Helps destroy acetaldehyde and free radicals produced by smoking and drinking
- Helps protect against heart disease
- Involved in communication between cells
- Is an antioxidant
- Prevents hair loss
- Promotes hair growth
- Promotes metabolism of fats and production of muscle
- Reduces inflammation

Recommended Dosage

It is rare to be deficient in cysteine. However, if you believe you need to supplement your cysteine levels, ask your doctor how much you should take. Cysteine can also be used to treat acetaminophen poisoning. Your doctor should be notified when cysteine is taken for this purpose.

Food Sources of Cysteine

• Beans	• Fish	• Red peppers
• Brewer's yeast	• Garlic	• Seafood
• Broccoli	• Legumes	• Seeds
• Brussels sprouts	• Meat	• Soy
• Dairy products	• Nuts	• Whey
• Eggs	• Onions	• Whole grains

Side Effects and Contraindications

Do not take D-cysteine, D-cystine, or 5-methyl cysteine because they can be toxic. Cysteine supplements must be taken with vitamin C. This will prevent an increase of kidney stone production. You cannot use cysteine if you have an active peptic ulcer. Also, do not take cysteine if you are diabetic because it may cause your glucose levels to change. After taking cysteine supplements, some people may experience any of the following symptoms.

- Abdominal pain
- Abnormal taste
- Anorexia
- Asthma
- Blurred vision
- Constipation
- Diarrhea
- Dizziness
- Dry mouth
- Flushes
- Headache
- Indigestion
- Nausea
- Rashes
- Shortness of breath
- Skin rash
- Sweating
- Vomiting

5-HYDROXYTRYPTOPHAN (5-HTP)

A by-product of tryptophan, 5-hydroxytryptophan (5-HTP) is a nonessential amino acid that increases the body's level of serotonin. Most of the problems it has been marketed to help—such as depression, sleeplessness, and night terrors—can occur because of low levels of serotonin. Most people are not deficient in 5-HTP and do not need take supplements.

Functions of 5-HTP in Your Body

- Manufactures serotonin, a neurotransmitter that affects many functions, including appetite, mood, and body temperature
- May improve sleep quality
- May decrease anxiety

Recommended Dosage

50 to 300 milligrams daily. Magnesium prolongs the benefits of 5-HTP.

Side Effects and Contraindications

If you are taking an SSRI or another antidepressant, you should not take 5-HTP. If you are taking medication for Parkinson's disease, you should not take 5-HTP. Consult your healthcare provider before taking 5-HTP if you are diabetic or have high blood pressure, heart disease, or an autoimmune disorder.

■ Diseases/Disorders that Can Be Treated with 5-HTP

- Addiction
- Anxiety
- Carbohydrate cravings
- Chronic headaches
- Depression

- Fibromyalgia
- Hyperactivity
- Insomnia
- Mood disorders
- Obesity

- Obsessive compulsive disorder
- Pain management
- Premenstrual syndrome (PMS)
- Stress

Food Sources of 5-HTP

- Avocados
- Poultry
- Red meat

GAMMA-AMINOBUTYRIC ACID

Gamma-aminobutyric acid (GABA) is derived from the amino acid glutamic acid. It is found in large amounts in your hypothalamus, the area of your brain responsible for regulating appetite and body temperature. If you take GABA supplements, it is important that you also take vitamin B_6 to act as a cofactor. Otherwise, your body cannot metabolize the GABA properly.

■ Functions of GABA in Your Body

- Aids your body in secreting growth hormone
- Helps control hypoglycemia
- Is an inhibitory neurotransmitter
- Lowers blood pressure
- Muscle relaxant
- Prevents anxiety
- Produces a calming effect on the brain
- Promotes sleep

Food Sources of GABA

- Beans
- Brewer's yeast
- Brown rice
- Dairy products
- Eggs
- Fish
- Legumes
- Meat
- Nuts
- Seafood
- Seeds
- Soy
- Wheat bran
- Whey
- Whole grains

■ Symptoms of GABA Deficiency

☐ Anxiety

☐ Racing mind

■ Recommended Dosage

- If you weigh less than 125 pounds, take 375 milligrams three times a day.
- If you weigh more than 125 pounds, take 750 milligrams three times a day.

■ Side Effects and Contraindications

Some people experience a tingling sensation in the face and a slight shortness of breath after taking GABA. Typically, however, this only lasts for a few minutes. GABA is best taken at night since it may make you drowsy. If you have kidney or liver disease, contact your physician before you take GABA.

GLUTAMATE

Glutamate, which is also known as glutamic acid, is a nonessential amino acid and the brain's major excitatory neurotransmitter. It can be converted into both glutamine and GABA by the body, and is made from aspartic acid, ornithine, arginine, proline, and alpha-ketoglutarate.

■ Functions of Glutamate in Your Body

- Acts as brain detoxifier of ammonia
- Involved in pain control

- Involved with sensory perception, memory, orientation in time and space, cognition, and motor skills
- Plays a role in the body's ability to adapt to environmental and genetic influences

■ Causes of Glutamate Toxicity

- Epilepsy
- Gout
- Schizophrenia

■ Side Effects and Contraindications

Do not use glutamic acid if you are sensitive to monosodium glutamate (MSG) because it may exacerbate the symptoms.

Food Sources of Glutamate

- Bacon
- Duck
- Granola
- Turkey
- Chicken
- Eggs
- Ham
- Wheat germ
- Cottage cheese
- Fish
- Sausage
- Yogurt

GLUTAMINE

Glutamine is one of the twenty amino acids used to make protein in your body. It is also involved in many metabolic processes. A conditionally essential amino acid, glutamine can be produced by the body but can also become depleted when used in overabundance, such as during intense physical activity or stress.

■ Functions of Glutamine in Your Body

- Balances blood sugar
- Fights cold and flu
- Helps the brain dispose of ammonia
- Improves mental alertness
- Increases energy
- Increases growth hormone

- Is a fuel source for your immune system
- Is a precursor for GABA
- Is an inhibitory neurotransmitter
- Needed for a healthy gut
- Needed for DNA synthesis
- Needed for the metabolism and maintenance of muscle
- Neutralizes toxins
- Promotes a healthy acid-alkaline balance
- Promotes growth
- Promotes healthy acid-alkaline balance in your body
- Promotes weight loss
- Promotes wound healing and tissue repair
- Protects the body from stress
- Stops food cravings
- Supports glutathione (see page 133)

■ Recommended Dosage

500 to 3,000 milligrams daily

■ Side Effects and Contraindications

If you have a sensitivity to monosodium glutamate (MSG), use glutamine with caution because your body metabolizes glutamine into glutamate. If you are taking medications for seizures, only take glutamine under the direction of your doctor.

Food Sources of Glutamine

Beans	Eggs	Nuts	Soy
Brewer's yeast	Fish	Parsley	Spinach
Brown rice	Legumes	Seafood	Whey
Dairy products	Meat	Seeds	Whole grains

GLUTATHIONE

Glutathione is a *tripeptide*—a compound composed of three amino acids—that is made of cysteine, glutamic acid, and glycine. It is responsible for the health of most of the cells in your body. Around the age of forty, your glutathione levels begin to diminish, and you may need to begin taking supplements.

■ Functions of Glutathione in Your Body

- Decreases sugar cravings
- Displaces glutamate from its binding site
- Enhances liver and brain detoxification of toxic chemicals and heavy metals
- Helps to recycle other antioxidants, such as vitamins C and E
- Involved in protein and prostaglandin (fatty acid compounds) synthesis
- Is a neuromodulator (transmits information between neurons)
- Is a neurotransmitter
- Is a very powerful antioxidant
- Part of amino acid transport
- Stimulates production of interleukin 1 and 2, which help regulate your immune system
- Used in DNA synthesis and repair

■ Symptoms of Glutathione Deficiency

☐ Asthma

☐ Faster progression of human immunodeficiency virus (HIV)

☐ Hemolytic anemia (destruction of red blood cells)

☐ Immune disorders

■ Causes of Glutathione Deficiency

- Acetaminophen (such as Tylenol)
- Cigarette smoking
- Excessive intake of alcohol
- Overly processed chemical-laden foods (such as luncheon meats that contain nitrites or nitrates)

■ Nutrients that Increase Glutathione Levels

- Alpha-lipoic acid
- Glutamine
- Methionine
- Milk thistle
- S-adenosyl methionine (SAMe)
- Vitamin C
- Vitamin E
- Whey protein

■ Recommended Dosage

Taking 500 to 3,000 milligrams of N-acetylcysteine (NAC) daily will increase your glutathione levels.

Most forms of glutathione are not effective if taken by mouth because they are broken down by digestive enzymes. Instead, they can be given to you by your physician intravenously. Glutathione can be taken orally, however, if in a specific form called N-acetylcysteine (NAC). This amino acid linkage is not broken down by digestive enzymes.

■ Side Effects and Contraindications

The cysteine in NAC can precipitate and cause kidney stones to form. Take extra vitamin C with NAC to avoid this. Also, if you are taking NAC for prolonged periods of time, you may need to take extra copper and zinc. NAC can bind these minerals and make them unavailable for usage in your body.

Food Sources of Glutathione

- Asparagus
- Avocado
- Fish
- Meat
- Walnuts

GLYCINE

Glycine is a nonessential amino acid and one of the building blocks of protein. Unlike most of the other amino acids, glycine does not come in D- and L- forms. Although most people do not need to take glycine supplementation because the body can produce it, some doctors have had success when prescribing it for certain health conditions.

■ Functions of Glycine in Your Body

- Calms aggression
- Decreases sugar cravings
- Enhances the neurotransmitters (messengers) in your brain
- Helps detoxify heavy metals and other toxins from your body
- Helps form collagen
- Involved in the metabolism of bile salts
- Is an inhibitory neurotransmitter
- Is important to manufacture glucose from glycogen in your liver
- Needed for prostate gland function
- Needed to maintain the nervous system
- Promotes health of various organs, including gland, prostate, and spleen
- Used for the formation of glutathione
- Used in metabolism of proteins
- Used in the synthesis of DNA, hemoglobin, glutathione, and RNA

■ Recommended Dosage

500 to 3,000 milligrams daily

■ Side Effects and Contraindications

If you are taking clozapine or another atypical antipsychotic medication, you should not take glycine.

■ Diseases/Disorders that Can Be Treated with Glycine

- Bipolar disorder
- Epilepsy
- Prostate enlargement (prevention)
- Schizophrenia
- Spasticity (involuntary muscle contractions)

Food Sources of Glycine

- Dairy products
- Fish
- Meat
- Wheat germ

Branched-Chain Amino Acids

The essential amino acids leucine, isoleucine, and valine are called *branched-chain amino acids (BCAAs)*. The main functions of all three are to stimulate protein synthesis and decrease protein breakdown, but they are each metabolized differently in the body. Leucine metabolizes fats, valine metabolizes carbohydrates, and isoleucine metabolizes both fats and carbohydrates. BCAAs are found in all food sources that contain protein and most people consume enough in their diet, but an injury or stress may result in an increased need for these amino acids.

The recommended dosage of BCAAs is one to five grams a day, depending on the reason for which they are being taken. Your healthcare provider can prescribe a specific dosage. The three BCAAs should be taken together, rather than individually, because supplementation of a single BCAA can cause a deficiency in the other two. Also, BCAA supplementation can reduce the effectiveness of medications used to treat Parkinson's disease, such as levodopa.

Food Sources of Leucine

- Asparagus
- Avocado
- Broccoli
- Cereals (especially millet)
- Cheese
- Corn
- Eggs
- Fish
- Gelatin
- Grains
- Green peas
- Lentils
- Meats
- Milk
- Mushrooms
- Nuts
- Potatoes
- Seeds
- Spinach
- Sweet potatoes
- Swiss chard
- Tomatoes
- Wheat germ

Food Sources of Valine

- Avocado
- Beets
- Broccoli
- Cereals (especially buckwheat, millet, and oatmeal)
- Cheese
- Chocolate
- Corn
- Green peas
- Milk
- Peanuts
- Potatoes
- Spinach
- Sweet potatoes
- Swiss chard

Food Sources of Isoleucine

- Avocado
- Beans (especially soy)
- Cereals (especially millet)
- Cheese
- Corn
- Eggs
- Grains
- Green peas
- Lentils
- Meats
- Milk
- Nuts
- Potatoes
- Seeds
- Spinach
- Swiss chard

HISTIDINE

Histidine is a standard amino acid. Most adults can manufacture histidine within their bodies. However, it is considered an essential amino acid because it cannot be produced in children, who must consume it through either diet or supplementation. Also, you may need to ingest additional histidine during periods of accelerated growth.

Functions of Histidine in Your Body

- Dilates vessels
- Helps absorb and transport zinc
- Helps to chelate (improve availability of) minerals
- Is a mild anti-inflammatory
- May be an antioxidant
- Needed for the maintenance of the myelin sheaths in your nervous system
- Produces histamine
- Provides the effects (itching, swelling, etc.) of an allergic reaction

Symptoms of Histidine Deficiency

☐ Cataracts
☐ Eczema
☐ Indigestion
☐ Joint pains

■ Symptoms of Histidine Toxicity

- Copper deficiency
- High LDL (bad) cholesterol

■ Recommended Dosage

Have your doctor perform an amino acid analysis test. From your results, he will be able to recommend a daily dosage.

Food Sources of Histidine

• Bananas	• Cheese	• Grains	• Potatoes
• Beans	• Chicken	• Meats	• Seeds
• Brewer's yeast	• Eggs	• Milk	• Soy beans
• Cereals	• Fish	• Nuts	• Turkey

LYSINE

The body uses the essential amino acid lysine to make protein, so it is important that you consume this nutrient daily. Found in both meat and dairy products, lysine helps your body produce antibodies, hormones, and enzymes.

■ Function of Lysine in Your Body

- Aids in the production of antibodies
- Helps fight herpes outbreaks (cold sores or genital herpes)
- Helps maintain bone health by enhancing calcium absorption
- Helps protect the lens of the eye
- Helps support immune defense
- Increases growth hormone
- Maintains nitrogen balance
- Needed for making enzymes

- Needed for production of hormones
- Regulates the mammary glands, ovaries, and pineal gland
- Required for growth and tissue repair
- Used in collagen production

■ Symptoms of Lysine Deficiency

☐ Anemia	☐ Fatigue	☐ Irritability
☐ Apathy	☐ Fever blisters	☐ Loss of energy
☐ Bloodshot eyes	☐ Hair loss	☐ Muscle loss
☐ Carnitine deficiency	☐ Inability to concentrate	☐ Stomach ulcers
☐ Depression		☐ Stunted growth
☐ Edema (swelling)	☐ Infertility	☐ Weakness

■ Recommended Dosage

500 to 1,600 milligrams daily

Food Sources of Lysine

• Asparagus	• Chicken	• Legumes	• Seafood
• Avocado	• Chocolate	• Lentils	• Seeds
• Beans	• Corn	• Lima beans	• Soy
• Beef	• Dairy products	• Meat	• Spinach
• Brewer's yeast	• Eggs	• Mushrooms	• Whey
• Broccoli	• Fish	• Nuts	• Whole grains
• Cheese	• Green peas	• Potatoes	• Yeast

■ Side Effects and Contraindications

Lysine should not be taken for more than six months because it can cause an imbalance of arginine. If you have diabetes or are allergic to eggs, milk, or wheat, do not take lysine supplements.

■ Diseases/Disorders that Can Be Treated with Lysine

For people with the herpes virus, lysine can be used to limit occurrence and severity of outbreaks. During a herpes outbreak, increase your lysine intake to 3,000 milligrams a day until it has resolved.

METHIONINE

Methionine is an essential amino acid that is coded for in the genetic code and used to make protein. Although it must be consumed because your body cannot manufacture it on its own, most people do not need to take methionine supplementation because it is available in many common foods. If you do begin a methionine regiment, be sure you are also getting enough folate, vitamin B_6, and vitamin B_{12}.

■ Functions of Methionine in Your Body

- Detoxifies the body of heavy metals
- Facilitates the breakdown of fats
- Needed for the absorption, transportation, and availability of selenium and zinc
- Needed for the formation of carnitine, choline, collagen, creatine, epinephrine, lecithin, melatonin, nucleic acids, and serine
- Normalizes homocysteine
- Prevents fat accumulation in your liver and arteries

Food Sources of Methionine

• Avocado	• Eggs	• Peanuts	• Sunflower seeds
• Cheese	• Fish	• Pork	
• Cottage cheese	• Lentils	• Pumpkin	• Wheat germ
	• Meat	• Sausage	• Whey
• Duck	• Milk	• Seafood	• Wild game

◼ Symptoms of Methionine Deficiency

☐ Apathy

☐ Edema (swelling)

☐ Fat loss

☐ Lethargy

☐ Liver damage

☐ Loss of pigmentation in hair

☐ Muscle loss

☐ Skin lesions

☐ Slow growth in children

☐ Weakness

◼ Recommended Dosage

250 to 2,000 milligrams daily

◼ Side Effects and Contraindications

If you are taking methionine, you must also take B$_6$ and folic acid to prevent a build-up of homocysteine. High levels of homocysteine can put you at risk for heart disease and Alzheimer's disease. Also, high intake of methionine may counter the effects of levodopa, a drug used to treat Parkinson's disease.

PHENYLALANINE

Phenylalanine converts to tyrosine in the liver. Tyrosine is then converted into the neurotransmitters L-dopa, norepinephrine, and epinephrine. Although phenylalanine is essential for human health, too much of this amino acid can be toxic and extremely dangerous. However, it can also be a hazard to your health to have low phenylalanine levels, which can result from excessive intake of caffeine.

◼ Functions of Phenylalanine

• Aids in thyroid hormone formation

• Improves alertness, ambition, and mood

• Regulates the release of cholecystokin (CCK), the hormone that signals the brain to feel satisfied after eating

■ Symptoms of Phenylalanine Deficiency

☐ Apathy

☐ Cataracts

☐ Confusion

☐ Depression

☐ Edema (swelling)

☐ Fat loss

☐ Increased eating

☐ Lethargy

☐ Liver damage

☐ Loss of pigmentation in hair

☐ Low levels of proteins

☐ Muscle loss

☐ Skin lesions

☐ Weakness

■ Symptoms of Phenylalanine Toxicity

☐ Agitation

☐ Headaches

☐ Increased blood pressure

☐ Insomnia

☐ Nerve damage

■ Recommended Dosage

500 to 3,000 milligrams daily

■ Side Effects and Contraindications

Phenylalanine should not be taken if you have the disease phenylketonuria (PKU) or are taking MAO inhibitors or tricyclic antidepressants. Phenylalanine should be used with caution if you have high blood pressure. It is best taken with food. Do not take tyrosine when taking phenylalanine.

Food Sources of Phenylalanine

- Almonds
- Avocado
- Bananas
- Beans
- Brewer's yeast
- Cheese
- Chocolate

- Corn
- Dairy products
- Eggs
- Fish
- Green peas
- Legumes
- Lentils

- Lima beans
- Meat
- Nuts
- Pickled herring
- Potatoes
- Pumpkin seeds

- Sesame seeds
- Soy
- Spinach
- Sweet potatoes
- Swiss chard
- Whey
- Whole grains

PROLINE

Proline, a nonessential amino acid that is used as a building block for protein, can be manufactured in your body from ornithine or glutamic acid. It is needed for the formation of collagen, a process that also requires vitamin C be present. Collagen is then used in the construction of arteries, ligaments, and tendons.

■ Functions of Proline in Your Body

- Component of collagen
- Improves skin texture
- Strengthens cartilage, connective tissue, joints, and tendons

■ Symptoms of Proline Deficiency

☐ Early signs of aging   ☐ Sagging skin   ☐ Stiff joints

■ Recommended Dosage

Have your doctor perform an amino acid analysis test. From your results, he will be able to recommend a daily dosage.

Food Sources of Proline

• Cottage cheese	• Eggs	• Ricotta cheese
• Dairy products	• Luncheon meats	• Turkey
• Duck	• Pork	• Wheat germ

SERINE

The nonessential amino acid serine is used by your body to make protein. It is made from glycine with folic acid and vitamin B_6. Serine is used in many bodily functions, including the metabolism of fats and fatty acids, the growth of muscle and tissue, and the maintenance of the immune system.

■ Functions of Serine in Your Body

- Aids in muscle growth
- Helps maintain a healthy immune system
- Helps manufacture the nerve cell sheath
- Needed for DNA synthesis
- Needed for the metabolism of fats and fatty acids
- Plays a part in the production of immunoglobulins and antibodies
- Stabilizes cell membranes
- Used in the formation of neurotransmitters

■ Serine Deficiency

Some people are born with a metabolic disorder that results in serine deficiency. Although this disease can be extremely serious, it is also very rare, and often goes undetected. There are many neurological symptoms of this disorder, including cerebral palsy, congenital microcephaly (an abnormally small and underdeveloped brain at birth), epilepsy, and seizures. However, serine deficiency is treatable.

■ Recommended Dosage

Have your doctor perform an amino acid analysis test. From your results, he will be able to recommend a daily dosage.

Food Sources of Serine

- Dairy products
- Eggs
- Pork
- Soy products
- Tuna fish
- Turkey

TAURINE

In adults, taurine is a conditionally essential amino acid made from methionine and cysteine. In children, it is an essential amino acid and must be ingested. It is necessary for normal brain development. Taurine requires zinc to function properly, and stress can deplete your body of taurine.

■ Functions of Taurine in Your Body

- Aids in glucose metabolism by increasing the activity of the insulin receptor
- Aids wound healing
- Boosts antioxidant defense
- Detoxifies toxic substances
- Helps modulate calcium movement
- Improves fat metabolism in the liver
- Improves lung health
- Improves sensitivity to insulin
- Is a natural diuretic
- Is an inhibitory neurotransmitter
- Lowers blood pressure
- Lowers LDL (bad) cholesterol
- Lowers triglyceride levels
- Needed for kidney function
- Needed for the formation of bile acids
- Prevents blood clots
- Protects cell membranes from damage
- Stabilizes heart rhythm
- Stabilizes membranes
- Strengthens the heart muscle
- Supports immune system

■ Symptoms of Taurine Deficiency

☐ Anxiety

☐ Hyperactivity

☐ Impaired brain function

☐ Seizures

■ Recommended Dosage

1 to 4 grams daily. Increase your taurine intake when you are stressed or ill.

■ Side Effects and Contraindications

Taurine should not be taken with aspirin or any salicylates.

■ Diseases/Disorders that Can Be Treated with Taurine

- Chemotherapy and radiation
- Congestive heart failure
- Diabetes
- Epilepsy
- Iron-deficiency anemia
- High blood pressure
- High LDL (bad) cholesterol
- Macular degeneration
- Muscle fatigue
- Psoriasis
- Tendency of blood to clot
- Wound healing

Food Sources of Taurine

- Brewer's yeast
- Dairy products
- Eggs
- Fish
- Meat
- Seafood

THREONINE

Threonine, an essential amino acid, is used as a building block to construct many of your body's proteins, as well as the important amino acids glycine and serine. It is also vital for proper functioning of the cardiovascular, central nervous, and immune systems.

■ Functions of Threonine in Your Body

- Helps metabolize fat
- Needed for proper digestion
- Needed for the formation of tooth enamel, collagen, and elastin
- Prevents the build-up of fat in the liver
- Stabilizes blood sugar

Food Sources of Threonine

- Beans
- Brewer's yeast
- Corn
- Cottage cheese
- Dairy products
- Eggs
- Fish
- Green peas
- Legumes
- Meat
- Nuts
- Potatoes
- Seafood
- Sesame seeds
- Soy products
- Spinach
- Watercress
- Whey
- Whole grains

■ Symptoms of Threonine Deficiency

☐ Depression
☐ Immunosuppression
☐ Indigestion

☐ Irritability
☐ Mental health deterioration
☐ Reduced growth

■ Recommended Dosage

Have your doctor perform an amino acid analysis test. From your results, he will be able to recommend a daily dosage.

TRYPTOPHAN

Tryptophan, an essential amino acid used to make protein, works best if taken with vitamin B_6 and carbohydrates. It is a precursor to serotonin, which may be why some people have found it effective as a sleep aid. Tryptophan is now available without a prescription.

■ Functions of Tryptophan in Your Body

- Acts as a mood stabilizer
- Boosts the release of growth hormone
- Breaks down into serotonin, a calming neurotransmitter
- Helps with insomnia
- Is an inhibitory neurotransmitter
- Needed for the production of vitamin B_3 (niacin)
- Suppresses appetite

■ Symptoms of Tryptophan Deficiency

☐ Decreased zinc levels

☐ Impaired growth

☐ Pellagra (a vitamin deficiency disease)

☐ Weight loss

■ Recommended Dosage

5 to 50 milligrams daily

■ Side Effects and Contraindications

If you are taking SSRIs or MAO inhibitors for depression, you should not take tryptophan supplements.

■ Diseases/Disorders that Can Be Treated with Tryptophan

• Depression

• Insomnia

• Obsessive compulsive disorder

• Parkinson's disease

• Schizophrenia

• Serotonin deficiency syndrome (which can contribute to anxiety, depression, insomnia, and migraines)

Food Sources of Tryptophan

• Beans	• Dairy products	• Grains	• Nuts
• Brown rice		• Lentils	• Pork
• Cereals	• Eggs	• Meats	• Seeds
• Chicken	• Fish	• Milk	• Turkey

TYROSINE

Tyrosine is a conditionally essential amino acid that is used by your body to make protein. In your body, it becomes the important neurotransmitters dopamine, epinephrine, L-dopa, and norepinephrine.

Food Sources of Tyrosine

- Almonds
- Avocados
- Bananas
- Beans
- Brewer's yeast
- Cheese
- Corn
- Cottage cheese
- Dairy products
- Eggs
- Fish
- Legumes
- Lima beans
- Meat
- Milk
- Nuts
- Pickled herring
- Potatoes
- Pumpkin seeds
- Seafood
- Seeds
- Soy
- Spinach
- Whey
- Whole grains

Functions of Tyrosine in Your Body

- Aids in making thyroxin, one of the thyroid hormones
- Helps form melanin, a skin pigment
- Helps you deal with stress
- Is an inhibitor neurotransmitter

Symptoms of Tyrosine Deficiency

- ☐ Aggression
- ☐ Anxiety
- ☐ Apathy
- ☐ Blood sugar imbalance
- ☐ Depression
- ☐ Edema (swelling)
- ☐ Fat loss
- ☐ Fatigue
- ☐ Lethargy
- ☐ Liver damage
- ☐ Loss of pigmentation in hair
- ☐ Low blood pressure
- ☐ Low serum levels of essential proteins
- ☐ Mood disorders
- ☐ Muscle loss
- ☐ Skin lesions
- ☐ Stress
- ☐ Weakness

Recommended Dosage

500 to 2,000 milligrams daily

Side Effects and Contraindications

Some people experience hypertension (high blood pressure), hypotension (low blood pressure), or migraine headaches when taking tyrosine supplementation. Do not take tyrosine if you are taking an MAO inhibitor medication.

5

Herbs

An herb is a plant grown for culinary or medicinal purposes. In this chapter, we will explore the healing powers of some common herbs, each of which can help you achieve optimal health in a different way. One decreases your cholesterol levels and risk of heart disease; one improves your memory and brain function; and one allows you to better cope with stress. Some herbs even contain *phytochemicals,* nutrients found in plants that may reduce the risk of cancer. This chapter will describe the most popular, healthful herbs and their healing potential.

Plants have been harvested for their medical properties for many thousands of years. More recently, some pharmaceutical companies began to isolate the most active ingredients in various herbs and sell them individually. Most people now agree, however, that the ingredients left behind when these extracts are taken are important. These other ingredients may have any of a number of purposes, such as curbing or augmenting the main ingredient's full effect. Some herbalists even believe that medicinal plants should only be used as they are found in nature.

Regardless of whether you choose pharmaceutical grade herbal supplements or naturally grown whole herbs, you must utilize them correctly and appropriately. Because herbs are natural, they are often considered safer than prescription drugs. Yet they can have serious, harmful effects—especially if taken without consideration for the proper guidelines and precautions, or if taken with certain medications. (See "Mixing Supplements, Drugs, and Food" on page 9.) Always read all directions before taking an herbal supplement. You should also consult your doctor before starting any supplement regimen—particularly if you have kidney or liver disease or are pregnant or nursing.

At the same time, unlike prescription drugs, the contents of supplements are not regulated by the US government. Always read the full ingredient list before ingesting any herb. Look specifically for the elements discussed starting on page 152 in the section "Buying Herbal Supplements."

BUYING HERBAL SUPPLEMENTS

Dietary supplements are not regulated by the Food and Drug Administration (FDA), so it is up to you (and your doctor) to be fully aware of what you are putting into your body. Familiarize yourself with the following tests, which will help you determine a product's quality and potential effectiveness. Every herbal supplement you take should pass each test. First check the side of the product's packaging for the applicable information. If the facts are not there or are unclear, you can call the company or visit its website. If the answers to your questions remain unavailable after checking these sources, I would avoid the products of that company. After all, most companies that properly examine their products will make the results easily available to their customers.

Authenticity

Only buy herbal supplements that have clearly labeled lists of ingredients and amounts. Unfortunately, these lists are not always reliable. Some companies use visual clues to label the herbs in their products, which can lead to mistakes because many herbs look alike. Dishonest companies may even knowingly turn a blind eye to this problem, due to the high cost of certain medicinal herbs. More reliable companies use tests, such a technique called thin layer chromatography (TLC), to scientifically identify the product's compounds and verify that the correct herb is being packaged.

Potency

A supplement's potency refers to its concentration of active ingredients. This detail is very important. After all, low potency usually means that the product will provide you with no results—and some herbal supplements are very expensive. There are tests the company can perform to determine a product's potency. One such test is the high-performance liquid chromatography (HPLC), which separates and identifies the product's molecules.

You can perform your own potency test. Drop an herbal supplement into a glass of water and watch what happens. The herbs should dissolve. An herb that doesn't dissolve will probably not be well absorbed by your body.

Purity

An herbal supplement is not pure if it contains any extraneous material or if its composition has been altered in any way. You can request that a company provide you with laboratory certificates ensuring that its product's purity has been tested.

Examining and tasting the product may allow you to determine its pureness. The following are some examples of qualities that would suggest your supplement is impure.

- If it has a gritty texture when chewed, it probably contains improper ingredients.

- If it is darker in color than usual or tastes particularly bitter, the herbs may have been burnt—which destroys the active materials and their effectiveness.

- If it tastes sweet or is sticky to the touch, a high percentage of the supplement may be made with sugar rather than the proper ingredients.

Safety

It is very important that the safety of a product has been thoroughly tested. Some companies do not perform these tests. Other companies perform these tests on a random sampling of their products. The companies from which you should buy herbal supplements have tested every batch of herbs they are putting on the market. When a product passes this inspection, the company is usually given a Certificate of Analysis (COA). You can request proof of this certificate before purchasing a company's products.

USING HERBS

There are a variety of different ways to utilize medicinal herbs. We will explore several examples here. I suggest experimenting with each of the following options before determining which you will use regularly.

Compresses

You can make a *compress* by soaking a clean cloth in an herbal solution. (For instructions on making herbal solutions, see "Decoctions and Infusions" on page 154.) Wring it out to remove the excess liquid. Then apply the cloth to your body. If you have a specific pain, apply the cloth to that area of your body, such as your head or back. The herbs will be absorbed into your skin and your blood vessels will transport them through your body.

Decoctions and Infusions

A *decoction* is an herbal solution. To make one, first break up pieces of bark, nuts, roots, or seeds of a plant. Simmer (cook just below boiling point) the pieces in water for fifteen to thirty minutes, keeping the pot or kettle covered. Then strain the plant pieces from the water.

An *infusion* is similar to a decoction but is made using the flowers, leaves, or stems of a plant. Also, the pieces are simmered in water for only ten minutes. (Again, keep the pot or kettle covered. Then strain the plant pieces from the water.)

These herbal solutions can be stored for up to two days in the refrigerator. They can be used to make compresses or drinks.

Extracts

Herbs are available as *extracts*—concentrated forms obtained by mixing herbs with a solvent such as alcohol and/or water. The potency of an herbal extract is expressed a ratio. For example, *tinctures,* which are made using a water and alcohol mixture as the solvent, are usually made at a 1:5 concentration. This means that there is five times the amount of alcohol and water than herbal material. A fluid extract is usually 1:1. A solid extract is usually at least four times stronger than the same amount of fluid extract and forty times as potent as a tincture if produced from herbs of the same quality.

Poultices

A *poultice* is a mixture of herbs applied to a cloth with oil or warm water. The cloth is then placed on your skin for relief from inflammation or soreness. You may want to reheat it when it cools off. Poultices are usually effective for twenty-four hours.

Tablets and Capsules

Herbs can be bought in tablet or capsule form. You can either take them with a glass of water or dissolve them in hot water before drinking. Many people consider tablets and capsules to be the most convenient way to take herbs.

Teas

You can make herbal tea by cooking herbs in boiling water for ten to fifteen minutes. Then, allow the herbs to steep in the water for five minutes. You can add honey for flavor but do not use milk. Although most herbs become less powerful when boiled, these teas are often helpful for daily invigoration and wellness. (For a more powerful herbal drink, see "Decoctions and Infusions" on page 154.)

Most people find it beneficial to drink one cup of herbal tea, three times a day. It can be drank hot or cold. To change the taste, experiment using more or less plant pieces.

ALOE VERA

Aloe vera is usually utilized for skin burns, infections, and wounds and applied as a topical ointment, gel, or spray. The gel-like center of the plant's leaves is extracted and used for this purpose. It can also be taken orally, although this has been studied less than its topical treatment. The liquid found in between the gel and outer leaf can be dried and ingested.

Functions of Aloe Vera

- Antibiotic and antiseptic properties (kills germs and bacteria)
- Encourages healing
- Improves ability to heal from wounds
- Reduces inflammation
- Relieves pain from certain skin conditions
- Strengthens immune system
- Works as a laxative

Recommended Dosage

- As a topical cream, Aloe vera can be applied liberally with no side effects.
- When taken orally, up to 150 milligrams of Aloe vera can usually be taken without causing any discomfort.

Side Effects and Contraindications

There are no noted side effects when using Aloe vera as a topical cream, but it should not be used on deep surgical wounds. When taken orally, Aloe vera can cause diarrhea and nausea. In addition, abusing Aloe vera (orally) can result in dangerous electrolyte imbalances such as low potassium levels. (See Chapter 2 for information on electrolyte imbalances.)

■ **Diseases/Disorders that Topical Aloe Vera Can Treat or Protect Against**

- Aphthous stomatitis
- Burns
- Dandruff
- Eczema
- Genital herpes
- Herpes simplex
- Psoriasis
- Skin infections
- Various wounds

■ **Diseases/Disorders that Oral Aloe Vera Can Treat or Protect Against**

- AIDS
- Asthma
- Constipation
- Diabetes
- Immune weakness
- Inflammation
- Inflammatory bowel disease
- Peptic ulcer disease

Herbs to Treat Inflammation

Herbs can help the body heal a variety of ailments. The herbs on the following list, for example, have anti-inflammatory properties. They can help decrease both inflammation and the associated pain. For suggestions on buying herbal supplements, as well as various ways to utilize them, see pages 152 to 155.

COX-2 is the enzyme that produces prostaglandins, a hormone that is responsible for inflammation and pain. Therefore, inhibition of COX-2 can greatly reduce these problems. However, most COX-2 inhibitor medications —such as Vioxx—can have extremely serious adverse effects, namely on blood pressure and the cardiovascular system. You will see that some of the following herbs are labeled natural COX-2 inhibitors. Like COX-2 inhibitor medications, these botanicals block the action of COX-2, but they have a decreased tendency to cause unwanted side effects. The other herbs on the list help inflammation in other ways, but can be just as effective.

- Aloe vera (*Aloe barbadensis*)
- Boswellia (*Boswellia serrata*)
- Bromelain (*Ananas comosus*). Natural COX-2 inhibitor.
- Capsaicin (cayenne; *Capsicum annuum*). Natural COX-2 inhibitor.

ASHWAGANDHA ROOT

Grown in India, Pakistan, and Sri Lanka, Ashwagandha root (*Withania somnifera*) is part of the nightshade family. It is known to improve resistance to emotional and physical stress.

■ Functions of Ashwagandha Root

- Activates your immune system
- Antibacterial
- Anti-inflammatory
- Antioxidant
- Enhances endurance and strength

- Carnosol/carnosic acid (rosemary; *Rosmarinus officinalis*). Natural COX-2 inhibitor.

- Carvacrol (oregano; *Oreganum vulgare*). Natural COX-2 inhibitor.

- Cayenne pepper (*Capsicum annuum*)

- Chinese skullcap (*Scutellaria baicalensis*). Natural COX-2 inhibitor.

- Curcumin (turmeric; *Curcuma longa*). Natural COX-2 inhibitor. Do not take with non-steroidal anti-inflammatory medications.

- Feverfew (*Tanacetum parthenium*). Natural COX-2 inhibitor.

- Ginger (*Zingiber officinale*). Natural COX-2 inhibitor. Do not take with coumadin or nonsteroidal anti-inflammatory pain medications (NSAIDs).

- Ginkgo (*Ginkgo biloba*). Do not take with blood thinners.

- Green tea (*Camellia sinensis*). Natural COX-2 inhibitor.

- Licorice root (*Glycyrrhiza glabra*). Do not take if you have high blood pressure.

- Quercetin. Natural COX-2 inhibitor.

- Thymol (thyme: *Thymus bulgaris*). Natural COX-2 inhibitor.

- Trans-resveratrol (purple grape). Natural COX-2 inhibitor.

- Willow bark (*Salix* species). Natural COX-2 inhibitor.

- Helps preserve adrenal size
- Helps you deal with stress
- Increases libido and sexual performance
- Increases muscle mass
- Lowers cholesterol
- Protects your liver

■ Recommended Dosage

- Capsule form: 500 to 2,000 milligrams daily
- Dried root prepared in tea: 3 to 4 grams daily

■ Side Effects and Contraindications

- Diarrhea
- Nausea
- Vomiting

■ Diseases/Disorders that Ashwagandha Root Can Treat or Protect Against

- Amnesia
- Back pain
- Constipation
- Depression
- Fever
- Inflammation
- Memory loss
- Mood swings
- Stress
- Swelling
- Weakness

BILBERRY

Bilberry (*Vaccinium myrtillus*) is a member of the same genus as the blueberry. One of its most important functions is enhancing eye health. The active component of bilberry is an *anthocyanin*—a plant pigment that provides color. This herb also contains tannins and vitamins A and C.

■ Functions of Bilberry

- Antibacterial
- Antiviral
- Helps your eyes adapt to the dark
- Improves circulation
- Improves failing eyesight

- Reduces the effects of diabetic retinopathy (damaged blood vessels in eyes as a result of long-term diabetes)
- Slows the progression of cataracts

■ Recommended Dosage

60 to 280 milligrams daily

■ Side Effects and Contraindications

Bilberry may interfere with iron absorption. If you are anemic, discuss bilberry supplementation with your doctor before starting a regimen.

■ Diseases/Disorders that Bilberry Can Treat or Protect Against

- Constipation
- Eye fatigue and strain
- Macular degeneration
- Poor circulation

BLACK COHOSH

Black cohosh grows in North America. It is known as a pain reliever and is particularly helpful for muscle soreness. Black cohosh is often recommended to women going through menopause. It is believed that black cohosh may lessen the duration and severity of certain menopausal symptoms, including hot flashes and night sweats. However, do not use black cohosh if you are taking antidepressants or are pregnant or if you have breast cancer.

■ Functions of Black Cohosh

- Lowers blood pressure
- Lowers LDL (bad) cholesterol
- May relieve mild depression
- Relieves muscle soreness
- Relieves some menopausal symptoms, such as hot flashes and vaginal dryness

■ Recommended Dosage

40 to 60 milligrams daily for no longer than six months

■ Side Effects and Contraindications

- Diarrhea
- Dizziness
- Headaches
- Impaired circulation
- Menopausal symptoms
- Nausea
- Vertigo
- Vomiting

■ Diseases/Disorders that Black Cohosh Can Treat or Protect Against

- Arthritis
- Cardiovascular disorder
- Fibrocystic breast disease
- Menopausal symptoms
- Muscle pain
- Premenstrual syndrome (PMS)
- Uterine fibroids

CAT'S CLAW

Cat's claw (*Uncaria tomentosai*) is a vine that grows in the Amazon Rainforest and other tropical areas of Central and South America. Its nickname is derived from its claw-like thorns. This woody vine can grow to over 100 feet. There are actually two different species of cat's claw. The second, *Uncaria guianensis,* is useful for treating osteoarthritis. In this section, we will explore *Uncaria tomentosa.*

■ Functions of Cat's Claw

- Boosts immune system
- Can cleanse/treat the gastrointestinal tract
- Can possibly inhibit growth of cancer cells
- Improves mental abilities
- Improves white blood cell function
- Inhibits autoimmune diseases (such as Crohn's and rheumatoid arthritis)
- Is an anti-inflammatory
- Is an antioxidant
- Relieves swelling of joints and muscle pain
- Reduces free radicals

■ Recommended Dosage

200 milligrams once a day

■ Side Effects and Contraindications

- Allergies that can cause kidney inflammation and rashes
- Altered heart rhythm
- Ataxia (loss of coordination)
- Diarrhea
- Hormonal change
- Nausea
- Stomach discomfort

■ Diseases/Disorders that Cat's Claw Can Treat or Protect Against

- AIDS
- Cancer
- Crohn's disease
- Diarrhea
- Inflammation
- Intestinal disorders
- Leaky bowel syndrome
- Ulcers

CAYENNE

Cayenne (*Capsicum annuum*) is popular as both a whole pepper and as a hot cooking spice. However, cayenne also has a number of healing abilities, including the potential to improve your entire circulatory and digestive systems. It also alters substance P—a compound that transfers pain messages to the brain—which can reduce pain and inflammation. It is very potent and, consequently, it is very important to wash your hands after using it, as well as to avoid contact between it and eyes, open wounds, or mucous membranes.

■ Functions of Cayenne

- Anti-inflammatory
- Antioxidant
- Diminishes awareness of pain
- Helps your body digest
- Improves blood flow and circulation
- Lowers LDL (bad) cholesterol
- Strengthens heart, kidneys, and lungs

■ Symptoms of Cayenne Toxicity

☐ Gastroenteritis   ☐ Kidney damage   ☐ Liver damage

■ Recommended Dosage

- As a capsule: 20 to 100 milligrams, three times a day.
- As a topical cream: Apply a thin coat three or four times a day for three weeks. Do not apply to broken skin.

■ Side Effects and Contraindications

- As a capsule: may cause nausea or vomiting if taken in too high a dose.
- As a topical cream: may cause burning or itching in some individuals. This usually subsides after several uses.

■ Diseases/Disorders that Cayenne Can Be Used to Treat or Protect Against

- Cluster headaches
- Cramps
- Heart disease
- Indigestion
- Inflammation
- Nerve pain
- Obesity
- Osteoarthritis
- Psoriasis
- Rheumatoid arthritis
- Shingles
- Sore throat

CHAMOMILE

Chamomile (*Matricaria recutita*) is one of the oldest and best-known medicinal herbs. It has been used for its calming and anti-inflammatory effects and as a pain reliever and sleep aid for ages. Yet it has many other healthful functions, including as a digestive aid and anti-inflammatory.

■ Functions of Chamomile

- Acts as a sleep aid/sedative
- Aids digestion
- Decreases inflammation
- Has calming effects
- Has anti-spasmodic effects

- Is a muscle relaxant
- Is an anti-inflammatory
- Relieves pain
- Relieves stress

■ Recommended Dosage

Chamomile is usually made into a tea and drank three to four times daily. It can also be applied as a topical cream, with the same frequency.

■ Side Effects and Contraindications

A sleep aid, chamomile may make users quite drowsy. Do not drink alcohol or other sedatives after ingesting chamomile. Also, chamomile may hinder blood from clotting and should not be taken with any other anticoagulants or by anyone who has difficult clotting blood.

■ Diseases/Disorders that Chamomile Can Treat or Protect Against

- Anxiety
- Colds
- Constipation
- Headache
- Indigestion
- Insomnia
- Irritable bowel syndrome (IBS)
- Menstrual cramps
- Sinusitis
- Stomach ache
- Stress

ECHINACEA

The North American plant Echinacea is mostly notable in its ability to improve your immune system and help you ward off colds and resist infections. There are three types of Echinacea that are commonly used for medicinal purposes: angustifolia, pallida, and purpurea.

■ Functions of Echinacea

- Boosts immune system
- Fights colds and flu
- Helps heal damaged skin
- Is an anti-inflammatory
- Protects skin from the sun

■ Recommended Dosage

- When taken for general well being, take 250 to 500 milligrams orally every day for no longer than eight weeks in a row.

- When taken to fight a cold for which the symptoms have already begun, take 1 to 2 grams orally every day. Start as soon as possible after noticing the symptoms. Continue treatment for three weeks before halting Echinacea consumption for one week.

- When taken to heal a burn or wound, apply topically to injured area daily. If improvement is not seen after one week, discontinue treatment.

■ Side Effects and Contraindications

Some people experience dizziness or nausea when taking echinacea. Do not use this herb if you are allergic to sunflowers, daisies, marigolds, chrysanthemums, or dandelions. Do not use echinacea if you have an autoimmune disease (such as lupus, multiple sclerosis, or rheumatoid arthritis) or tuberculosis.

■ Diseases/Disorders that Echinacea Can Treat or Protect Against

- Allergies
- Bronchial asthma
- Burns
- Cancer
- Candidiasis
- Colic
- Common colds
- Compromised immune system
- Eczema
- Flu
- Herpes
- Infections
- Sore throat
- Upper respiratory infections
- Urinary tract infections
- Wounds

ELEUTHERO

Eleuthero (*Eleutherococcus senticosus*) is an herb that is commonly used to increase energy. For many years, it was called Siberian ginseng. That name is now illegal in the United States because it implies that the herb is part of the Panax genus (like the American and Asian ginseng), while it actually belongs to the genus Eleutherococcus. Regardless of the controversy over its name, this herb is used to treat a variety of ailments.

■ Functions of Eleuthero

- Acts as a stimulant
- Acts as an adaptogen (strengthens the body's resistance to stress)
- Aids the immune system (increases T-cell and natural killer cell activity)
- Can be used be athletes during training
- Decreases inflammation
- Helps you deal with stress
- Improves endurance
- Improves learning ability
- Increases mental awareness
- Increases physical performance and stamina
- Increases tolerance to excess heat, noise, and workload
- Is an antioxidant
- Promotes healing

■ Recommended Dosage

500 to 1,000 milligrams daily

■ Side Effects and Contraindications

Some people experience headaches or agitation when taking eleuthero supplementation. If one of these side effects occur, consult your doctor regarding continued use. Do not take eleuthero if you have a history of heart disease.

■ Diseases/Disorders that Eleuthero Can Treat or Protect Against

- Anxiety
- Common cold
- Exhaustion
- Kidney disease
- Inflammation
- Insomnia
- Joint pain
- Liver disease
- Low energy
- Premenstrual syndrome (PMS)
- Stress

Ephedra:
A Potentially Dangerous Herb

Many of the herbs in this chapter can have serious side effects, but most of these can be avoided if you prudently adhere to the medical advice offered by your doctor and pharmaceutical company. Unfortunately, there are other herbs that can have more common and more serious consequences. Some are even banned in the United States by the Food and Drug Administration (FDA). One such herb is ephedra. At the height of its popularity, ephedra—and one of its main active ingredients, ephedrine—was responsible for over half the herb-related deaths in the country.

Although originally used for a variety of purposes, ephedra was mainly being sold as a stimulant and appetite suppressant in the mid-1990s. Many body builders and dieters utilized the herbal supplement, which stimulates the metabolism; burns stored fat; and creates a speedy, energetic feeling in the user. It was advertised as a natural supplement, which led many people to conclude that the pills were safe.

A short time later, a growing number of ephedra-related deaths began to surface in the news. The fatalities were largely linked to the dangerous effects ephedra can have on the heart, which include heart attacks, strokes, and cardiac arrest. Some ephedra-taking athletes, provided with extra energy that allowed them to practice far beyond what was healthy, died of heatstroke. Many other users experienced a number of less serious side effects, including increased anxiety, insomnia, irritability, and nausea.

Interestingly, studies have shown that ephedra, when properly used, is actually fairly safe. The Chinese have been using the herb for thousands of years. However, the supplement has very high potential for addiction and overuse. It was also found to be ineffective at promoting long-term weight loss!

The FDA first became concerned with ephedra in 1997, but it was the high-profile death of Baltimore Orioles pitcher Steve Bechler in 2003 that set the wheels in motion to ban the product. As of April 2004, the sale of ephedra in the United States is illegal. There have also been lawsuits filed against certain companies that sold ephedra, claiming that unsubstantiated statements were made in the marketing of these diet pills. Several of these lawsuits have already been settled—in favor of the plaintiffs.

EVENING PRIMROSE OIL

The evening primrose (*Oenthera biennis*) is an interesting plant. Its flowers live for only one day. Throughout the summer, this North American plant has flowers that bloom every morning, and die every night. In addition, extracted from its seeds is oil that has some important health benefits, including being an excellent source of certain essential fatty acids (which were discussed in Chapter 3).

■ Functions of Primrose

- Acts as an anti-inflammatory
- An excellent source of the omega-6 fatty acid gamma linolenic acid (GLA). (See page 112 to read about GLA.)
- Can help you lose weight
- Can restrain thrombosis (unhealthy blood clots that can lead to heart attack or stroke) from forming
- Lowers blood pressure levels

■ Recommended Dosage

Most people need approximately 3,500 milligrams of primrose oil daily, but the exact dosage depends on the reason for which you are taking it. Consult your doctor for his or her recommendation.

■ Side Effects and Contraindications

- Bloating
- Diarrhea
- Headaches
- Indigestion
- Nausea
- Vomiting

■ Diseases/Disorders that Primrose Can Treat or Protect Against

- Allergies
- Arthritis
- Asthma
- Chronic headaches
- Diabetes
- Eczema
- High blood pressure
- Hypertension
- Menopausal symptoms
- Multiple sclerosis
- Premenstrual syndrome (PMS)
- Psoriasis

GARLIC

For thousands of years, garlic (*Allium sativum*) has been known to have a variety of medicinal benefits. It contains amino acids, vitamins, trace minerals, flavonoids, enzymes, and 200 additional compounds. Garlic's main active ingredient is allicin, an antibacterial compound that is produced when the garlic is crushed or chopped. Because allicin is most effective immediately after its production, garlic should be eaten soon after it is prepared.

▪ Functions of Garlic

- Balances blood sugar
- Boosts natural killer cell activity (which helps prevent cancer)
- Boosts your immune system
- Decreases LDL (bad) cholesterol
- Increases nitric oxide
- Lowers blood pressure
- Lowers triglycerides
- May lower risk of prostate cancer
- Natural blood thinner
- Raises HDL (good) cholesterol

▪ Recommended Dosage

Garlic products are described in terms of fresh or whole garlic equivalent. An average daily dose is 1,500 to 1,800 milligrams of fresh garlic equivalent, which equals approximately one half a clove of fresh garlic.

▪ Side Effects and Contraindications

Garlic is a blood thinner. If you are taking a blood thinner, therefore, check with your physician before ingesting large amounts of garlic. Do not take large doses of garlic if you are pregnant because they may cause uterine contractions.

■ Diseases/Disorders that Garlic Can Treat or Protect Against

- Atherosclerosis
- Cancer (colon, esophageal, and stomach)
- Heart disease
- High blood pressure
- High cholesterol levels

GINKGO

Ginkgo (*Ginkgo biloba*) is an herbal extract that comes from the leaves of the ginkgo tree. This tree, also called the maidenhair tree, grows in China. Ginkgo is said to improve circulation and cognitive abilities.

■ Functions of Ginkgo

- Decreases blood clotting (antagonist of platelet-aggregating factor)
- Decreases inflammation
- Enhances learning and memorization
- Helps prevent memory loss and improve brain function
- Improves circulation
- Improves mood
- Increases acetylcholine synthesis
- Increases oxygen to the brain by increasing blood supply (by dilating vessels)
- Increases serotonin receptors
- Increases uptake of glucose
- Is an antioxidant and prevents membrane damage

■ Recommended Dosage

60 to 120 milligrams daily

■ Side Effects and Contraindications

People who experience headaches, nausea, vomiting, or dizziness when taking ginkgo should stop taking it. Also, you should not take ginkgo if you are on blood thinners, pregnant, or taking an MAOI inhibitor. If you are taking cyclosporine, papverine, thiazide diuretics, or trazodone, consult your doctor before taking ginkgo.

◼ Diseases/Disorders that Ginkgo Can Treat or Protect Against

- Alzheimer's disease
- Asthma
- Depression
- Diabetic retinopathy (damaged blood vessels in eyes as a result of long-term diabetes)
- Glaucoma
- Headaches
- Heart disease
- Impotence
- Macular degeneration
- Memory loss
- Peripheral vascular disease, claudication, or decreased circulation, all of which can result in leg pains
- Raynaud's disease (restricted blood flow to extremities)
- Tinnitus (ringing in ears)

GINSENG

Ginseng (*Panax*) is a family of herbs that are believed to have strong medicinal benefits. These herbs are often found in energy drinks and other health products, but usually not in effective dosages. Supplements, on the other hand, offer ginseng's full benefits. There are two popular types of ginseng: American and Asian. Ancient Chinese and Korean medicine believed that Asian ginseng contributed to the body's yang energy and that American ginseng contributed to the body's yin energy. However, the two forms have many similar medicinal effects.

AMERICAN GINSENG

American ginseng (*Panax quinquefolium*) can enhance your immune system while also improving your memory and mental capabilities. It is also speculated that American ginseng may be effective in treating breast cancer when prescribed in tandem with chemotherapy.

◼ Functions of American Ginseng

- Helps control menopausal symptoms
- Helps you deal with stress

- Increases energy
- Is an adaptogen (strengthens the body's resistance to stress)
- Is an antioxidant
- Lowers blood sugar levels
- Lowers insulin levels
- May improve memory
- Strengthens the immune system

Recommended Dosage

125 to 500 milligrams daily for one month, followed by two weeks abstinence. If you are taking American ginseng to lower your blood sugar, consume thirty to forty minutes before meals.

Side Effects and Contraindications

Although American ginseng can be very useful for people with diabetes
because it can lower blood sugar levels, this process should be monitored by a doctor. Ginseng should always be taken with food so that it
doesn't lower your blood sugar level too dramatically. Do not take ginseng with blood thinners because it can stop your blood from clotting
appropriately. If you are taking haloperidol, morphine, or an MAO
inhibitor, see your doctor before taking ginseng. It can also cause the following side effects.

- Anxiety
- Headaches
- Insomnia
- Restlessness

ASIAN GINSENG

Asian ginseng (*Panax ginseng*), also called Chinese ginseng and Korean
ginseng, is available in two forms: red and white. They are prepared differently. White ginseng is dried, while red ginseng is steamed. Although
both are common and available, the red form is preferred for medicinal
purposes because the active ingredients are broken down when white ginseng is dried out. (Although red ginseng is dried, too, the steaming
process done first prevents this breakdown.)

■ Functions of Asian Ginseng

- Decreases bloating and fullness
- Decreases depression
- Enhances heart function
- Helps increase physical endurance
- Helps relieve insomnia and restlessness
- Helps relieve stress and anxiety
- Helps with forgetfulness
- Helps with glucose metabolism
- Improves mood
- Increases energy
- Increases mental abilities
- Is an adaptogen (strengthens the body's resistance to stress)
- Relieves lethargy and fatigue
- Stimulates immune function
- Supports adrenal glands

■ Recommended Dosage

125 to 500 milligrams daily for one month, followed by two weeks abstinence

■ Side Effects and Contraindications

Do not take ginseng with blood thinners because it can stop your blood from clotting appropriately. If you are taking haloperidol, morphine, or an MAO inhibitor, see your doctor before taking ginseng. It can also cause the following side effects.

- Anxiety
- Headaches
- Insomnia
- Restlessness

GOLDENSEAL

Goldenseal (*Hydrastis canadensis*), one of today's most popular herbs, has many different medicinal uses. These uses are derived from its many constituents, including the alkaloids berberine and hydrastine. It is important to note, however, that prolonged use of goldenseal can decrease your body's absorption of the B vitamins. Therefore, do not take goldenseal daily for more than two weeks.

Functions of Goldenseal

- Boosts immune system
- Can treat sore or inflamed gums
- Cleans and treats mucous membranes
- Eliminates toxins from your body
- Fights fungi, infection, and yeast
- Flushes and cleans your systems
- Has antibacterial properties
- Helps digestion
- Is an antibiotic
- Is an anti-inflammatory
- Kills pathogens in your body
- Promotes functioning capacities of many major organs
- Relieves congestion
- Stimulates antibodies

Recommended Dosage

Goldenseal can be taken orally—usually as either a capsule, tea, or liquid extract—or used as a topical cream. You should take or use 250 to 500 milligrams, two or three times a day. Do not use for longer than two weeks. Then, allow a break of at least two weeks.

Side Effects and Contraindications

Do not take goldenseal if you are pregnant or nursing or have heart disease, diabetes, or high blood pressure. Side effects of goldenseal are uncommon. However, prolonged use can decrease your body's absorption of the B vitamins, as well as the effectiveness of doxycycline and other tetracycline antibiotics. Also, large doses of goldenseal *can* be toxic. If you experience any of the following side effects, stop all consumption and use of goldenseal.

- Anxiety
- Diarrhea
- Hypertension
- Nausea
- Respiratory failure
- Seizures

■ Diseases/Disorders that Goldenseal Can Treat or Protect Against

- Alcohol-related liver disease
- Allergies
- Arthritis
- Atherosclerosis
- Bladder infection
- Canker sores
- Cardiac arrhythmias
- Colds
- Constipation
- Diarrhea
- Eczema
- Indigestion
- Inflammation
- Psoriasis
- Sore throat
- Sores
- Stomach problems
- Vaginitis
- Wounds
- Yeast infections

GREEN TEA

Although green tea has been popular in Eastern countries such as China, India, and Japan for much of recorded history, it has also become increasingly popular in the Western world. Recognized for its varied medicinal benefits, green tea is particularly praised for its high content of antioxidants. It is from the *Camellia sinensis* plant, as are black tea and oolong tea, but is steamed rather than fermented. This allows it to retain its healthful qualities, unlike the other two teas. Green tea can be taken as a capsule or drank as a tea.

■ Functions of Green Tea

- Has a high content of antioxidants
- Improves alertness
- Improves heart health
- Inhibits growth of cancerous cells
- Kills unhealthy bacteria in both body and mouth

- Lowers LDL (bad) cholesterol
- May encourage weight loss
- Regulates blood sugar level
- Restricts growth of unhealthy blood clots

■ Side Effects and Contraindications

Green tea contains caffeine, so some drinkers experience insomnia or restlessness. However, the amount of caffeine contained in a glass of tea is minimal compared that in to coffee or soda. The only other problems recorded are from drinkers who had allergic reactions. The most common effects experienced were anxiety; constipation or diarrhea; headache; loss of appetite; and nausea.

■ Diseases/Disorders that Green Tea Can Treat or Protect Against

- Allergies
- Arteriosclerosis
- Arthritis
- Asthma
- Atherosclerosis
- Cancer (prevention and treatment of cancers including bladder, breast, colon, liver, lung, pancreas, prostate, skin, small intestine, and stomach)
- Cardiovascular disease
- Diabetes
- Diarrhea
- High cholesterol levels
- Infection
- Irritable bowel syndrome (IBS)
- Obesity

HAWTHORN

Hawthorn (*Crataegus laevigata*) has been found to be very helpful in the treatment of cardiovascular illnesses, such as arrhythmias, congestive heart failure, and heart pain. It is also believed to be an antioxidant.

■ Functions of Hawthorn

- Dilates blood vessels and improves blood flow
- Is an antioxidant

- Keeps heart rhythm regular
- Lowers cholesterol levels
- Normalizes blood pressure
- Prevents heart from racing
- Stabilizes collagen

■ Side Effects and Contraindications

- Dizziness
- Fatigue
- Nausea

■ Diseases/Disorders that Hawthorn Can Treat or Protect Against

- Anemia
- Arthritis
- Congestive heart failure
- Coronary heart disease
- High blood pressure
- Irregular heart beat

MILK THISTLE

Silybum marianum is extracted from the seeds of the milk thistle plant and has many important health benefits. Most notably, this milk thistle extract has been used to treat kidney and liver disease. I recommend taking milk thistle capsules because this herb does not dissolve well in water and is usually ineffective in the form of tea. You can also take silymarin, an antioxidant bioflavonoid extract found in milk thistle that has also been shown to promote liver health.

■ Functions of Milk Thistle

- Decreases blood sugar
- Decreases the oxidation of LDL (bad) cholesterol
- Diminishes oxidation
- Helps prevent damage due to excessive alcohol ingestion
- Helps protect kidneys from the effects of cisplatin
- Increases growth of new tissue to repair damaged areas
- Increases HDL (good) cholesterol
- Increases production of glutathione

- Is an antioxidant
- Lowers LDL (bad) cholesterol
- Maintains bile flow
- Protects against iron damage in the liver
- Protects your liver from damage due to toxins
- Reduces inflammation

■ Recommended Dosage

Capsules are usually more effective than tea because milk thistle does not dissolve well in water.

- If you have diabetes, take 250 milligrams of milk thistle, split into two doses, daily.
- If you have liver disease, take 400 milligrams of milk thistle, split into two doses, daily.
- If you want to increase your glutathione levels, take 150 to 300 milligrams of milk thistle, split into two doses, daily.

■ Side Effects and Contraindications

- Diarrhea
- Nausea
- Reduced effectiveness of birth control pills
- Stomach pain

■ Diseases/Disorders that Milk Thistle Can Treat or Protect Against

- Cirrhosis
- Constipation
- Diarrhea
- Gall bladder disease
- Hepatitis
- Inflammation
- Kidney disease
- Liver disease
- Prostate disease

ST. JOHN'S WORT

Although it is not know exactly *how* St. John's wort works, it has achieved a fair amount of attention for its ability to treat mild cases of depression. However, it is important to realize that cases of moderate or severe depression should always be treated with the help of a doctor, who will recommend the best medicinal route.

■ Functions of St. John's Wort

- Contains hypericin, which increases the body's level of dopamine (a neurotransmitter involved with feelings of pleasure)
- Contains hyperforin, which increases the body's dopamine, gamma-aminobutyric acid (GABA), glutamate, noradrenaline, and serotonin levels. (It is thought that the increase of these neurotransmitters is the main reason that St. John's wort relieves mild depression.)
- Has antibacterial properties
- Is an anti-inflammatory
- May inhibit vital infections

■ Recommended Dosage

To treat mild depression, take 900 to 1,200 milligrams, split into two or three doses, of St. John's wort daily. It is usually consumed in capsule form, and takes an average of two to six weeks of daily consumption to begin working effectively. It is available as a topical cream for burns and sores.

■ Side Effects and Contraindications

- Anxiety
- Dry mouth
- Dizziness
- Headache
- Mild palpitations

- May reduce effectiveness of medications such as anticoagulants, antidepressants, and oral contraceptives
- Sexual dysfunction
- Stomach ache

■ Diseases/Disorders that St. John's Wort Can Treat or Protect Against

- Alcoholism (may reduce cravings by treating depression)
- Anxiety
- Burns
- Herpes
- HIV and AIDS. However, it also counteracts certain medications

prescribed for this virus. Consult your doctor before ingesting.

- Inflammation
- Mild depression
- Nerve pain
- Premenstrual syndrome (PMS)
- Wounds

SAW PALMETTO

Saw palmetto (*Serenoa repens*) is an herb grown in Florida that has nutritious properties and can help strengthen your immune system. It may effectively fight certain cancers, but more testing is needed before this information can be considered valid. Saw palmetto is primarily beneficial because it can help men maintain a healthy prostate. However, ask your doctor before taking this herb if you have any sex hormone-related disease or disorder or are taking birth control.

■ Functions of Saw Palmetto

- Can be used to lower high testosterone levels in women
- May be effective in treating male pattern baldness
- Strengthens immune system
- Treats enlarged prostate gland
- Works as an anti-inflammatory

■ Recommended Dosage

Some people need to take saw palmetto for up to thirty dates before any effects are seen.

- If you have an enlarged prostate, take 160 milligrams of saw palmetto, twice daily.
- If you are a woman and want to decrease your testosterone, take 250 milligrams of saw palmetto, twice daily.

■ Side Effects and Contraindications

- Altered hormonal activity
- Cramping
- Decreased sexual drive
- Diarrhea
- Headache
- Nausea

■ Diseases/Disorders that Saw Palmetto Can Treat or Protect Against

- Hair loss
- Hormone imbalance
- Symptoms of an enlarged prostate gland

VINPOCETINE

Vinpocetine is from the periwinkle plant. It is very important to your overall health because of its ability to increase the flow of glucose to your brain, as well as increase your brain's metabolism of oxygen. This results in improved memory and brain function.

■ Functions of Vinpocetine

- Decreases the deformity of red blood cells
- Helps with hair loss
- Improves your brain's utilization of oxygen
- Increases memory by increasing blood flow, increasing the rate at which your brain cells create energy, and speeding up your brain's use of glucose (its main fuel source)
- Increases serotonin (a neurotransmitter that effects behavior and emotions)
- Inhibits platelet aggregation (which causes blood to be less sticky and therefore decreases unhealthy clotting)

■ Recommended Dosage

10 to 40 milligrams daily

■ Side Effects and Contraindications

- Chest pains
- Dizziness
- Dry mouth
- Headaches
- Nausea
- Skin problems such as hives, itchiness, or rashes
- Tightness in chest

■ Diseases/Disorders that Vinpocetine Can Treat or Protect Against

- Depression
- Headache
- Macular degeneration
- Memory loss
- Meniere's Syndrome
- Migraine headaches
- Mood changes
- Seizure disorder
- Sensorineural hearing loss (damage to inner ear nerves)
- Sleep disorders
- Stroke
- Tinnitus (ringing in ears)
- Vertigo

OTHER MEDICINAL HERBS

There are many, many herbs with various medicinal properties. Some useful and popular examples that were not covered elsewhere in this chapter are discussed here.

■ Astragalus

Astragalus (*Astragalus membranaceus*) is a plant that belongs to the pea family. It contains an isoflavone (4'-hydroxy-3'-methoxyisoflavone) that can enhance metabolism and digestion, as well as treat related problems. Astragalus also contains triterpenoid saponins, substances that are believed to lower cholesterol levels and have antioxidant effects. Furthermore, Astragalus contains polysaccharides that strengthen the immune system. Astragalus is usually used to treat peripheral vascular disease (a condition that limits blood flow to the limbs) and hypertension.

■ Bacopa

Bacopa (*Bacopa monnieri*) has been used for many years in Ayurvedic medicine (traditional Indian medicine) to revitalize nerves, brain cells, and the mind. Bacopa helps to strengthen the adrenal glands and purify the blood. Studies have shown that it may have beneficial effects on anxiety and mental fatigue.

■ Baikal Skullcap

Also known as Chinese skullcap, Baikal skullcap (*Scutellaria baicalensis*) is a member of the mint family. It has been used in China for many years to treat a number of health problems, including high blood pressure, hepatitis, constipation, and various viruses. It is, however, particularly well known for treating conditions associated with inflammation. Its anti-inflammatory qualities are from the isoflavones it contains—baicalein, baicalin, and wogonin.

■ Beta-Sitosterol

Beta-sitosterol is a plant extract. Studies reveal that it improves urinary symptoms related to prostate enlargement. Beta-sitosterol can be used alone or in conjunction with medications such as alpha-adrenergics blockers and 5-alpha reductase inhibitors, which are commonly prescribed as treatment for an enlarged prostate. (See also Benign Prostatic Hypertrophy in Part 2.) It has also been shown that beta-sitosterol can have a positive impact on hair loss. (See also Hair Loss in Part 2.) Some scientists believe that beta-sitosterol may inhibit the growth of prostate and breast cancer cells. As of this time, more research is needed to confirm this theory.

■ Boswellia

Boswellia (*Boswellia serrata*) has been used to treat inflammatory conditions for many centuries. Its main active components are called boswellic acids, which are strong inhibitors of the inflammatory mechanisms 5-LOX and TNF-alpha. In addition, boswellia decreases the activity of human leukocyte elastase (HLE), an inflammatory enzyme associated with rheumatoid arthritis, pulmonary emphysema, cystic fibrosis, chronic bronchitis, and acute respiratory distress syndrome. Clinical trials with Boswella have resulted in markedly improved comfort for sufferers of arthritis, chronic colitis, and asthma.

■ Curcumin

Curcumin is a phytonutrient derived from the spice turmeric. Turmeric, the main element of curry, is a member of the ginger family. Curcumin has many medicinal benefits. It has a long history of relieving inflammation by inhibiting certain enzymes and other substances within the inflammatory pathway. It can lower LDL (bad) cholesterol and total cholesterol. Curcumin may also prove to have an anti-cancer effect. Furthermore, clinical trials have shown that curcumin may help maintain cognition and treat inflammatory bowel diseases. It has also been shown to reduce both duodenal and gastric ulcers.

■ Dandelion

Dandelion (*Taraxacum officinale*) has been used to increase the flow of bile and aid in the digestion of fats. It has also been used therapeutically to restore appetite, calm the stomach, and as a diuretic. If you have gallstones or obstructed bile ducts, do not take dandelion without first consulting your healthcare practitioner.

■ Fenugreek

Fenugreek (*Trigonella foenum-graecum*) is an herb that can lower blood sugar levels. This effect is due to its soluble fiber and fatty acids components. A recent study was completed on the effect of fenugreek on diabetics with heart disease. It was found that this herb not only lowered blood sugar levels but also lowered both total cholesterol and triglyceride levels.

■ Feverfew

Feverfew (*Tanacetum parthenium*) is an herb used to treat migraine headaches. It inhibits the production of prostaglandins. This reduces inflammation, decreases histamine release, and reduces fever. This herb needs to be taken for at least a month to effectively prevent migraine headaches. If you are allergic to plants in the daisy family (such as chamomile or ragweed), do not take feverfew. It also has the potential to interact with anticoagulant drugs such as coumadin.

■ Gotu Kola

Gotu kola (*Centella asiatica*) is an ancient medicinal herb. There are varieties found in several different countries, but the strongest type, Centella, is found only in Madagascar. Centella affects the development of connective tissue by enhancing and strengthening its structural components. It also aids in wound healing by increasing keratinization—the process by which skin grows back after damage by sores or ulcers. Similary, Centella also strengthens veins by repairing the surrounding connective tissue, decreasing the fragility of the capillaries, and effectively treating cellulite.

■ Gugulipid

Gugulipid (*Commniphora mukul*) is from guggul resin, which is derived from the mukul myrrh tree native to Arabia and India. It is used to lower both cholesterol and triglyceride levels. Gugulipid has also been shown to effectively treat rheumatoid arthritis. This herb may exacerbate pre-existing stomach conditions. Consult your doctor before combining gugulipid with any medication.

■ Gurmari

Gurmari (*Gymnema sylvestre*) is an Indian plant from which extracts have been shown to enhance the action of insulin. The dosage of this extract (standardized to contain 24-percent gymnemic acid) is 200 milligrams taken twice a day. If you are on medication to lower your blood sugar, be careful to monitor your blood sugar levels when you take gurmari. You may need to take less than the recommended dosage of your medication.

■ Jujube

Jujube (*Zizyphus jujuba*) is a fruit that grows on trees in China. In Chinese medicine, it is the most commonly used herb to treat insomnia because it both induces sleep and improves sleep quality. Jujube can also boost the immune system. It has a muscle-relaxing effect and has been used to treat abnormal heart rhythms and convulsions.

■ Licorice

Licorice (*Glycyrrhiza glabra* or *Glycyrrhiza uralensis*) is a plant extract that has been used to treat coughs, colds, congestion, rashes, arthritis, consti-pation, cancer, and hepatitis, and helps heal stomach and mouth ulcers. It may even be able to kill *nitrosamines*—carcinogens found in food.

There are two types of licorice available. Deglycyrrhizinated licorice (DGL) is used to treat stomach ailments. Glycyrrhizia-containing licorice is used to treat adrenal problems. You should take 200 milligrams. Consult your healthcare practitioner before taking if you have hypertension, glau-coma, diabetes, kidney or liver disease, or heart disease. You should also consult your healthcare practioner if you are on the medication digitalis.

■ Modern Sage

Modern sage (*Salvia officinalis*), a member of the mint family, is often used to treat inflammation. It has been shown to be effective for digestive com-plaints, flatulence, inflammation of the intestines, diarrhea, and problems related to menopause. It is also an antibacterial, antifungal, and astrin-gent. Modern sage can become toxic if used for long periods of time.

■ Olive Leaf Extract

Olive leaf extract (*Olea europa*) contains the plant chemical oleuropein, which effectively fights viral and bacterial infections. Oleuropein also lowers blood pressure, dilates the arteries of the heart, and inhibits the oxidation of LDL (bad) cholesterol. Olive leaf extract can be hard on the stomach, so always take it with food.

◼ Passion Flower

Passion flower (*Passiflora incarnata*) is a vine native to North and South America that contains glycosides and flavonoids. It helps to calm, shift mood, and aid in concentration. It also contains a flavonoid (chrysin) that has anti-anxiety properties. In addition, passion flower can be used to treat insomnia and does not produce confusion upon awakening. High dosages of passion flower should be avoided since it can cause irregular heartbeat in some people. You should also not take it if you are taking a MAO inhibitor for depression.

◼ Perilla Seed Extract

Perilla (*Perilla frutescens*) is a unique herb that reduces allergic reactions by supporting a healthy immune response in individuals who may be sensitive to particular foods or environmental factors. Dried perilla seed and leaf extracts are also used in Chinese medicine to alleviate chest fullness, support healthy mucus secretion, and promote healthy breathing. Studies have also shown that perilla seed extract has both an anti-inflammatory function and antioxidant potential.

The recommended dosage of perilla is approximately 100 to 150 milligrams per day. It may interact with aspirin, nonsteroidal anti-inflammatory drugs (NSAIDs), ginkgo, garlic, and possibly other herbs. Discontinue use ten days before surgery.

◼ Rhodiola

Rhodiola (*Rhodiola rosea*) is an herb used to increase immunity and decrease inflammation. It affects the activities and levels of the important neurotransmitters serotonin and norepinephrine, and can therefore be used to treat fatigue, stress, sleep disturbances, poor appetite, decline in work performance, irritability, hypertension, and headaches.

◼ Theanine

Theanine is an amino acid derived from herbal green tea. Studies show that theanine decreases anxiety, helps promote relaxation, supports brain health by improving focus and attention, and boosts cognition. In animal studies, theanine increases serotonin levels, which could be responsible for these effects. It also promotes the activity of an enzyme that breaks down beta-amyloid proteins—which are linked to the development of

Alzheimer's disease. Theanine may also lower blood pressure and help with the tendency to gain abdominal fat. Recommended dosage is 100 to 400 milligrams a day.

■ Valerian

Valerian (*Valeriana officinalis*) is an herb valued for its calming and sedative effects. It has been shown to reduce the time it takes to fall asleep and decrease the number of nighttime awakenings. Likewise, valerian has been shown to improve sleep quality and mood, calm fear and restlessness, and even curb aggression.

Valerian has been used to alleviate pain from rheumatoid arthritis, neuralgia, migraines, and intestinal cramping, as well as to settle nervous stomachs and heal ulcers. It has even been found to slow the rate of the heart while increasing the strength of the beats. Also efficient as a smooth muscle relaxer, valerian has been used to treat premenstrual syndrome and menstrual cramps.

Be aware that valerian can cause sedation. It may be contraindicated if you are taking other sedatives, antihistamines, antidepressants, or anti-anxiety agents. Although the plant itself has a sweet (sometimes overpowering) smell, the dried root smells akin to dirty gym socks.

6

Other Nutrients

This chapter will look at certain nutrients that have not yet been discussed. Although they may not fit into the categories of the previous chapters, these nutrients are all important to your nutritional health and overall well being. Please consult your physician before taking any supplement if you have kidney or liver disease, are pregnant, or are nursing.

ALPHA-GLYCERYL PHOSPHORYL CHOLINE

Alpha-glyceryl phosphoryl choline (Alpha-GPC or GPC) is a derivative of soy lecithin (a phospholipid found in certain plant and animal foods that acts as an antioxidant). It is a direct precursor to choline, which is critical to your health because it makes *acetylcholine,* an important neurotransmitter involved with communication in your brain. GPC is preferable to choline or lecithin supplements because it allows a greater amount of choline to be absorbed by your intestines.

■ Functions of Acetylcholine-Sensitive Neurons

- Allow REM sleep
- Control arousal
- Improve learning and memory
- May increase growth hormone release
- Responsible for motor activity

■ Recommended Dosage

- For healthy young people: 300 milligrams daily.
- To treat memory loss: 1,200 milligrams daily for one month. Then reduce dosage to 600 milligrams daily.

■ GPC Supplementation

In the United States, GPC is available as a dietary supplement. In Europe, however, it is only available by prescription.

ALPHA-LIPOIC ACID

Alpha-lipoic acid is a nutrient that is both fat and water soluble. It can also be called lipoic acid and α-lipoic acid. It is essential to good health, including mental alertness and memory. Unfortunately, your body makes less alpha-lipoic acid as you age.

■ Functions of Alpha-Lipoic Acid

- Acts as a metal chelator for (causes a reaction with) cadmium, copper, and iron
- Helps insulin work more effectively
- Helps prevent cataracts
- Improves your immune system
- Increases glutathione (a tripeptide discussed on page 133) by 30 to 70 percent
- Is a cofactor of (required for activity by) mitochondrial enzymes (which are needed for energy production)
- Lowers levels of calcium and copper if you have too much
- Modulates gene expression to help insulin work more effectively in the body
- Neutralizes free radicals
- Protects collagen in the skin from cross-linking, which can cause sagging and wrinkles
- Recycles coenzyme Q_{10}, glutathione, vitamin C, and vitamin E
- Slows brain aging

- Stimulates the sprouting of new nerve fibers on nerve cells
- Stops activation of NF-kappa B (a protein complex that, if overactivated, can cause cancer, heart disease, and a variety of other illnesses) in your cells
- Stops the adhesion of macrophages (large white blood cells that can cause heart disease) to your artery wall

Recommended Dosage

Take 50 to 300 milligrams daily. I recommend capsules or tablets of alpha-lipoic acid. Although it is present in some foods, it is impossible to eat enough to be therapeutic. Consider, for example, that 100 pounds of spinach has the same amount of alpha-lipoic acid as a 100-milligram capsule of lipoic acid.

Diseases/Disorders that Can Be Treated or Prevented with Alpha-Lipoic Acid

• AIDS	• Eczema	• Memory disorders
• Alzheimer's disease	• Heart disease	• Multiple sclerosis
• Atherosclerosis	• Hepatitis C	• Parkinson's disease
• Burns	• Immunosuppression	• Psoriasis
• Cataracts	• Lou Gehrig's disease	• Rheumatoid arthritis
• Circulatory disorders	• Lupus	• Scleroderma
• Diabetes mellitus	• Macular degeneration	• Skin cancer
• Diabetic neuropathy		• Stroke

COENZYME Q_{10}

Coenzyme Q_{10} (CoQ_{10}) is a fat-soluble nutrient that is found in many foods and is made in nearly all of your body's tissues. It has the important responsibility of producing cellular energy. However, your body makes less and less CoQ_{10} as you age. You can take supplements to counter this effect. I highly recommended these supplements to most women because there are now several studies that show a correlation between CoQ_{10} depletion and breast cancer. If you are taking a blood thinner, this enzyme should not be used without the close supervision of your doctor.

■ Functions of Coenzyme Q$_{10}$

- Enhances the regeneration of vitamin E
- Is a coenzyme in the energy-producing metabolic pathways of all your cells
- Is an antioxidant
- Lowers blood pressure
- Reduces platelet stickiness (discouraging potentially harmful blood clots)

■ Symptoms of Coenzyme Q$_{10}$ Deficiency

- ☐ Excessive free radicals
- ☐ General fatigue
- ☐ Muscle weakness
- ☐ Weakness

■ Causes of Coenzyme Q$_{10}$ Deficiency

- Adriamycin intake
- Beta blockers intake
- Chlorpromazine intake
- Clonidine intake
- Deficiency of vitamins B$_1$, B$_5$, B$_6$, and B$_{12}$
- Desipramine intake
- Doxepin intake
- Fluphenizine intake
- Excess exercise
- Fluvastatin intake
- Folic acid deficiency
- Gemfibrozil intake
- Genetic mutations
- Glucophage intake
- Glyburide intake
- Haloperidol intake
- Hydralazine intake
- Hydrochlorothiazide intake
- Hyperthyroidism
- Imipramine intake
- Malabsorption due to coeliac disease/sprue (an inherited auto-immune disorder)
- Malabsorption due to steatorrhea (fatty stools)
- Medicines and over-the-counter supplements that are usually used for weight loss and decrease fat absorption
- Phenothiazines intake
- Protryptyline intake
- Statin drugs (HMG-CoA-reductase inhibitors including Lipitor, Mevacor, Zocor, and Pravachol)
- Taurine deficiency
- Tolazamide intake
- Trimipramine intake

■ Recommended Dosage

30 to 360 milligrams daily, depending on diagnosis. However, do not use more than 100 milligrams daily without consulting your healthcare provider.

■ Side Effects and Contraindications

The following side effects can occur from taking CoQ_{10} supplements. However, they are usually less severe if you take the supplement after meals.

- Abdominal discomfort
- Appetite loss
- Diarrhea (when doses taken are greater than 100 milligrams)
- Heartburn
- Increase in liver enzymes (when doses taken are greater than 300 milligrams)
- Insomnia (when doses taken are greater than 100 milligrams)
- Irritability
- Mild nausea
- Palpitations
- Photophobia (sensitivity to light)

■ Diseases/Disorders that Can Be Treated or Prevented with Coenzyme Q_{10}

- Alzheimer's disease
- Arrhythmia (abnormal heart rhythm)
- Asthma
- Breast cancer
- Chronic fatigue syndrome (CFS)
- Chronic obstructive pulmonary disease (COPD)
- Congestive heart failure
- Coronary heart disease
- Diabetes
- Dilated cardiomyopathy (heart disease)
- Fibromyalgia
- High blood pressure
- Migraine headaches
- Mitral valve prolapse (heart disease)
- Parkinson's disease
- Periodontal disease
- Pulmonary fibrosis
- Side effects of adriamycin treatment
- Sun-damaged skin
- Weight loss

Food Sources of Coenzyme Q_{10}

- Anchovies
- Beef heart
- Broccoli
- Mackerel
- Nuts
- Pork
- Salmon
- Sardines
- Spinach

ENZYMES

Enzymes are proteins that are catalysts for chemical activity. In fact, they are involved with nearly all of the biochemical reactions in your body. The molecules on which enzymes provide their reactions are called *substrates;* once the reaction has occurred, these molecules become *products.* The enzyme itself remains unchanged during this process.

There are over 3,000 different enzymes, and each is responsible for a different vital function. Therefore, the malfunction or depletion of any single enzyme can have serious health consequences.

Although some enzymes are produced in your body, there are other essential enzymes that must be ingested. For example, the specific enzyme needed to break down a particular food is often only available in that food. For that reason, it can be unhealthy to eat certain foods when they have been stripped of their enzymes. ("The Purpose of this Book" on page 3 explained that many of the foods we eat today are deprived of their natural nutrients.)

■ Functions of Enzymes

Enzymes are involved with many, many bodily functions. The list below is not intended to be complete. It will, however, illustrate the importance of enzymes.

- Allow metabolism to occur at its proper speed
- Are antioxidants
- Break down food particles and large molecules into smaller, usable pieces
- Convert stored food into energy
- Help form necessary blood clots
- Help remove waste from the body

■ Enzyme Deficiencies

Since enzymes have so many varied responsibilities, deficiencies can be very dangerous. Your body makes certain enzymes, but others must be eaten in enzyme-rich food such as raw vegetables and fruit. Enzymes in food can be damaged or depleted when exposed to prolonged heat (over 117°F). Once eaten, enzymes can be destroyed by a very acidic or alkaline environment.

■ Enzyme Supplementation

Enzyme supplements can be destroyed by heat. You can keep enzymes that are in tablet or liquid form in the refrigerator. Powder and capsule forms of enzymes need to be kept in a cool but dry place, so the refrigerator is not ideal. The applicable dosage of an enzyme depends on the specific enzyme and the reason you are taking it. Read the information that comes with the bottle and consult your doctor.

The groups of digestive enzymes (listed below) are very important because they allow your body to properly digest foods including starches, fats, and proteins. I suggest taking a supplement that contains amylase, lipase, and protease. If you are eating processed or cooked foods, take the supplement while you are eating. Otherwise, take the supplement after the meal.

■ Digestive Enzymes

- Amylase: breaks down starches into simple sugars. Amylase is produced in your pancreas and salivary glands, and can also be ingested in breads. It reduces arteriosclerotic plaques, which can decrease your risk of coronary heart disease.

- Lipase: breaks down fats, particularly triglycerides. Lipase is secreted by the pancreas and helps protect you against coronary heart disease.

- Protease: breaks down proteins into smaller proteins or amino acids so they can be absorbed by the intestine. Protease is produced in your pancreas and stomach, and can be ingested in milk. It is thought to reduce both the pain and risk of certain cancers. Bromelain is one type of protease that contains several other substances as well. It is found in pineapples and is helpful in treating a variety of health disorders.

Food Sources of Enzymes

Because even moderate heat can destroy enzymes, I recommend eating these foods raw.

• Avocados	• Brussels sprouts	• Papaya
• Bananas	• Cabbage	• Pineapple
• Broccoli	• Mangos	• Wheatgrass

FIBER

Fiber is a food substance found in plants that contains no nutrients or calories. It occurs in both a soluble and insoluble form, both of which help with digestion and neither of which can be digested or absorbed by your body. Soluble fibers bind to fats in foods and prevent their absorption, which helps lower cholesterol and blood sugar. Insoluble fibers help food move through your body and be excreted more quickly. Fiber is suspected to help prevent certain cancers.

■ Functions of Fiber

- Improves absorption of certain vitamins and minerals

- Improves digestion

- Increases HDL (good) cholesterol

- Lowers blood pressure

- Lowers blood sugar levels

- Lowers cholesterol levels

- Lowers triglycerides

- Prevents constipation

Food Sources of Soluble Fiber

• Apples	• Blackberries	• Flaxseed	• Pears
• Apricots	• Broccoli	• Grapefruit	• Prunes
• Bananas	• Brussels sprouts	• Nuts	• Psyllium
• Barley		• Oat bran	• Split peas
• Beans (kidney, lime, navy, and pinto)	• Cabbage	• Okra	• Sweet potatoes
	• Carrots	• Oranges	
	• Chick peas		

Food Sources of Insoluble Fiber

- Bananas
- Beans
- Broccoli
- Brown rice
- Brussels sprouts

- Cauliflower
- Celery
- Corn
- Crackers
- Grains

- High-fiber cereal
- Lentils
- Pasta
- Potato (with skin)

- Prunes
- Spinach
- Wheat bran
- Whole wheat bread

INDOLE-3-CARBINOL

Indole-3-carbinol (I-3-C) is developed from the breakdown of glucobrassicin, a compound that occurs when cruciferous vegetables (those in the cabbage family) are broken or cooked.

Functions of Indole-3-Carbinol

Indole-3-carbinol helps prevent the development of estrogen-enhanced cancers (such as breast, cervical, and uterine). Some doctors believe that I-3-C also protects against prostate cancer, as well as cancers caused by pesticides and other toxins. It is an antioxidant, and inhibits oxidation and the formation of free radicals.

Recommended Dosage

300 to 500 milligrams daily

Food Sources of Indole-3-Carbinol

- Broccoli
- Brussels sprouts

- Cabbage
- Cauliflower

- Kale
- Turnips

MELATONIN

Melatonin is a hormone produced in the pineal gland that is associated with sleep. It is also an antioxidant, and new research has suggested that it may help significantly in the treatment of breast cancer. The amount of melatonin your body produces decreases as you age, and depends on the activity of an enzyme called serotonin-N-acetyltransferase (NAT). Your body's production of NAT, on the other hand, depends on its storage of vitamin B_6.

■ Functions of Melatonin

- Acts as an antioxidant
- Decreases platelet stickiness
- Decreases your risk of heart disease by decreasing atherosclerosis
- Helps you get to sleep and stay asleep
- Promotes healthy cholesterol levels
- Relieves jet lag
- Strengthens the immune system

■ Causes of Melatonin Deficiency

- Acetaminophen intake
- Alcohol intake
- Alprazolam intake
- Aspirin intake
- Atenolol intake
- Benserazideintake
- Bepridil intake
- Caffeine intake
- Clonidine intake
- Dexamethasone intake

- Deficiency of vitamin B_{12}
- Diazepam intake
- Diltiazem intake
- Felodipine intake
- Flunitrazepam intake
- Fluoxetine intake
- Ibuprofen intake
- Indomethacin intake
- Interleukin-2 intake
- Isradipine intake
- Luzindole intake

- Methylcobalamin intake
- Metoprolol intake
- Nicardipine intake
- Nifedipine intake
- Nimodipine intake
- Nisoldipine intake
- Nitrendipine intake
- Prazosin intake
- Propranolol intake
- Reserpine intake
- Ronidazole intake
- Tobacco intake

■ Causes of Increased Melatonin Levels

- Food such as bananas, barley, ginger, oats, rice, sweet corn, and tomatoes
- Medications such as clorgyline, desipramine, fluvoxamine, thorazine, and tranylcypromine
- Melatonin supplementation
- St. John's wort supplementation

■ Recommended Dosage

1 to 6 milligrams daily. If taken as a sleep aid, melatonin should be taken thirty minutes before bedtime and while in a dark room. You should begin with 1 milligram and gradually ingest more if you find it necessary. Larger dosages can be used to treat breast cancer. Consult your physician regarding this melatonin for this purpose.

■ Side Effects and Contraindications

Melatonin is an immune stimulator. Consequently, you should not take it if you have an autoimmune disease. Furthermore, you should not take melatonin if you are pregnant, on prescription steroids, or have depression, mental illness, leukemia, or lymphoma.

METHYLSULFONYLMETHANE

Methylsulfonylmethane (MSM) is a natural substance that you make in your body as well as ingest in certain foods. It is used to treat pain and inflammation. MSM supplies the mineral sulfur—an important compound that is vital to life—to your body. However, it is *not* sulfa. If you are allergic to sulfa, you probably *can* take MSM. Discuss this with your doctor before beginning supplementation.

MSM is formed from the oxidation of the sulfur compound dimethyl sulfoxide (DMSO). Although DMSO has similar pain-relieving attributes to MSM, DMSO may cause side effects that range from nasal congestion to shortness of breath to body odor. Therefore, MSM is a more highly recommended route to improving your sulfur level.

■ Ways in Which MSM Provides Pain Relief

- Has an immune normalizing effect (which can help treat certain autoimmune diseases)
- Increases blood supply
- Inhibits pain impulses along nerve fibers
- Lessens inflammation
- Reduces muscle spasms
- Softens scar tissue

■ Recommended Dosage

500 to 10,000 milligrams twice daily. MSM can be taken as a capsule, powder, or tablet, or applied as a lotion or gel. All forms are fine. However, if you find yourself needing a high dosage of MSM, you may want to ingest the powder, which contains the highest concentration of the substance. When first starting oral supplementation, arrange dosage to take with meal to avoid possible heartburn. Most people need to take MSM for at least two weeks—and sometimes for as long as two months—before seeing any results.

MSM supplements should not contain fillers. To determine the purity of a certain MSM supplement, you can request a company's laboratory certificate. You can also perform your own experiment. Drop the supplement in a glass of water. Any particles floating at the top once the supplement dissolves are filler.

■ Diseases/Disorders that Can Be Treated or Prevented with MSM

- Acne
- Allergies
- Bursitis
- Carpal tunnel syndrome
- Chronic back pain
- Chronic headaches
- Fibromyalgia
- Heartburn
- Inflammation after an injury
- Joint pain
- Muscle pain
- Osteoarthritis
- Rheumatoid arthritis
- Temporomandibular joint disorder (TMJ)
- Tendonitis

Food Sources of MSM

- Alfalfa sprouts
- Brussels sprouts
- Cabbage
- Cauliflower
- Corn
- Horseradish
- Kale
- Kohlrabi
- Leeks
- Milk
- Mustard greens
- Onion
- Peppers
- Radish
- Tea
- Tomatoes
- Watercress

OLIGOMERIC PROANTHOCYANIDINS

Oligomeric proanthocyanidins (OPCs) are a class of flavonoids—plant substances—that are powerful antioxidants (which help to eliminate unhealthy free radicals). Your body cannot make them. The richest sources of OPCs are extracts of red wine, grape seeds, and pine bark.

■ Functions of OPCs

All forms of OPCs have some similarities. They all have anti-carcinogenic properties and act as anti-inflammatories. However, extracts from different sources can also have different effects on your body.

Grape Seed Extract

- Boosts immune system
- Is an antioxidant
- Lowers LDL (bad) cholesterol
- Prevents damage to DNA

Pine Bark Extract

- Boosts immune system
- Helps treat venous (veins and blood flow) inadequacies
- Is an antioxidant
- Protects your cells from oxidative damage
- Treats certain skin conditions

Red Wine Extract

- Decreases cholesterol
- Is an antioxidant
- Lowers apolipoprotein B (which carries LDL cholesterol to your tissues)
- Prevents platelet stickiness (discouraging potentially harmful blood clots)
- Reduces triglycerides

■ Recommended Dosage

50 to 200 milligrams daily

■ Diseases/Disorders that Can Be Treated or Prevented with OPCs

- Allergies
- Alzheimer's disease
- Arthritis
- Cancer
- Certain skin disorders
- Chronic fatigue syndrome
- Glaucoma
- High cholesterol
- Varicose veins
- Weight loss

PHOSPHATIDYLCHOLINE

Phosphatidylcholine is a phospholipid and a major component of lecithin. Often, the word "lecithin" is used as a synonym for "phosphatidyl-choline." It is a good source of choline. This substance is isolated from egg yolk, soy beans, and certain meats in order to manufacture supplements.

■ Recommended Dosage

3 to 6 grams daily. However, alpha-glyceryl phosphoryl choline (see page 187) is a preferred supplement because it allows a greater amount of choline to be absorbed by your body.

■ Diseases/Disorders that Can Be Treated or Prevented with Phosphatidylcholine

- Decreased liver function
- Fibrocystic breast disease
- Fibroids
- Helps convert estradiol (E2) to estriol (E3) (female hormones)
- High homocysteine
- Memory loss

Other Nutrients

Although you have read about some very important nutrients in this chapter, there are many others that can help as you strive to achieve optimal health. In conjunction with the supplements already discussed, the nutrients listed here have the ability to help you fight disease and maintain wellness.

Chlorella

Chlorella is a green algae that contains excellent essential nutrients. Its main components are protein, carbohydrates, and unsaturated (good) fats, and it contains vitamins A, B_2, B_6, C, E, and K. Chlorella is also abundant with minerals such as calcium, magnesium, iron, zinc, phosphorus, and iodine.

Chlorella has many medical benefits. It can boost immunity function, reduce high blood pressure, decrease risk of diabetes and anemia, reduce symptoms of PMS and menopause, and promote healthy cell growth and wound healing. Some people are allergic to chlorella, so begin use with caution. If you develop nausea or other gastrointestinal distress, stop taking chlorella.

Chondroitin Sulfate

Chondroitin sulfate is part of a large protein molecule that is found naturally in cartilage. Although it is commonly sold as a supplement, it is usually less effective than the similar glucosamine sulfate (also found in cartilage and discussed on page 202) because its large size doesn't allow it to be easily absorbed and utilized. Yet, its sulfur molecules *are* able to be absorbed. As a result, sufferers of osteoarthritis often report pain relief after taking chondroitin sulfate. It can take several months to become effective.

Colostrum

Colostrum, a nutrient with immune-enhancing benefits, is secreted by humans and animals in breast milk. It is also taken as a supplement because it has certain curative properties. Individuals with short bowel syndrome, chemotherapy-induced mouth ulcers, and inflammatory bowel disease often report success after taking colostrum supplementation. Colostrum may also protect the stomach and bowel from damage caused by anti-inflammatory medications.

Cordyceps

Cordyceps (*Cordyceps sinsensis*) is a mushroom that has long been used, particularly in traditional Chinese medicine, for ailments ranging from asthma to coughs to female hormonal problems. Its use has since extended to include treating bronchitis, hepatitis B, and hepatic cirrhosis, and acting as a replacement to certain immunosuppressive medications. Some studies have also found that cordyceps provides increased energy levels and improved lung capacity. For that reason, this herbal supplement is popular among athletes.

Glucosamine

Glucosamine is an amino acid that occurs naturally in all tissues. It is vitally important to the preservation of cartilage, for two reasons: First, it is a main component of the connective tissue. Second, it is an aid in the process of transporting sulfur (another main component of cartilage) into the tissue.

As people age, they often gradually lose the ability to produce adequate levels of glucosamine. It is theorized that this is a main cause of osteoarthritis. Studying the effect of glucosamine supplements on arthritis sufferers, researchers have found that pain was relieved and mobility was improved. Although it has not yet been proven, some people believe that this supplement can actually slow down the progression of the disease. Glucosamine sulfate is the form most highly recommended for relief from osteoarthritis.

Don't take any form of glucosamine if you are allergic to shellfish. Consult use with your healthcare provider if you have diabetes, because glucosamine can alter blood sugar levels. Also, taking glucosamine with a diuretic reduces the effectiveness of this supplement, so you may need to increase the dosage to compensate.

Glycerophosphocholine

Glycerophosphocholine (GPC) is a compound related to phosphatidylcholine. It is only available with a prescription in Europe; it is available without a prescription in the United States. GPC stimulates the production of new acetylcholine, the neurotransmitter that helps maintain memory and allows learning. It also has an effect on nerve growth factor, a substance that regulates acetylcholine receptors. Studies have shown that this supplement can forestall, stabilize, and even reverse some memory loss that occurs in the early stages of dementia.

Ipriflavone

The synthetic ipriflavone is similar in structure to soy isoflavonoids. It is approved in some countries as a prescription drug for the treatment and prevention of osteoporosis, while it is available over the counter in the United States. Ipriflavone works by enhancing the effects of calcitonin (a thyroid hormone that regulates calcium) on calcium metabolism. The recommended dosage is 200 milligrams three times a day.

Malic Acid

Malic acid is found naturally in the body, but can also be consumed in apples, currants, and most tart fruits (as well as in some supplements). It is essential to life, as it is involved in several energy-producing reactions including the Krebs cycle and mitochondrial respiration. Despite its importance, healthy people do not usually need to take malic acid supplementation. However, a deficiency is associated with physical exhaustion, muscle pain, and fibromyalgia, and a malic acid supplementation program can help treat these conditions. Cisplatin, a chemotherapy medication, and certain other drugs can reduce the level of malic acid in the body.

Ornithine Alpha-Ketoglutarate

Ornithine alpha-ketoglutarate (OKG) is a combination of two amino acids, ornithine and glutamine. It increases the release of muscle-building hormones, prevents the breakdown of muscle, enhances muscle growth, and improves immune function. Clinical trials have shown that OKG supplementation also improves wound healing.

Policosanol

Policosanol is a mixture of fatty alcohols isolated from the wax of sugar cane and yams. Its main compound is octanosol. Studies have shown that policosanol lowers LDL (bad) cholesterol and raises HDL (good) cholesterol. It can also help prevent atherosclerosis. Policosanol reduces platelet aggregation of the blood and, therefore, its ability to clot, so consult use with your healthcare provider if you are taking a blood thinner.

Quercetin

Quercetin is a plant flavonoid. An anti-inflammatory, quercetin can be used to reduce arthritis pain. It can also help treat prostatitis and respiratory illnesses associated with inflammation such as asthma and bronchitis. Quercetin inhibits the release of histamine, which decreases the severity of allergic reactions, and is an antioxidant. Studies have also shown that men who intake more flavonoids, particularly quercetin, suffer fewer strokes and heart attacks than those who do not. In addition, quercetin has been found to protect the kidneys against the aging process. It can be found in apples and red onions as well as nutritional supplements.

Red Yeast Rice

Red yeast rice is the fermented product of rice on which red yeast (*Monascus purpureus*) has been grown. Red yeast is a natural statin drug. It forms naturally occurring HMG-CoA reductase inhibitors known as monacolins, which lower cholesterol. In fact, monacolin-K (which is also called lovastatin) is the ingredient in the cholesterol medication Mevacor. Red yeast rice also contains sterols (beta-sitosterol, campesterol, stigmasterol, sapogenin), isoflavones, and monounsaturated fatty acids, which also have a cholesterol-lowering effect on the body.

Similarly to a statin drug, red yeast rice can deplete the body of coenzyme Q_{10}. Therefore, after taking red yeast rice, the body's supply of coenzyme Q_{10} must be replenished. Consult your healthcare practitioner regarding the recommended dosage of coenzyme Q_{10} for you.

Tea tree oil

Tea tree oil is made from the leaves of the *Melaleuca alternifolia,* a small tree that grows in Australia. With antiseptic and antifungal properties, tea tree oil can be applied topically to treat sunburn, sores, cuts, arthritis, bruises, insect bites, warts, acne, fungal infections, mouth ulcers, and dandruff. Do not take tea tree oil internally because it can cause nerve damage. It should also not be applied in the ears, eyes, or other mucous membrane.

PHOSPHATIDYLSERINE

Phosphatidylserine is a *phospholipid*—it contains both phosphorus and fat molecules—and is one of the key building blocks in your brain. It is also present in every cell in your body and has many important functions.

■ Functions of Phosphatidylserine in Your Body

- Benefits heart rhythm
- Critical for neurotransmission (electrical signals sent between neurons)

- Immune function
- Incorporates membrane proteins
- Influences the fluidity of nerve-cell membraces
- Needed for electrical activity of your brain
- Reduces cortisol (a stress hormone)
- Testicular function
- Used in bone formation

■ Diseases/Disorders that Can Be Treated with Phosphatidylserine

- Alzheimer's disease
- Anxiety
- Depression
- Improving learning, concentration, and work skills
- Memory decline
- Parkinson's disease
- Stress

■ Recommended Dosage

100 to 500 milligrams daily

PROBIOTICS

Probiotics are the friendly bacteria in your intestines that increase your defenses against disease. Overuse of antibiotics and poor nutritional intake can create an overgrowth in your bowel of unhealthy bacteria while also killing the healthy probiotics. This can cause problems ranging from the development of food allergies to a decline of your immune system. Probiotic supplementation after antibiotic treatment is complete helps limit the negative effects of antibiotics by decreasing the unhealthy bacteria and encouraging the repopulation of healthy bacteria. However, if you are taking an antibiotic, wait three hours before taking probiotics.

■ Functions of Probiotics

- Help manufacture biotin, folic acid, and niacin
- Increase your immune system (increase white blood cells, phagocytosis, and gama-interferon)
- Make lactase, an enzyme needed to help the digestion of milk products
- Play a major role in digestion

■ Probiotic Health

The health of your probiotics is crucial to your overall well-being. Unfortunately, many of us do not take particularly good care of them. For example, many people today regularly overuse antibiotics. Antibiotics kill probiotics while they wipe out the harmful bacteria.

Your diet is also important. Probiotics are healthier when your diet consists of complex carbohydrates such as legumes, vegetables, and whole grains. A diet that mainly consists of dairy products, fats, and sugars, on the other hand, provides the probiotics with a very unhealthy living environment.

PYCNOGENOL

Pycnogenol is the trademarked name for a mixture of forty different antioxidants from the bark of the maritime pine tree (*Pinus maritime*). This supplement provides a variety of health benefits. It also may improve the effectiveness of Adderall in treating attention deficit disorder (ADD).

■ Functions of Pycnogenol

- Elevates your body's production of glutathione (see page 133) and vitamin E
- Helps regulate nitric oxide production
- Improves endurance
- Improves the circulation in your capillaries
- Increases the lifespan of vitamin C in your body
- Is an antioxidant
- Protects against platelet stickiness
- Relieves inflammation
- Stimulates natural killer cells that help your body fight off cancer

■ Recommended Dosage

25 to 250 milligrams a day

■ Diseases/Disorders that Can Be Treated or Prevented with Pycnogenol

- Attention-deficit disorder (ADD) when used in conjunction with Adderall
- Heart disease
- Rotator cuff tendonitis
- Varicose veins

RESVERATROL

Resveratrol is a *polyphenol*—a plant substance that can fight certain diseases. As explained below in the list "Functions of Resveratrol," it may help you avoid a large variety of serious illnesses. In the past, it was even theorized that this substance was the answer behind the "French paradox"—the contradiction between the low occurrence of cardiovascular disease in the French people and their relatively high-fat diets. However, most people now generally agree that there is not enough resveratrol in wine to account for this difference. Some people claim that procyanidins, another group of polyphenols, are responsible, while other people believe that the French Paradox is actually a myth born out of incorrect statistics.

■ Functions of Resveratrol

- Decreases platelet stickiness
- Helps prevent Alzheimer's disease
- Helps prevent cancer
- Induces phase II detoxification enzymes (which convert toxic substances into less toxic ones that the body can then excrete)
- Inhibits COX-2 enzyme induction (which can relieve inflammation)
- Inhibits oxidation of LDL (bad) cholesterol
- Inhibits mitochondrial ROS (damaging molecules that can lead to disease) formation
- Is a phytoestrogen (a plant substance that can reduce the risk of some cancers)
- Is an anti-inflammatory
- Is an antioxidant

- Opens arteries by increasing nitric oxide, allowing blood to flow more easily
- Reduces risk of certain cardiovascular diseases
- Stops the proliferation of cells that narrow your arteries

■ Recommended Dosage

20 to 40 milligrams daily. Because resveratrol oxidizes easily, you should store it in a cool, dry place.

Food Sources of Resveratrol

- Grape skins   • Mulberries   • Peanuts   • Red wine

PART 2

Health Conditions

Your body's complex inner workings have the ability to heal many ailments. Today, however, pharmaceutical medications are often prescribed frequently and indiscriminately. While these conventional treatments may provide quick relief, they usually do not treat the cause of the problem.

The natural products discussed in Part 1 can not only help you achieve optimal health, but also help your body fight various diseases and disorders. Unlike many pharmaceuticals, nutrients boost your immune system while also regulating your other bodily systems and helping them work more effectively and efficiently. Part 2 explores many common—and some less common—health problems and the appropriate natural remedies.

There are times—such as most emergency situations and acute conditions—in which pharmaceuticals are the best option. Unfortunately, their prescription is not reserved for these times. The following pages provide powerful and competent alternatives to the conventional therapies. However, my intentions are not to have the natural ways completely replace the pharmaceuticals. Sometimes the natural and the conventional must even be combined to achieve the best results. With the help of a healthcare provider, every patient will need to determine—and possibly experiment with—his or her individual treatment plan. But when at all possible, I strongly encourage the use of natural healing over pharmaceuticals to avoid unhealthy and far-reaching side effects.

Each description begins with an explanation, symptoms, and causes of the disease or disorder. This is followed by a list of suggested supplements that can help you avoid or recover from the problem. The list also includes recommended adult dosages and, in many instances, important considerations when taking the supplement. See Part 1 for any questions you may have regarding the supplements and their effects.

There are a number of different therapeutic options given for most of the following conditions. You may find that some treatments are most effective when combined. However, they do not all have to be used simultaneously. This section is not a cookbook with ingredient lists to which you must carefully adhere. After all, one size does not fit all when it comes to your medical treatment. As always, working with a health professional trained in nutrition and anti-aging medicine is suggested. (Contact information for finding a functional medicine or anti-aging healthcare provider can be found in the Resource section.)

Supplements should always be taken with a full glass of water. It is also important that you note the following precautions, along with the considerations given for each supplement. The dosages given are intended for adults without kidney or liver disease. If you have kidney or liver disease, you may need to take lower dosages of most supplements, and should consult your doctor before embarking upon any nutritional program. Similarly, if you are pregnant or nursing, consult your doctor before following any of these protocols. If you are taking coumadin or any other blood thinner, your dosage of certain nutrients must be lower than what is suggested. Please ask your physician for help determining the appropriate dosage. If you are having surgery, do not take any nutrients (except for the surgery pre- and post-operative protocol that your doctor gives you) for two weeks before and one week after your surgery date.

The following list of conditions covers a wide range of disorders, but it is, by no means, comprehensive of what can be treated through natural means. Your healthcare provider should be able to help you with information regarding any disorders that are not listed here.

ACNE

An inflammatory skin condition, acne is characterized by clogged pores, blackheads, and pimples. It is caused by a problem with the oil-secreting sebaceous glands, which lubricate the skin and are found in large numbers on the face, chest, and back. When the sebaceous glands produce too much oil (called *sebum*) and combine with dead skin cells, the pores become clogged, bacteria multiply, and the skin becomes inflamed and forms pimples. A blackhead forms when the sebum combines with skin pigments and is trapped in the pores.

The exact cause of acne is not known, but there are a number of factors that can contribute to this condition. One major factor is hormone imbalance, which is why so many teenagers, who experience increased hormone production during puberty, suffer from acne. Because hormonal changes also occur before and after menstruation—as well as before, during, and after pregnancy and menopause—some women experience outbreaks (usually short-lived) during these times. Other factors can include a family history of acne, emotional stress, allergies, and an over-consumption of junk food, saturated fats, and hydrogenated fats. The use of certain drugs, such as steroids, oral contraceptives, and lithium, can also contribute to this skin condition.

Along with treating acne by following the supplement program presented below, wash the skin once or twice a day with a mild cleanser. Avoid scrubbing the skin or washing more frequently, as this can worsen the condition. Use oil-free skin products and cosmetics that are labeled "water-based" or "non-comedogenic," which means that they do not contain mineral oil, which can clog pores, and do not aggravate acne.

SUPPLEMENTS TO TREAT ACNE

Supplements	Dosage	Considerations
B-complex vitamins	50 to 100 mg once a day	I suggest taking a multi-vitamin.
Copper	2 to 3 mg once a day	Your copper-to-zinc ratio is very important for your health. Also, do not take copper supplement cupric oxide, which has a very low bioavailability.
Dandelion	100 mg once a day	If you have gallstones or obstructed bile ducts, consult your healthcare practitioner before taking.
EPA/DHA (fish oil)	1,000 to 3,000 mg once a day	Choose a source that contains vitamin E to prevent oxidation.
Evening primrose oil	500 to 1,000 mg once a day	
Glucosamine	1,000 mg once a day	Don't take if you are allergic to shellfish. Consult use with your healthcare provider if you have diabetes because glucosamine can alter blood sugar levels.
Milk thistle	200 mg once a day	Reduces efficiency of certain blood pressure medication.
Probiotics	20 billion units once a day	If taking an antibiotic, wait three hours before taking probiotics.
Taurine	1,000 to 2,000 mg once a day	Take between meals. Discontinue use if you suddenly have feelings of chest or throat tightness or if you break out in hives. Do not take with aspirin.
Tea tree oil	Apply directly to blemishes once or twice a day.	Do not ingest or use in ears, eyes, or other mucous membranes.

Vitamin A and mixed carotenoids	5,000 to 15,000 IU— half vitamin A and half mixed carotenoids— once a day	Use caution when taking vitamin A supplements because they have the potential to be toxic. Do not take for extended periods of time. Do not take more than 8,000 IU a day if you have liver disease, are a smoker, or are exposed to asbestos.
Vitamin C	500 to 1,500 mg twice a day	Do not take high dosages if you are prone to kidney stones or gout.
Vitamin D	Have your blood levels measured by your health-care provider, who will then determine proper dosage.	
Vitamin E	400 IU once a day	Take mixed tocopherols, the more active type of vitamin E. Consult healthcare provider first if you are taking a blood thinner.
Zinc	25 to 75 mg once a day	The best zinc supplements are zinc picolinate and zinc citrate. If you are taking zinc and iron supplements, take one in the morning and one in the evening. (Taking them together reduces the efficiency of both.)

ADD/ADHD

Attention Deficit Disorder/Attention Deficit Hyperactivity Disorder (ADD/ADHD) is usually characterized by an inability to maintain focus or pay attention. People with ADD/ADHD may also exhibit uncontrollable hyperactivity. It is often inherited, but can be caused by environmental factors such as brain injury, high fever, and toxic exposure. Diet, food allergies, metal toxicities, pre-natal fatty acid deficiencies, zinc deficiencies, and zinc-to-copper imbalances can also play a role.

Stimulants are the conventional medicinal treatment for ADD/ADHD. Unfortunately, these pharmaceuticals reduce the overall blood flow to the brain and disturb glucose metabolism. On the other hand, a nutritional approach, such as that described starting on page 214, strives to actually increase academic and social abilities. Also, sugar, food additives, and food colorings should be avoided.

SUPPLEMENTS TO TREAT ADD/ADHD

Supplements	Dosage	Considerations
American ginseng	200 mg once a day	Always take with food. Do not take if you are taking a blood thinner.
B-complex vitamins	50 mg twice a day	I suggest taking a multi-vitamin.
Boron	5 to 10 mg once a day	
Carnitine	2,000 to 4,000 mg once a day	
EPA/DHA (fish oil)	500 to 1,000 mg once a day	Choose a source that contains vitamin E to prevent oxidation.
5-Hydroxy-tryptophan (5-HTP)	100 to 200 mg once a day	Do not take with vitamin B_6. Consult your healthcare provider regarding use if you are taking antidepressants. Do not take at the same time as antidepressants or any serotonin-affecting drugs.
Gamma-linolenic acid (GLA)	240 to 720 mg once a day	It is important to maintain the proper ratio of omega-6 fatty acids to omega-3 fatty acids. (See page 110.)
Ginkgo biloba	60 mg twice a day	Do not take if you are taking a blood thinner.
Magnesium	250 to 500 mg once a day	Consult healthcare provider for dosage if you have kidney disease. Discontinue use and see your doctor if you experience abdominal pain. Take a lower dose if it causes diarrhea.
Phosphatidylserine	100 to 500 mg once a day	
Probiotics	20 billion units once a day	If taking an antibiotic, wait three hours before taking probiotics.
St. John's wort	300 to 1,200 mg once a day	Do not take with antidepressants, indinavir, cyclosporine, theophylline, warfarin, or ethinylestradiol. If you are exposed to the sun, it may cause a skin rash. May lessen effects of birth control.
Selenium	100 mcg once a day	
Vitamin B_9 (folic acid)	500 to 1,000 mcg once a day	High doses can deplete your body of other vitamins in the B complex.
Vitamin B_{12} (cobalamin)	500 to 1,000 mcg once a day	High doses can deplete your body of other vitamins in the B complex.

| Zinc | 25 to 50 mg once a day | The best zinc supplements are zinc picolinate and zinc citrate. If you are taking zinc and iron supplements, take one in the morning and one in the evening. (Taking them together reduces the efficiency of both.) |

ADRENAL FATIGUE AND EXHAUSTION

The adrenal glands—triangle-shaped glands that sit on top of the kidneys—are chiefly responsible for regulating the body's short-term stress response through the production of hormones such as cortisol and dehydroepiandrosterone (DHEA). Many believe that under long-term stress, the adrenal glands become overworked, begin to function improperly, and eventually become unable to respond to stress. This condition—referred to as *adrenal fatigue, adrenal exhaustion,* and *hypoadrenia*—can lead to a wide range of symptoms, including weakness, fatigue, depression,

Symptoms of Adrenal Fatigue and Exhaustion

As explained above, unrelieved stress can lead to fatigue and exhaustion of the adrenal glands. This, in turn, can cause the following symptoms and disorders.

- Absent-mindedness
- Allergies
- Autoimmune disorders
- Bone loss
- Constipation and diarrhea
- Cravings for salt
- Cravings for spices
- Cravings for sugar
- Depression
- Dizziness
- Fatigue that worsens in evenings and with stress
- Frustration
- Headaches
- Hormone imbalance
- Hypoglycemia
- Immune system suppression
- Inability to concentrate
- Insomnia
- Irritability
- Lightheadedness
- Moodiness
- Muscle loss
- Nervousness
- Pale, cold, clammy skin
- Restlessness
- Tachycardia (fast heart rate) and/or palpitations
- Weakness

muscle and bone loss, suppression of the immune system, hormonal imbalance, autoimmune disorders, and many other problems. (See the inset on page 215 for more possible symptoms of adrenal fatigue.)

It is believed that adrenal fatigue is largely a disorder of the modern world. The adrenal glands evolved to handle only short-term stress, but today's world creates constant stress through job problems; lack of sleep; poor diet, including dieting, skipped meals, and high caffeine intake; chemical toxins; and widespread use of prescription drugs without supplementation of the nutrients that become depleted. This continuous stress taxes the adrenal glands until they become first fatigued, and then exhausted. The end result is often an inability to produce DHEA, a precursor hormone to estrogen, progesterone, and testosterone.

Prayer, meditation, yoga, qigong, relaxation therapies, adequate sleep, regular exercise, and a sound diet are all vital to repair of the adrenal glands and normal adrenal function. There are also a number of supplements that can help relieve the symptoms of adrenal fatigue, as well as restore healthy function of the glands.

SUPPLEMENTS FOR ADRENAL SUPPORT

Supplements	Dosage	Considerations
Ashwagandha root	160 mg twice a day	
Carnitine	1,000 to 3,000 mg once a day	The most effective form for this purpose is acetyl-L-carnitine (ALCAR).
Cordyceps	400 mg twice a day	
DHEA	As prescribed by your doctor.	
Ginseng	200 mg twice a day	Always take with food. Do not take if you are taking a blood thinner. Use with caution if you have high blood pressure.
Glycyrrhiza	600 mg twice a day	
Rehmannia root	2,000 mg twice a day	
Rhodiola	50 mg twice a day	
Vitamin B_6 (pyridoxine)	100 mg twice a day	Do not take more than 500 mg a day. If you are taking L-dopa for Parkinson's disease, do not take B_6 without first consulting your doctor.

| Vitamin C | 500 to 1,000 mg twice a day | Do not take high dosages if you are prone to kidney stones or gout. |

SUPPLEMENTS FOR STRESS ACCOMPANIED BY ANXIETY AND JITTERINESS		
Supplements	Dosage	Considerations
Ashwagandha root	1,000 mg once a day	
Bacopa	5 to 13 mg of 1:2 liquid extract once a day	
B-complex vitamins	50 mg twice a day	I suggest taking a multi-vitamin.
Chromium	300 mcg once a day	Combining with the protein picolinate allows your body to absorb chromium more efficiently. However, some chromium picolinate supplements contain more chromium than necessary. Ask your healthcare provider for a recommendation on chromium consumption.
EPA/DHA (fish oil)	2,000 mg once a day	Choose a source that contains vitamin E to prevent oxidation.
Gamma-amino-butyric acid (GABA)	300 to 1,200 mg once a day	GABA may make you drowsy, so begin by taking before bed.
Holy basil	Use as directed by practitioner.	
Inositol	50 to 100 mg once a day	May stimulate uterine contractions. Women who wish to become pregnant should consult their doctor regarding its use.
Magnesium	400 to 600 mg once a day	Consult healthcare provider for dosage if you have kidney disease. Discontinue use and see your doctor if you experience abdominal pain. Take a lower dose if it causes diarrhea.
Rehmannia root	2,000 mg twice a day	
Taurine	2,000 mg once a day	Take between meals. Discontinue use if you suddenly have feelings of chest or throat tightness or if you break out in hives. Do not take with aspirin.

SUPPLEMENTS FOR STRESS ACCOMPANIED BY FATIGUE

Supplements	Dosage	Considerations
Ashwagandha root	1,000 mg once a day	
Bacopa	5 to 13 mg of 1:2 liquid extract once a day	
B-complex vitamins	50 mg twice a day	I recommend taking a multi-vitamin.
Cordyceps	400 mg twice a day	
Ginseng	200 mg twice a day	Always take with food. Do not take if you are taking a blood thinner. Use with caution if you have high blood pressure.
Holy basil	Use as directed by practitioner.	
Rhodiola	50 mg twice a day	

ALLERGIES

See Food Allergies.

ALOPECIA

See Hair Loss.

ALZHEIMER'S DISEASE

Alzheimer's disease, the most common form of dementia, is a progressive deterioration of the brain. It affects memory and thought, as well as communication and the ability to make decisions. Although the symptoms are usually mild at the onset of the disease, they often progress to such an extent that work and socializing become impossible.

Alzheimer's usually afflicts people who are over the age of sixty. The most common symptoms are memory loss, inability to recognize family or friends, difficulty speaking and remembering words, personality changes, and difficulty making decisions. If you fear that yourself or someone you love may have Alzheimer's, see a doctor for a diagnosis. This disease is incurable, but its progress can often be slowed down. The following supplements can help.

SUPPLEMENTS TO TREAT ALZHEIMER'S DISEASE

Supplements	Dosage	Considerations
Acetyl-L-Carnitine	1,500 to 3,000 mg once a day	
Alpha-lipoic acid	200 to 400 mg once a day	Improves blood sugar levels so diabetics may be able to take less medication.
B-complex vitamins	50 mg twice a day	I suggest taking a multi-vitamin.
Bilberry	200 mg once a day	May cause low blood sugar levels.
Carotenoids	10,000 to 20,000 IU once a day	Do not take for extended periods of time. Do not take high dosages if you have liver disease, are a smoker, or are exposed to asbestos.
Coenzyme Q_{10}	100 to 300 mg once a day	May reduce the effects of blood thinners. Dosages over 100 mg may cause diarrhea.
EPA/DHA (fish oil)	1,000 to 2,000 mg once a day	Choose a source that contains vitamin E to prevent oxidation.
Ginkgo biloba	120 to 240 mg once a day	Do not use if taking a blood thinner.
Huperzine A	50 mcg once a day	This Chinese herb should not be taken with other medications for Alzheimer's disease.
Inositol	500 mg twice a day	May stimulate uterine contractions. Women who wish to become pregnant should consult their doctor regarding its use.
Magnesium	400 to 600 mg once a day	Consult healthcare provider for dosage if you have kidney disease. Discontinue use and see your doctor if you experience abdominal pain. Take a lower dose if it causes diarrhea.
NADH	5 mg twice a day	Reduced and more active form of niacin.
Phosphatidylcholine (Lecithin)	200 to 600 mg once a day	Use with caution if you have malabsorption problems, as this could exacerbate them.
Phosphatidylserine	300 to 500 mg once a day	This product is particularly helpful to prevent Alzheimer's, as well as toward the onset of the disease.
Selenium	200 mcg once a day	
Vinpocetine	10 to 40 mg once a day	Do not take if you are taking a blood thinner.

Vitamin B$_9$ (folic acid)	1,000 mcg once a day	High doses can deplete your body of other vitamins in the B complex.
Vitamin B$_{12}$ (cobalamin)	5,000 to 10,000 mcg once a day	High doses can deplete your body of other vitamins in the B complex.
Vitamin C	1,000 to 2,500 mg twice a day	Do not take high dosages if you are prone to kidney stones or gout.
Vitamin D	Have your blood levels measured by your health-care provider, who will then determine proper dosage.	
Vitamin E	400 IU once a day	Take mixed tocopherols, the more active type of vitamin E. Consult healthcare provider first if you are taking a blood thinner.

SUPPLEMENTS TO IMPROVE MEMORY		
Supplements	Dosage	Considerations
Acetyl-L-Carnitine	1,000 to 2,000 mg once a day	
Alpha-lipoic acid	100 to 200 mg once a day	Improves blood sugar levels so diabetics may be able to take less medication.
B-complex vitamins	50 mg twice a day	I suggest taking a multi-vitamin.
Coenzyme Q$_{10}$	100 to 200 mg once a day	May reduce the effects of blood thinners.
EPA/DHA (fish oil)	1,000 to 2,000 mg once a day	Choose a source that contains vitamin E to prevent oxidation.
Ginkgo biloba	100 to 250 mg once a day	Do not take if you are taking a blood thinner.
N-acetylcysteine (NAC)	1,000 mg once a day	When taking NAC supplements, also take extra vitamin C, copper, and zinc.
Phosphatidylcholine (Lecithin)	1,000 to 4,000 mg once a day	Use with caution if you have malabsorption problems, as this could exacerbate them.
Phosphatidylserine	200 to 300 mg once a day	
Resveratrol	20 mg a day	
Selenium	100 to 200 mcg once a day	

Vinpocetine	5 mg three times a day	Do not take if you are taking a blood thinner.
Vitamin A and mixed carotenoids	5,000 IU—half vitamin A and half mixed carotenoids—once a day	Use caution when taking vitamin A supplements because they have the potential to be toxic. Do not take for extended periods of time. Do not take high doses if you have liver disease, are a smoker, or are exposed to asbestos.
Vitamin B$_9$ (folic acid)	800 mcg once a day	High doses can deplete your body of other vitamins in the B complex.
Vitamin B$_{12}$ (cobalamin)	1,000 mcg once a day	High doses can deplete your body of other vitamins in the B complex.
Vitamin C	500 to 1,000 mg twice a day	Do not take high dosages if you are prone to kidney stones or gout.
Vitamin E	400 to 800 IU once a day	May need to take a lower dose if on a blood thinner.

ANOREXIA NERVOSA

Anorexia nervosa is an eating disorder that arises from a person's intense fear of being overweight. There are many ways that anorexic people control their weight, including starvation, obsessive exercising, purging, and taking diuretics. Although most anorexics have a low—usually unhealthily so—body weight, they often have a distorted self-image. A large majority of anorexics are female, but more and more males are affected each year.

This eating disorder is one of the most dangerous psychiatric disorders. It affects many people and has a variety of serious consequences. Hair can become brittle and fall out; skin can easily bruise; the immune system can weaken; the menstrual cycle can be disrupted; and nerves can deteriorate, causing severe pain during simple movement. There are dozens of other related symptoms that can occur as well. Anorexia can also have devastating effects on the heart and cardiovascular system, and can cause electrolyte imbalances. (The dangers of electrolyte imbalance were discussed in Chapter 2.) Cardiac arrest and even death can occur.

The harm to physical health is very serious, but anorexia can also cause behavioral problems including withdrawal from friends and activities, self-harming, and suicidal thoughts. The problem can extend into every part of the person's life. If you are or someone you know is anorexic, it is important that you seek professional help immediately.

SUPPLEMENTS TO TREAT ANOREXIA NERVOSA		
Supplements	Dosage	Considerations
Amino acid supplements	Individualized compounds are composed from results of amino acid testing.	
Carnitine	500 mg once a day	
Coenzyme Q_{10}	30 to 50 mg once a day	May reduce the effects of blood thinners.
EPA/DHA (fish oil)	500 to 1,000 mg once a day	Choose a source that contains vitamin E to prevent oxidation.
Gamma-linolenic acid (GLA)	480 to 720 mg once a day	It is important to maintain the proper ratio of omega-6 fatty acids to omega-3 fatty acids. (See page 110.)
Magnesium	400 mg once a day	Consult healthcare provider for dosage if you have kidney disease. Discontinue use and see your doctor if you experience abdominal pain. Take a lower dose if it causes diarrhea.
Taurine	500 mg once a day	Take between meals. Discontinue use if you suddenly have feelings of chest or throat tightness or if you break out in hives. Do not take with aspirin.
Vitamin A and mixed carotenoids	5,000 IU—half vitamin A and half mixed carotenoids—once a day	Use caution when taking vitamin A supplements because they have the potential to be toxic. Do not take for extended periods of time. Do not take high doses if you have liver disease, are a smoker, or are exposed to asbestos.
Zinc	25 to 50 mg once a day	Take zinc picolinate or zinc citrate. If you are taking zinc and iron supplements, take one in the morning and one in the evening.

ANXIETY

Anxiety can be a normal state of mind that allows you to react appropriately to uncomfortable or dangerous situations. However, several million Americans find themselves burdened by excessive apprehension, fear, and stress. When this reaction is disproportionate to the situation, it may be the result of an anxiety disorder. The three main causes of these disorders are genetics, life experiences, and brain chemistry.

Increased blood pressure, heart rate, and sweating are common ways that feelings of anxiety are exhibited. Anxiety can also manifest itself in chest pains, muscle tension, panic attacks, and shortness of breath, as well as a variety of other symptoms. See a doctor if any of these problems interfere with your daily life or become crippling. If your anxiety is not hindering your normal activities but is causing you discomfort, the following nutrients may be sufficient in treating the problem. Avoiding alcohol, caffeine, and sugar may also help. However, you may still want to consider seeing a doctor, who can help you discover the root of your anxiety.

SUPPLEMENTS TO TREAT ANXIETY		
Supplements	Dosage	Considerations
B-complex vitamins	50 mg twice a day	I suggest taking a multi-vitamin.
Calcium	600 mg twice a day	Although most people are deficient in calcium, there is a danger in taking too much calcium. Do not ingest more than 1,000 to 1,200 mg of calcium a day.
Gamma-amino butyric acid (GABA)	375 to 750 mg three times a day	Must be taken with vitamin B_6, which will act as a cofactor and allow your body to metabolize GABA. May make your drowsy, so take before going to bed.
Glutamine	1,000 mg once a day	If you have a sensitivity to monosodium glutamate (MSG), use glutamine with caution. If you are taking medications for seizures, only take glutamine under the direction of your doctor.
Glycine	1,000 mg once a day	Do not take with clozapine or other atypical antipsychotic medications.
Inositol	12 g once a day (under medical supervision)	May stimulate uterine contractions. Women who wish to become pregnant should consult their doctor regarding its use.
Magnesium	300 to 600 mg once a day	Consult healthcare provider for dosage if you have kidney disease. Discontinue use and see your doctor if you experience abdominal pain. Take a lower dose if it causes diarrhea.
Theanine	200 to 400 mg once a day	

ARTERIOSCLEROSIS

See Atherosclerosis.

ARTHRITIS

Arthritis occurs when there is damage to the joints. It can cause pain, stiffness, and swelling to the affected area. Sufferers often experience diminished mobility of the affected limb. The type of arthritis is determined by its cause. Conventional forms of treatment include physical therapy and medication. *See also* Gout; Inflammation; Osteoarthritis; Rheumatoid Arthritis.

ASTHMA

Asthma is a condition in which a person's *airways*—the tubes through which air travels to and from the lungs—become periodically inflamed. The inflammation causes the tubes to narrow, restricting the amount of air that can be inhaled. Asthma sufferers exhibit symptoms such as coughing, shortness of breath, and wheezing.

Asthma can have mild to serious—even life-threatening—effects. During an asthma attack, a person cannot inhale the proper amount of air and cannot breathe normally. The degree to which air is restricted and the length of the attacks determine the severity of the illness. Also, some people with asthma have, besides these acute attacks, permanent respiratory problems that may restrict their daily activities.

Attacks can be triggered by allergens, such as animal dander, chemicals, environmental pollution, or smoke. Treatment should begin by identifying and removing, if possible, any applicable triggers. On the other hand, asthma attacks can also be caused by adrenal disorders, anxiety, changes in temperature, exercise, stress, and other unavoidable factors. When the triggers cannot be removed, treatment usually consists of controlling and monitoring the attacks. The doctor will be able to help the asthma patient prepare for attacks as well as identify when an asthma attack is coming. This can often prevent the more serious symptoms.

SUPPLEMENTS TO TREAT ASTHMA

Supplements	Dosage	Considerations
B-complex vitamins	100 mg once a day	I suggest taking a multi-vitamin.
Carotenoids	50 to 5,000 IU once a day	Do not take for extended periods of time. Do not take high dosages if you have liver disease, are a smoker, or are exposed to asbestos.
Curcumin	100 to 1,000 mg once a day	
EPA/DHA (fish oil)	2,000 mg once a day	Choose a source that contains vitamin E to prevent oxidation.
Gingko biloba	80 to 240 mg once a day	Do not use if on a blood thinner.
Grape seed extract	300 mg three times a day	
Magnesium	400 to 600 mg once a day	Consult healthcare provider for dosage if you have kidney disease. Discontinue use and see your doctor if you experience abdominal pain. Take a lower dose if it causes diarrhea.
Methylsulfonyl-methane (MSM)	3,000 to 15,000 mg once a day	When beginning supplementation, ingest with meals to avoid possible heartburn. May cause stomach upset in dosages larger than 6,000 mg.
N-acetylcysteine (NAC)	1,000 to 2,000 mg once a day	When taking NAC supplements, also take extra vitamin C, copper, and zinc.
Probiotics	20 billion units once a day	If taking an antibiotic, wait three hours before taking probiotics.
Quercetin	100 to 900 mg once a day	
Selenium	400 mcg once a day	
Taurine	1,000 to 3,000 mg once a day	Take between meals. Discontinue use if you suddenly have feelings of chest or throat tightness or if you break out in hives. Do not take with aspirin.
Vitamin B_9	1,000 mg once a day (folic acid)	High doses can deplete your body of other vitamins in the B complex.
Vitamin B_{12} (cobalamin)	5,000 mcg once a day	High doses can deplete your body of other vitamins in the B complex.
Vitamin C	1,000 mg twice a day	Do not take high dosages if you are prone to kidney stones or gout.

Vitamin E	400 to 800 IU once a day	Take mixed tocopherols, the more active type of vitamin E. Consult healthcare provider first if you are taking a blood thinner.
Zinc	25 mg once a day	The best zinc supplements are zinc picolinate and zinc citrate. If you are taking zinc and iron supplements, take one in the morning and one in the evening. (Taking them together reduces the efficiency of both.)

ATHEROSCLEROSIS

Atherosclerosis, or *arteriosclerosis,* is a buildup of fat deposits on the walls of your arteries. These deposits cause cartilage in the arteries to lose elasticity and the artery walls to become hard and thick.

Atherosclerosis can lead to major health problems. The fat may continue to grow inside the artery until the deposits rupture. This causes the artery to narrow, which limits the amount of blood that can travel its path. Suddenly, vital organs may not be receiving the blood they need to function. Doctors may treat severely clogged arteries by performing an angioplasty. This procedure restretches and widens the narrow arteries so that the blood can flow more smoothly through the body.

On the other hand, the fat may not rupture. Instead, an *aneurysm*—a bulge in the wall of an artery—may form to accommodate the growing size of the deposits. Unfortunately, the aneurysm can burst and cause a stroke. There are several treatment options available for people with aneurysms. It is important to take care of the problem with the help of your doctor since both ruptured fat deposits and aneurysms can cause life-threatening problems, such as blood clots, cardiac arrest, heart attack, or stroke.

Risk factors for developing atherosclerosis include family history of heart disease, high cholesterol levels (see page 280), hypertension (see page 276), and smoking (see page 357). Yet these factors do not apply to a large percentage of people with atherosclerosis. Research is still being performed on the disease so that we can gain a more complete understanding of it. But there are precautions you can take. Along with the nutrients listed starting on page 227, a diet rich in olive oil and "good" fats wards off many deaths related to atherosclerosis.

SUPPLEMENTS TO PREVENT ATHEROSCLEROSIS

Supplements	Dosage	Considerations
B-complex vitamins	100 mg once a day	I suggest taking a multi-vitamin.
Carnitine	1,000 to 4,000 mg once a day	
Chromium	400 mcg once a day	Combining with the protein picolinate allows your body to absorb chromium more efficiently. However, some chromium picolinate supplements contain more chromium than necessary. Ask your health-care provider for a recommendation on chromium consumption.
Coenzyme Q$_{10}$	60 to 100 mg once a day	May reduce the effects of blood thinners.
Copper	2 to 4 mg once a day	Your copper-to-zinc ratio is very important for your health. Also, do not take copper supplement cupric oxide, which has a very low bioavailability.
EPA/DHA (fish oil)	500 to 2,000 mg once a day	Choose a source that contains vitamin E to prevent oxidation.
Fiber, soluble		Choose a fiber supplement with no added sugar. Supplement with several glasses of water.
Gamma-linolenic acid (GLA)	480 mg once a day	It is important to maintain the proper ratio of omega-6 fatty acids to omega-3 fatty acids. (See page 110.)
Magnesium	500 to 1,000 mg once a day	Consult healthcare provider for dosage if you have kidney disease. Discontinue use and see your doctor if you experience abdominal pain. Take a lower dose if it causes diarrhea.
Niacin	100 mg once a day	Do not drink alcohol or hot drinks within one hour of taking niacin.
Phosphatidylcholine (Lecithin)	2,000 to 4,000 mg once a day	Use with caution if you have malabsorption problems, as this could exacerbate them.
Taurine	1,000 to 2,000 mg once a day	Take between meals. Discontinue use if you suddenly have feelings of chest or throat tightness or if you break out in hives. Do not take with aspirin.
Vitamin B$_9$ (folic acid)	500 mcg once a day	High doses can deplete your body of other vitamins in the B complex.

Vitamin B$_{12}$ (cobalamin)	500 to 1,000 mcg once a day	High doses can deplete your body of other vitamins in the B complex.
Vitamin C	500 to 2,500 mg twice a day	Do not take high dosages if you are prone to kidney stones or gout.
Vitamin E	400 IU once a day	Take mixed tocopherols, the more active type of vitamin E. Consult healthcare provider first if you are taking a blood thinner.
Zinc	25 to 50 mg once a day	The best zinc supplements are zinc picolinate and zinc citrate. If you are taking zinc and iron supplements, take one in the morning and one in the evening. (Taking them together reduces the efficiency of both.)

ATTENTION DEFICIT DISORDER

See ADD/ADHD.

AUTOIMMUNE DISEASES

Your immune system is supposed to respond to injury, infection, and other irritation by inflaming and thus protecting the affected area. It does this with the release of antibodies, which combat the problem. The immune systems of people with autoimmune diseases, on the other hand, trigger this response without being prompted by outside stimuli. These antibodies are called autoantibodies, and they attack normal, healthy tissue.

There are many different autoimmune diseases. They are classified according to the single body part they affect or whether they are *systemic*. Systemic disorders affect the body as a whole, and the attack occurs to many of the body's organs. When a single organ or tissue is involved, the disease is referred to as *localized*. It is possible for a person to be affected by more than one autoimmune disease. At the same time, some share similar symptoms.

Most autoimmune diseases are usually either genetic or caused by a bacteria or virus. Treatment can vary depending on the type of autoimmune disease, but often consists of immunosuppresive drugs, anti-inflammatory medication, or an effort to alleviate symptoms and relieve pain. If you believe you may have an autoimmune disorder, you should see your physician. *See* Crohn's Disease; Hashimoto's Thyroiditis; Lupus; Multiple Sclerosis; Myasthenia Gravis; Rheumatoid Arthritis; Scleroderma; Sjögren's Syndrome.

■ Symptoms of an Autoimmune Disease

- Clear, watery discharge from nose or eyes
- Cough or wheezing
- Dark circles under eyes
- Easy bruising
- Extreme dryness of eyes, nasal passages, or mouth
- Foot pain, inflammation, and/or stiffness
- Heart palpitations after eating particular foods
- Localized or general itching
- Loss of hair (on head and/or rest of body)
- Migraine headaches
- Moody, irritable behavior
- Muscle weakness
- Muscles fatigue quickly
- Nails loosened, pitted, and/or discolored
- Pain and/or stiffness throughout body
- Postnasal drip with certain foods
- Severe fatigue
- Sensitivity to light (skin or eyes)
- Severe pain, redness, and/or swelling of the joints
- Sneezing
- Swollen face or body
- Weight loss

BALDING

See Hair Loss.

BENIGN PROSTATIC HYPERTROPHY (BPH)

Benign prostatic hypertrophy (BPH) is a noncancerous condition in which the prostate of an aging man becomes enlarged. The prostate may then push against the urethra and bladder. Symptoms include frequent, difficult, or painful urination. Although it is unknown *why* the prostate becomes enlarged, it is known that it becomes more common with age. Men fifty-one to sixty years of age have a 40- to 50-percent chance of having benign prostate enlargement. Men over the age of 80 have an 80-percent chance.

These urination problems usually begin quite mildly, but you should see your doctor if they occur. He will perform a rectal exam to determine whether the problem is actually BPH. This is very important, because the symptoms can also be indicative of a more serious problem. To patients with BPH, doctors will often suggest to wait and see if their situations improve without any medication treatment. Many patients have found it helpful to take the nutrients in the table below. If the symptoms do not go away or if they become more uncomfortable, there are two popular options available. The first is medication. There are several different kinds of applicable medications. However, some cause (mostly sexual) side effects—and the BPH symptoms tend to come back when medication is stopped. The most successful treatment is surgery. Yet doctors often consider surgery a last resort because it does pose a small degree of risk to the patient. Your doctor will be able to suggest which option is most appropriate to your situation.

SUPPLEMENTS TO TREAT BENIGN PROSTATIC HYPERTROPHY

Supplements	Dosage	Considerations
Amino acids: alanine, glutamic acid, and glycine	As measured by your doctor.	
B-vitamin complex	25 to 50 mg twice a day	I suggest taking a multi-vitamin.
Copper	1 to 2 mg once a day	Your copper-to-zinc ratio is very important for your health. Also, do not take copper supplement cupric oxide, which has a very low bioavailability.
Flaxseed	1,000 mg once a day	May interfere with anticoagulants, work as a laxative, or affect blood sugar levels.
Gamma-linolenic acid (GLA)	500 mg once a day	It is important to maintain the proper ratio of omega-6 fatty acids to omega-3 fatty acids. (See page 110.)
Lycopene	10 mg once a day	If eaten in food, best absorbed when cooked with fat.
Saw palmetto	320 mg once a day	Use with caution if taking a blood thinner.
Selenium	100 to 200 mcg once a day	
Soy isoflavones	50 to 300 mg once a day	
Stinging needles	100 mg (of 10:1 extract) once a day	

Vitamin A and mixed carotenoids	5,000 to 10,000 IU— half vitamin A and half mixed carotenoids —once a day	Use caution when taking vitamin A supplements because they have the potential to be toxic. Do not take for extended periods of time. Do not take high dosages if you have liver disease, are a smoker, or are exposed to asbestos.
Vitamin C	1,000 mg once a day	Do not take high dosages if you are prone to kidney stones or gout.
Vitamin E	400 to 800 IU once a day	Take mixed tocopherols, the more active type of vitamin E. Consult healthcare provider first if you are taking a blood thinner.
Zinc	35 to 50 mg once a day	The best zinc supplements are zinc picolinate and zinc citrate. If you are taking zinc and iron supplements, take one in the morning and one in the evening. (Taking them together reduces the efficiency of both.)

Herbs to Help the Prostate Gland

Various prostate problems affect a large number of older men. The following herbs, which help keep this gland healthy, should be taken by most men, regardless of prostate history. Exercising regularly will also help maintain prostate health.

- Buchu
- Cernilton
- Couch grass
- Cramp bark
- Cranberry
- Dong quai (Do not use if you have diabetes.)
- Echinacea (Use short term to treat *prostatitis*—inflammation of the prostate.)
- Garlic
- Goldenseal (Do not use if you have high or low blood pressure, heart disease, diabetes, or glaucoma, or have had a stroke.)
- Juniper
- Marshmallow
- Pipsissewa
- Pycnogenol
- Pygeum (*Pygeum africanum*)
- Rosemary
- Saw palmetto
- Siberian ginseng
- Skullcap
- Stinging nettles (*Urtica dioica*)
- Valerian

BPH

See Benign Prostatic Hypertrophy.

CANCER

Cancer refers to an abnormal and uncontrolled growth of cells. The rene-gade cells form a mass—or *malignant tumor*—that can disrupt and poten-tially destroy the surrounding cells and tissue. They can then spread through a process called *metastasis*. This can occur in nearly any part of the body. The type of cancer is usually named after the location in the body where the tumor originated.

Some tumors are *benign*. They are comprised of similarly abnormal cells, but they do not invade the surrounding areas. Benign tumors needs to be regularly monitored by a doctor because they can become cancerous. Additionally, they can displace the body's regular tissues, which can be harmful if occurring in an area such as the brain. Your doctor can perform a biopsy to determine whether a tumor is malignant or benign.

The goal of cancer treatment is the complete removal of the malignant cells. Certain types of cancers are more treatable than others. There are many different treatment options, with the most common being surgery, chemotherapy, and radiation therapy (or some combination of these three procedures). Surgery is often the best option if the tumor has not yet begun to spread. However, if metastasis has already occurred, it can be difficult to eliminate all the cancerous cells this way. *Chemotherapy*, the use of one or more drugs to destroy the cancer cells, may be used instead. These drugs can be taken orally or intravenously. *Radiation* concentrates ionizing radiation on the infected area in an attempt to kill the cancer or at least alter the cells so that they can no longer multiply. Your doctor will advise you on the most effective way to treat your cancer.

Naturally, it is preferable to avoid cancer in the first place. Although it may be beyond your control, there are steps you can take to decrease your risk. Try to avoid *carcinogens*—cancer-causing agents such as smok-ing tobacco, asbestos, and prolonged exposure to the sun. Recent cancer journals suggest that diet plays an important role, as well. In fact, Dr. Bruce Ames stated that diet "is expected to contribute to about one-third

Cancer Prevention

As you read on page 232, cancer is a group of diseases caused by an uncontrolled growth of cells. The following is a list of recommendations for steps to take to avoid cancer. It is adapted from a list found on the websites of the American Institute for Cancer Research and the World Cancer Research Fund. This list was compiled from extensive research analyzation performed by scientists from these two foundations. Keep in mind that these suggestions are generalized, and each person has individual requirements for health. Therefore, you should see an anti-aging specialist and have your vitamin levels measured to determine a plan that will work specifically for you.

- Keep your weight at a healthy level for your height.
- Get daily exercise.
- Limit consumption of food and drinks high in sugar, low in fiber, and high in fat.
- Increase consumption of vegetables, fruits, whole grains, and beans.
- Avoid both red and processed meats.
- Don't eat too much salt.

- Keep alcohol intake to a minimum. Men should have no more than two drinks daily; women should have no more than one drink daily.
- Avoid both smoking and chewing tobacco.
- Mothers should breastfeed babies for six months after giving birth.
- Cancer survivors should keep their weight at a healthy level to lessen the chance of the cancer's return.

In addition to the above recommendations, the following foods were named by the National Foundation for Cancer Research as the "Top 10 Cancer Fighting Foods." Included after each food is the cancer-fighting agents it contains.

- Acorn squash (contain beta-carotene)
- Apples (contain phytochemicals)
- Berries (contain fiber, vitamin C, phytochemicals, potassium, and vitamin B_9 and are antioxidants)
- Crucifers (contain phytochemicals)
- Extra virgin olive oil (contains phytochemicals with antioxidants and vitamin E)
- Pumpkins (contain beta carotene)

- Mineral, seltzer, or spring water, as well as decaffeinated tea (all of which help with digestion and other bodily functions)
- Peppers (contain potassium, vitamin A, vitamin C, and vitamin B_9)
- Sweet potatoes (contain beta carotene)
- Tomatoes and tomato-based products (contain lycopene, which is an antioxidant)

of preventable cancers." He then pointed specifically to the harm caused by vitamin and mineral deficiencies. The following list of supplements will help you maintain good health and fight the negative effects of carcinogens.

SUPPLEMENTS TO HELP PREVENT CANCER		
Supplements	**Dosage**	**Considerations**
Alpha-lipoic acid	100 to 300 mg once a day	Improves blood sugar levels so diabetics may be able to take less medication.
Chlorella	1 tbsp once a day	Stop taking if experience nausea or gastrointestinal distress. Use with caution if you have allergic tendencies.
Coenzyme Q_{10}	100 to 400 mg once a day	May reduce the effects of blood thinners. You can also take 400 mg of coenzyme Q_{10} if you have breast cancer. May cause diarrhea in dosages above 100 mg once a day.
Conjugated linoleic acid (CLA)	100 to 300 mg once a day	
Curcumin	100 to 1,000 mg once a day	
EPA/DHA (fish oil)	2,000 mg once a day	Choose a source that contains vitamin E to prevent oxidation.
Indole-3-carbinol (I-3-C)	300 to 500 mg once a day	
Iodine	150 mcg once a day	Most table salts contain iodine, but sea salts do not.
Kaprex AI	1 softgel capsule twice a day	Made by Metagenics. Do not use if taking an anticoagulant.
Lycopene	10 to 20 mg once a day	If eaten in food, best absorbed when cooked with fat.
Magnesium	600 mg once a day	Consult healthcare provider for dosage if you have kidney disease. Discontinue use and see your doctor if you experience abdominal pain. Take a lower dose if it causes diarrhea.
Niacinamide	100 to 1,000 mg once a day	
Pycnogenol	20 mg to 40 mg once a day	May affect blood sugar levels.
Quercetin	300 to 900 mg once a day	

Selenium	100 to 200 mcg once a day	
Vitamin A and mixed carotenoids	5,000 IU—half vitamin A and half mixed carotenoids—once a day	Use caution when taking vitamin A supplements because they have the potential to be toxic. Do not take for extended periods of time. Do not take high doses if you have liver disease, are a smoker, or are exposed to asbestos.
Vitamin B₉ (folic acid)	100 to 800 mcg once a day	High doses can deplete your body of other vitamins in the B complex.
Vitamin C	500 to 1,000 mg twice a day	Do not take high dosages if you are prone to kidney stones or gout.
Vitamin D	Have your blood levels measured by your health-care provider, who will then determine proper dosage.	
Vitamin E	400 IU once a day	Take mixed tocopherols, the more active type of vitamin E. Consult healthcare provider first if you are taking a blood thinner.
Zinc	25 mg once a day	The best zinc supplements are zinc picolinate and zinc citrate. If you are taking zinc and iron supplements, take one in the morning and one in the evening. (Taking them together reduces the efficiency of both.)

CANDIDIASIS

Candida albicans, a yeast, is part of your *gut flora*—the microorganisms found in your mouth and digestive tract. It is found in your genital area, intestines, mouth, throat, and urinary areas, and does not usually have any ill effects. However, under certain conditions—such as having a compromised immune system, using certain detergents, chronic antibiotic use, taking oral birth control, consuming excess sugar, or having diabetes—it can grow uncontrolled, resulting in the infection candidiasis.

There are many symptoms of candidiasis. Men usually get red sores near their penis or foreskin while women may have vaginal burning, discharge, or itching. The most common symptoms include abdominal pain, anxiety, bloating, constipation, fatigue, insomnia, intestinal gas, muscle aches, and muscle weakness. However, you may also have chronic rashes or itching, food sensitivity, headaches, moodiness, rectal itching, sinusitis, or a white tongue. Men may also have prostate inflammation. If you suspect you have candidiasis, see your healthcare provider, who will test the infected area.

Candidiasis can be treated. Your symptoms—which often mimic the flu—may get worse for a week or two as the yeast die off. Then, about three weeks after beginning treatment, the budding yeast expire. This can cause the symptoms to resurface.

I recommend CandiBactin-AR and CandiBactin-BR. Both products are by Metagenics and contain several of the items on the list below. CandiBactin-AR contains lemon balm leaf, oregano leaf extract, red thyme oil, and sage leaf. Candibactin-BR contains barberry root extract, berberine sulfate, coptis root, and rhizome extract. Candicid Forte by Ortho Molecular contains many of these herbs, as well. You may also find it helpful to take probiotics (beneficial bacteria) as well as the other nutrients in the table "Supplements to Treat Candidiasis." Continue the regimen for two to six months. At that point, discontinue your use of glutamine. Continue to take probiotics once a day. When the problem has been resolved, try the supplements in the table "Supplements for Long-Term Management of Yeast Overgrowth."

SUPPLEMENTS TO TREAT CANDIDIASIS		
Supplements	Dosage	Considerations
Arginine	1 to 5 g once a day	Except under a doctor's supervision, do not take if you have kidney disease, liver disease, or herpes.
B-complex vitamins	50 mg twice a day	I suggest taking a multi-vitamin.
Candicid Forte or CandiBactin	2 capsules three times a day	These multi-vitamins contain many helpful nutrients, including red thyme oil, sage leaf, barberry root, and grape seed extract. (See Resources.)
Glutamine	5 to 10 g once a day	If you have a sensitivity to monosodium glutamate (MSG), use glutamine with caution. If you are taking medications for seizures, only take glutamine under the direction of your doctor.
Molybdenum	250 to 500 mcg once a day	Check your copper levels after molybdenum supplementation because the two minerals are antagonistic.

| Probiotics | 20 billion units once a day | If taking an antibiotic, wait three hours before taking probiotics. |
| Zinc | 25 mg once a day | The best zinc supplements are zinc picolinate and zinc citrate. If you are taking zinc and iron supplements, take one in the morning and one in the evening. (Taking them together reduces the efficiency of both.) |

SUPPLEMENTS FOR LONG-TERM MANAGEMENT OF YEAST OVERGROWTH

Supplements	Dosage	Considerations
Carnitine	1,000 to 3,000 mg once a day	
Chromium	300 mcg once a day	Combining with the protein picolinate allows your body to absorb chromium more efficiently. However, some chromium picolinate supplements contain more chromium than necessary. Ask your healthcare provider for a recommendation on chromium consumption.
Gamma-linolenic acid (GLA)	240 to 480 mg once a day	It is important to maintain the proper ratio of omega-6 fatty acids to omega-3 fatty acids. (See page 110.)
Magnesium	400 to 800 mg once a day	Consult healthcare provider for dosage if you have kidney disease. Discontinue use and see your doctor if you experience abdominal pain. Take a lower dose if it causes diarrhea.
Taurine	1 to 3 g once a day	Take between meals. Discontinue use if you suddenly have feelings of chest or throat tightness or if you break out in hives. Do not take with aspirin.
Vitamin C	500 mg twice a day	Do not take high dosages if you are prone to kidney stones or gout.
Vitamin E	400 IU once a day	Take mixed tocopherols, the more active type of vitamin E. Consult healthcare provider first if you are taking a blood thinner.

CATARACTS

A cataract is a clouding of the eye's natural lens, which lies behind the iris and the pupil. Lenses are composed largely of water and protein, with the protein being arranged in a precise way. When the protein starts to clump together, a cataract begins to form.

Cataracts can develop for a variety of reasons. Simple old age is probably the most common cause, with other causes including diabetes, long-term ultraviolet exposure, exposure to radiation, genetic factors, and eye injury and trauma. Some drugs, such as corticosteroids, can also induce cataract formation.

When cataracts first start to develop, they have little effect on vision. Sometimes, a newly forming cataract can even *improve* close vision, causing near-sightedness. Over time, though, as the cataract grows, vision becomes impaired. Images may become blurred or fuzzy. Night vision may be poor, and street lights may cause glare or appear to be surrounded by halos. Colors may seem to fade or change. Eventually, if the cataract is left untreated, blindness can result. In advanced cases, the lens can even rupture, leading to severe inflammation.

When a cataract has developed to the point where there is a good deal of vision loss, surgery can remove the clouded lens and replace it with a permanent plastic lens. In earlier stages, however, certain nutrients can slow the formation of cataracts and even prevent them from developing in the first place.

SUPPLEMENTS TO TREAT CATARACTS

Supplements	Dosage	Considerations
Alpha-lipoic acid	100 to 300 mg once a day	Improves blood sugar levels so diabetics may be able to take less medication.
B-complex vitamins	50 to 100 mg once a day	I suggest taking a multi-vitamin.
Beta carotene	5,000 to 10,000 IU once a day	Do not take for extended periods of time. Do not take high dosages if you have liver disease, are a smoker, or are exposed to asbestos.
Bilberry	60 to 240 mg once a day	May cause low blood sugar levels.
Carnosine eye drops	Use as directed.	

Copper	1 mg once a day	Your copper-to-zinc ratio is very important for your health. Also, do not take copper supplement cupric oxide, which has a very low bioavailability.
Lutein	6 mg to 12 mg once a day	
Manganese	2 mg once a day	Ingesting more than 4 mg a day can be toxic. Use with caution if you have liver disease.
N-acetylcysteine (NAC)	500 mg once a day	When taking NAC supplements, also take extra vitamin C, copper, and zinc.
Quercetin	500 to 1,000 mg once a day	
Selenium	100 to 200 mcg once a day	
Vitamin A and mixed carotenoids	5,000 to 10,000 IU— half vitamin A and half mixed carotenoids— once a day	Use caution when taking vitamin A supplements because they have the potential to be toxic. Do not take for extended periods of time. Do not take more than 8,000 IU a day if you have liver disease, are a smoker, or are exposed to asbestos.
Vitamin C	1,000 mg twice a day	Do not take high dosages if you are prone to kidney stones or gout.
Vitamin E	400 to 800 IU once a day	Take mixed tocopherols, the more active type of vitamin E. Consult healthcare provider first if you are taking a blood thinner.
Zinc	25 to 50 mg once a day	The best zinc supplements are zinc picolinate and zinc citrate. If you are taking zinc and iron supplements, take one in the morning and one in the evening. (Taking them together reduces the efficiency of both.)

CEREBROVASCULAR ACCIDENT

See Stroke.

CERVICAL CANCER

Cervical cancer occurs when a woman experiences an uncontrolled growth of cells in the cervix (the lower portion of the uterus). Symptoms include vaginal bleeding and discharge and pelvic pain. There are several different treatment options, including chemotherapy and radiation, and 70 percent of infected women are cured of the cancer after treatment.

Nearly all cases are the result of an infection by the human papillomavirus (HPV), a group of sexually transmitted viruses. However, not all cases of HPV lead to cervical cancer. Some strains of the virus manifest into warts, while others will lay dormant and result in no symptoms. (Some strains can also lead to penile cancer in men.) Gardasil is a new FDA-approved vaccine that protects against many strains of HPV. At the present time, it is only approved for women aged nine to twenty-six.

Cervical dysplasia manifests prior to the cancer's development. During this early stage, the cells begin to undergo the changes that will result in the malignant cells. This is the best time to catch the problem, which can be discovered during a Pap smear or colposcopy (examination of the cervix and vagina). The treatments available for cervical dysplasia—of which there are several methods—can often cure the disease, and many times it even resolves on its own. However, there is a 20-percent recurrence rate, so checkups are advised. Because the frequency of these examinations is decided on a case-by-case basis, this should be determined with the help of a healthcare provider.

SUPPLEMENTS TO PREVENT AND TREAT CERVICAL DYSPLASIA		
Supplements	Dosage	Considerations
Alpha-lipoic acid	100 to 300 mg once a day	Improves blood sugar levels so diabetics may be able to take less medication.
B-complex vitamins	50 mg twice a day	I suggest taking a multi-vitamin.
EPA/DHA (fish oil)	1,000 mg once a day	Choose a source that contains vitamin E to prevent oxidation.
Indole-3-carbinol (I-3-C)	200 to 400 mg once a day	
Quercetin	300 to 900 mg once a day	
Rutin	300 mg once a day	
Selenium	200 mcg once a day	

Vitamin A and mixed carotenoids	50,000 to 100,000 IU— half vitamin A and half mixed carotenoids —once a day	Only take these doses under a doctor's supervision. Do not take for extended periods of time. Do not take high dosages if you have liver disease, are a smoker, or are exposed to asbestos.
Vitamin B_9 (folic acid)	800 mcg once a day	High doses can deplete your body of other vitamins in the B complex.
Vitamin B_{12} (cobalamin)	1,000 to 5,000 mcg once a day	High doses can deplete your body of other vitamins in the B complex.
Vitamin C	500 to 1,000 mg once a day	Do not take high dosages if you are prone to kidney stones or gout.
Vitamin E	400 IU once a day	Take mixed tocopherols, the more active type of vitamin E. Consult healthcare provider first if you are taking a blood thinner.
Zinc	25 mg once a day	The best zinc supplements are zinc picolinate and zinc citrate. If you are taking zinc and iron supplements, take one in the morning and one in the evening. (Taking them together reduces the efficiency of both.)

CERVICAL DYSPLASIA

See Cervical Cancer.

CHOLESTEROL

See High Cholesterol.

CHRONIC FATIGUE SYNDROME

Chronic fatigue syndrome, or CFS, is a debilitating condition character-ized by a profound feeling of fatigue that is not improved by bed rest, and is greatly worsened by activity. In fact, increased fatigue sometimes lasts twenty-four hours after exertion. Other defining symptoms of this condi-tion include substantial impairment in memory and concentration, mus-cle pain, pain in multiple joints, unusual headaches, sore throat, and tender lymph nodes in the neck or armpit. Less common symptoms include abdominal pain, alcohol intolerance, bloating, chest pain, chronic cough, diarrhea, and dizziness. Generally, to be considered chronic fatigue syndrome, symptoms have to persist for six or more consecutive months. This condition affects more than one million people in the United States.

There are no physical signs that allow physicians to identify CFS. Instead, physicians must rule out other disorders that have similar symptoms. Moreover, there is no known cause of CFS, and no known cure. However, it is important to avoid substances like alcohol that can worsen fatigue, to explore the possibility of food allergies, and to use supplements—such as those below—that can foster overall good health and proper energy production. Detoxification can also be helpful.

SUPPLEMENTS TO TREAT CHRONIC FATIGUE SYNDROME

Supplements	Dosage	Considerations
Alpha-lipoic acid	50 to 1,000 mg once a day (above 600 mg see physician for treatment)	Improves blood sugar levels so diabetics may be able to take less medication.
B-complex vitamins	50 mg twice a day	I suggest taking a multi-vitamin.
Bromelain	2,400 mcg three to four times a day	
Carnitine	1,000 to 3,000 mg once a day	The most effective form for this purpose is acetyl-L-carnitine (ALCAR).
Coenzyme Q_{10}	200 mg once a day	May reduce the effects of blood thinners. May cause diarrhea in dosages above 100 mg once a day.
Copper	1 to 3 mg once a day	Your copper-to-zinc ratio is very important for your health. Also, do not take copper supplement cupric oxide, which has a very low bioavailability.
Curcumin	1,500 to 3,000 mg once a day	
EPA/DHA (fish oil)	1,000 to 3,000 mg once a day	Choose a source that contains vitamin E to prevent oxidation.
5-Hydroxy-tryptophan (5-HTP)	100 mg once a day	Do not take with vitamin B_6. Consult your healthcare provider regarding use if you are taking antidepressants. Do not take at the same time as antidepressants or any serotonin-affecting drugs.

Gamma-linolenic acid (GLA)	240 to 720 mg once a day	It is important to maintain the proper ratio of omega-6 fatty acids to omega-3 fatty acids. (See page 110.)
Glutamine	500 to 1,500 mg three times a day	If you have a sensitivity to monosodium glutamate (MSG), use glutamine with caution. If you are taking medications for seizures, only take glutamine under the direction of your doctor.
Magnesium citrate or malate	50 to 1,000 mg once a day	Do not use for longer than ten days unless otherwise directed by healthcare provider.
Malic acid	1,200 to 2,400 mg once a day	
Manganese	2 to 5 mg once a day	
Methylsulfonyl-methane (MSM)	3,000 to 15,000 mg once a day	Use with caution if you are allergic to sulfur. When beginning supplementation, ingest with meals to avoid possible heartburn. May cause stomach upset in dosages larger than 6,000 mg.
N-acetylcysteine (NAC)	500 to 1,000 mg once a day	When taking NAC supplements, also take extra vitamin C, copper, and zinc.
NADH	5 to 10 mg twice a day	Reduced and more active form of niacin.
Phosphatidylserine	200 to 300 mg twice a day	
Probiotics	20 billion units once a day	If taking an antibiotic, wait three hours before taking probiotics.
Quercetin	1,500 mg once a day	
Ribose	5 to 15 g once a day	
Selenium	100 to 200 mcg once a day	
UltraInflamX	Follow instructions on bottle.	Metagenics product. (See Resources.) Do not use if taking a diuretic.
Vitamin A and mixed carotenoids	5,000 IU—half vitamin A and half mixed carotenoids—once a day	Use caution when taking vitamin A supplements because they have the potential to be toxic. Do not take for extended periods of time. Do not take high dosages if you have liver disease, are a smoker, or are exposed to asbestos.
Vitamin C	500 to 3,000 mcg twice	Do not take high dosages if you are prone to kidney stones or gout.

Vitamin D	Have your blood levels measured by your health-care provider, who will then determine proper dosage.	
Vitamin E	400 to 1,000 IU once a day	Take mixed tocopherols, the more active type of vitamin E. Consult healthcare provider first if you are taking a blood thinner.
Vitamin K	100 to 1,000 mcg once a day	High dosages can cause toxicity. Consult your healthcare provider before taking if you are taking a blood thinner.
Zinc	25 to 50 mg once a day	The best zinc supplements are zinc picolinate and zinc citrate. If you are taking zinc and iron supplements, take one in the morning and one in the evening. (Taking them together reduces the efficiency of both.)

CLOSED HEAD INJURY

A closed head injury occurs when there is trauma to the brain without penetration of the skull. The soft tissue of the brain is delicate, and the skull usually serves to protect it. But when a moving head is abruptly stopped—as may occur in a car accident or fall—or when the head is forcibly struck, the brain may hit against the side of the rough, hard skull. The resulting damage, which can include bleeding, swelling, and tearing, can range from mild to serious.

Although doctors used to believe that a closed head injury was less severe than an open head injury (in which the skull has been penetrated), this is not necessarily the case. In fact, an open head injury may actually allow pressure in the brain caused by the accident to be relieved. A closed head injury, on the other hand, allows no outlet for this pressure. Instead, any swelling is constrained, which can cause further, exacerbated damage to both the brain and brain stem.

A person who has had a closed head injury may show no immediate signs of being hurt. The three major problems listed above—bleeding, swelling, and tearing—can go undetected after an accident for hours or even days. However, postponing their discovery can allow these problems to become worse, leading to more permanent damage or even death. If you have a head injury, see a doctor, regardless of whether you are aware of any effects. The following supplements should not be started until after any bleeding, swelling, and tearing has been resolved, unless otherwise directed by a healthcare provider.

SUPPLEMENTS TO TREAT A CLOSED HEAD INJURY		
Supplements	**Dosage**	**Considerations**
Calcium citrate	500 mg twice a day	
Coenzyme Q_{10}	120 mg once a day	May reduce the effects of blood thinners. May cause diarrhea in dosages above 100 mg once a day.
Copper	2 mg twice a day	Your copper-to-zinc ratio is very important for your health. Also, do not take copper supplement cupric oxide, which has a very low bioavailability.
EPA/DHA (fish oil)	3,000 mg once a day	Choose a source that contains vitamin E to prevent oxidation.
Flaxseed	1,000 mg once a day	
Magnesium citrate	600 to 800 mg once a day	Do not take if you have kidney disease. Do not use for longer than ten days unless otherwise directed by healthcare provider.
Multi-vitamin	1 tablet once a day or as directed	
Phosphatidylserine	300 mg once a day	
Vitamin B_5 (pantothenic acid)	100 mg twice a day	Stop taking B_5 supplements if you begin having chest pains or breathing problems.
Vitamin B_6 (pyridoxine)	100 mg twice a day	Do not take more than 500 mg a day. If you are taking L-dopa for Parkinson's disease, do not take B_6 without first consulting your doctor.
Zinc	25 mg twice a day	The best zinc supplements are zinc picolinate and zinc citrate. If you are taking zinc and iron supplements, take one in the morning and one in the evening. (Taking them together reduces the efficiency of both.)

COMMON COLD

The common cold is a viral infection of the upper respiratory tract. The most common of all diseases, colds are characterized by congestion, coughing, headache, runny nose, and sneezing. (Although some people exhibit a slight fever, a high temperature is usually indicative of influenza rather than a cold.) Most of these symptoms are the attempts of your immune system to fight the virus. They usually clear up in five to ten days, after which there is a several-week period of residual coughing and slight congestion.

Colds are extremely contagious, but there are steps you can take to protect yourself. Avoid close contact with infected people. Whenever possible, wash your hands, which can remove viruses before they enter your body. Do not touch your face until you have washed your hands. If you believe you have been exposed to a cold or if your symptoms have already begun, ingest the following supplements. They will help shorten the duration of your cold and lessen its severity.

SUPPLEMENTS TO TREAT THE COMMON COLD		
Supplements	Dosage	Considerations
Echinacea	Twice a day	Do not use long term.
Essential Defense	One to two tablets every hour or as needed	Metagenics product. (See Resources.)
N-acetylcysteine (NAC)	1,000 to 3,000 mg once a day	When taking NAC supplements, also take extra vitamin C, copper, and zinc.
Taurine	2,000 mg once a day	Take between meals. Discontinue use if you suddenly have feelings of chest or throat tightness or if you break out in hives. Do not take with aspirin.
Vitamin C	1,000 to 2,500 mg twice a day	Do not take high dosages if you are prone to kidney stones or gout.
Zinc	25 to 50 mg once a day	The best zinc supplements are zinc picolinate and zinc citrate. If you are taking zinc and iron supplements, take one in the morning and one in the evening. (Taking them together reduces the efficiency of both.)

CONCUSSION

See Closed Head Injury.

CONGESTIVE HEART FAILURE

Congestive heart failure, also called *congestive cardiac failure* or simply *heart failure,* is a condition in which the heart is unable to pump an adequate amount of blood throughout the body. The failing heart keeps working, but not as efficiently as it should.

The symptoms of congestive heart failure can include *edema*—fluid build-up that can result in swollen legs and ankles; shortness of breath; fatigue; and nocturnal cough. But because these can also be signs of other disorders, a physician is needed to confirm diagnosis.

Congestive heart failure can have many causes, including narrowing of the arteries that supply blood to the heart muscle (coronary artery disease), scar tissue due to past heart attacks, high blood pressure (hypertension), heart valve disease, primary disease of the heart muscle (cardiomyopathy), congenital heart defects, and infection of the heart valves and/or muscles of the heart. If a specific cause can be found, it is generally treated and, if possible, corrected. Other treatments may include rest, dietary modifications, changes in daily activities, and appropriate medications. Supplements that protect and enhance the health of the heart and blood vessels can also be an important part of congestive heart failure management.

SUPPLEMENTS TO TREAT CONGESTIVE HEART FAILURE

Supplements	Dosage	Considerations
Arginine	3,000 to 9,000 mg once a day	Except under a doctor's supervision, do not take if you have kidney disease, liver disease, or herpes.
Berberine	300 to 500 mg four times a day	
Carnitine	2,000 mg once a day	
Coenzyme Q_{10}	120 to 400 mg once a day	May reduce the effects of blood thinners. May cause diarrhea in dosages above 100 mg once a day.
EPA/DHA (fish oil)	2,000 to 3,000 mg once a day	For most patients EPA/DHA is very helpful but for some it can worsen condition, so only use under the guidance of your physician. Choose a source that contains vitamin E to prevent oxidation.

Hawthorn	160 to 900 mg once a day	If you are on a blood pressure medication, this herb may decrease the appropriate dosage. See your healthcare provider.
Magnesium	600 to 800 mg once a day	Consult healthcare provider for dosage if you have kidney disease. Discontinue use and see your doctor if you experience abdominal pain. Take a lower dose if it causes diarrhea.
Potassium	See your healthcare provider for dosage directions.	
Ribose	5 to 30 g once a day	D-ribose is most effective for this purpose.
Selenium	100 to 200 mcg once a day	
Vitamin B_1 (thiamine)	50 to 200 mg once a day	High doses can deplete your body of other vitamins in the B complex.
Vitamin E	400 IU once a day	Take mixed tocopherols, the more active type of vitamin E. Consult healthcare provider first if you are taking a blood thinner.

CROHN'S DISEASE

Crohn's disease is a chronic inflammatory bowel disease. It affects the gastrointestinal tract by causing inflammation and swelling. The cause is unknown, but many doctors believe that the inflammation is due to a misdirected attack by the immune system.

Crohn's disease can attack any part of the gastrointestinal tract, from the mouth to the anus. The name of the exact illness is derived from the location of the problem. Ileocolic Crohn's disease, the most prevalent type, affects the large intestine and the part of the small intestine that connects to the large intestine. Crohn's ileitis is less common, and affects the *ileum*—the part of the small intestine that connects to the colon. Only 20 percent of people with Crohn's disease have Crohn's colitis, which inflames the large intestine.

Crohn's disease is made up of periods of outbreaks followed by periods of remission. Symptoms of outbreaks include abdominal cramps, diarrhea, rectal bleeding, and weight loss. The skin around the anus is often the site of itchiness, fissures, or abscesses. Long term, Crohn's disease can damage other organs, such as the eyes and kidneys, and it also increases the risk of cancer of the inflamed areas.

There is no cure for Crohn's disease. Treatment aims to decrease the inflammation and shorten outbreaks, as well as prolonging periods of remission. Doctors usually prescribe anti-inflammatories or antibiotics. Some patients have the most success with *immunosuppressive drugs*—medication that suppresses the immune system. Although these drugs are often effective at restricting the immune system's attack on the body, however, they also limit the immune system when fighting actual infection or other problem. Therefore, their use can result in a host of other health issues. Use of supplements to treat Crohn's disease often allows less medication to be used. In some cases, the medication can even be discontinued. Before changing your dosage or stopping your medication, however, please see your healthcare provider.

SUPPLEMENTS TO TREAT CROHN'S DISEASE		
Supplements	Dosage	Considerations
EPA/DHA (fish oil)	1,000 to 5,000 mg once a day (may use up to 10,000 mg under the direction of your healthcare provider)	Choose a source that contains vitamin E to prevent oxidation.
Eleuthero	50 to 200 mg once a day	Do not use if you have a history of heart disease.
Gamma-linolenic acid (GLA)	240 to 720 mg once a day	It is important to maintain the proper ratio of omega-6 fatty acids to omega-3 fatty acids. (See page 110.)
Glucosamine	300 to 900 mg once a day	Don't take if you are allergic to shellfish. Consult use with your healthcare provider if you have diabetes because glucosamine can alter blood sugar levels.
Glutamine	1 to 5 g once a day	If you have a sensitivity to monosodium glutamate (MSG), use glutamine with caution. If you are taking medications for seizures, only take glutamine under the direction of your doctor.
Kaprex AI	1 softgel capsule twice a day	Made by Metagenics. (See Resources.) Do not use if taking an anticoagulant.

Magnesium	400 to 800 mg once a day	Consult healthcare provider for dosage if you have kidney disease. Discontinue use and see your doctor if you experience abdominal pain. Take a lower dose if it causes diarrhea.
Olive leaf extract	1 capsule one to three times daily	Take with food.
Probiotics	20 billion units once a day	If taking an antibiotic, wait three hours before taking probiotics.
Selenium	200 mcg once a day	
Vitamin C	500 to 1,500 mg twice a day	Do not take high dosages if you are prone to kidney stones or gout.
Vitamin E	400 IU once a day	Take mixed tocopherols, the more active type of vitamin E. Consult healthcare provider first if you are taking a blood thinner.

DEMENTIA

See Alzheimer's Disease.

DEPRESSION

Depression is a state of intense sadness, melancholy, or despair that lasts for a prolonged period of time—sometimes for months. In some cases, it does not seriously affect the individual's ability to function. When it does disrupt function, it is referred to as *clinical depression*. According to the National Institute of Mental Health, one in ten people suffer from a depressive illness of some type each year.

The symptoms of depression can include sadness, fatigue, irritability, apathy, feelings of isolation, loss of interest in favorite activities, hopelessness, insomnia, significant weight changes, aches and pains, and even thoughts of death or suicide. It has been found that symptoms vary according to age, gender, and culture. For instance, a depressed teen-age boy is more likely to experience irritability and grumpiness, while a grown man who is depressed is more likely to experience sleep problems, fatigue, and loss of interest in work and hobbies. Sometimes, there appears to be a cause of the depression, such as loss of a loved one or declining health. In other cases, no obvious cause can be found.

Nutritional deficiencies are associated with depression, so certain supplements can help treat this disorder. But because depression can not only have a great impact on daily life, but even lead to suicide, it is important to consult a physician if you suspect that you or a loved one suffers from this disorder. A doctor should also be consulted about the nutritional aspect of treatment, as certain medications may contraindicate the use of some supplements.

■ Nutritional Deficiencies Linked with Depression

- B vitamins, particularly B_1 (thiamine), B_2 (riboflavin), B_6 (pyridoxine), B_7 (biotin), B_9 (folic acid), and B_{12} (cobalamin)

- Calcium

- Copper

- Iron

- Magnesium

- Vanadium

- Zinc

Fatty acid deficiencies can also contribute to depression. Your doctor can have your fatty acid and mineral levels analyzed by a laboratory company such as Genova Diagnostics. (See Resources for contact information.) A laboratory company such as SpectraCell, on the other hand, can measure your vitamin levels. When treating depression nutritionally, it is important to see an anti-aging specialist who is fellowship trained. Both this specialist and your conventional doctor must work together to help treat this disease.

SUPPLEMENTS TO TREAT DEPRESSION		
Supplements	Dosage	Considerations
Alpha-lipoic acid	100 mg once a day	Improves blood sugar levels so diabetics may be able to take less medication.
Ashwagandha root	500 to 1,000 mg once a day	

Bacopa monniera	5 to 13 mg of 1:2 liquid extract once a day	
B-complex vitamins	50 mg twice a day	I suggest taking a multi-vitamin.
Calcium	500 mg twice a day	Although most people are deficient in calcium, there is a danger in taking too much calcium. Do not ingest more than 1,000 to 1,200 mg of calcium a day.
Carnitine	500 to 3,000 mg once a day	
Centella asiatica	9 to 150 mg once a day	
Chromium	400 mcg once a day	Combining with the protein picolinate allows your body to absorb chromium more efficiently. However, some chromium picolinate supplements contain more chromium than necessary. Ask your health-care provider for a recommendation on chromium consumption.
Coenzyme Q_{10}	60 to 100 mg once a day	May reduce the effects of blood thinners. May cause diarrhea in dosages above 100 mg once a day.
Copper	1 to 3 mg once a day	Your copper-to-zinc ratio is very important for your health. Also, do not take copper supplement cupric oxide, which has a very low bioavailability.
EPA/DHA (fish oil)	1,000 to 3,000 mg once a day	Choose a source that contains vitamin E to prevent oxidation.
5-Hydroxy-tryptophan (5-HTP)	100 mg once a day	Do not take with vitamin B_6. Consult your healthcare provider regarding use if you are taking antidepressants. Do not take at the same time as antidepressants or any serotonin-affecting drugs.
Ginseng	500 mg once a day	Always take with food. Do not take if you are taking a blood thinner. Use with caution if you have high blood pressure.
Inositol	1 to 10 g once a day	May stimulate uterine contractions. Women who wish to become pregnant should consult their doctor regarding its use.
Magnesium	600 to 800 mg once a day	Consult healthcare provider for dosage if you have kidney disease. Discontinue use and see your doctor if you experience abdominal pain. Take a lower dose if it causes diarrhea.

Multi-vitamin	1 tablet once a day or as directed	
Phosphatidylcholine	1,000 to 2,000 mg once a day	Use with caution if you have malabsorption problems, as this could exacerbate them.
Phosphatidylserine	300 mg once a day	
St. John's wort	900 to 1,800 mg once a day	Do not take with antidepressants, indinavir, cyclosporine, theophylline, warfarin, or ethinylestradiol. If you are exposed to the sun, it may cause a skin rash. May lessen effects of birth control.
Selenium	400 mcg once a day	
Tryptophan	1,500 mg twice a day	Do not take if you are on an antidepressant.
Tyrosine	1,000 to 4,000 mg once a day	Do not take if you are taking an MAO inhibitor medication.
Valerian	500 mg once a day	Do not take if you have liver disease or if you abuse alcohol.
Vitamin A and mixed carotenoids	5,000 IU—half vitamin A and half mixed carotenoids—once a day	Use caution when taking vitamin A supplements because they have the potential to be toxic. Do not take for extended periods of time. Do not take high dosages if you have liver disease, are a smoker, or are exposed to asbestos.
Vitamin B_9 (folic acid)	500 mcg twice a day	High doses can deplete your body of other vitamins in the B complex.
Vitamin B_{12} (cobalamin)	500 mcg twice a day	High doses can deplete your body of other vitamins in the B complex.
Vitamin C	500 mg twice a day	Do not take high dosages if you are prone to kidney stones or gout.
Zinc	25 to 50 mg once a day	The best zinc supplements are zinc picolinate and zinc citrate. If you are taking zinc and iron supplements, take one in the morning and one in the evening. (Taking them together reduces the efficiency of both.)

DERMATITITIS

See Eczema.

DIABETES MELLITUS

Diabetes mellitus—better known simply as diabetes—is a chronic disease characterized by abnormally high blood levels of the sugar glucose. There are two main types of diabetes. In *type 1 diabetes* (insulin-dependent diabetes), the pancreas produces little or no insulin, which is the hormone that lowers blood glucose levels. In *type 2 diabetes* (non-insulin-dependent diabetes), the body continues to produce insulin—sometimes at even higher-than-normal levels—but the cells of the body are unable to react properly to the hormone. The more common form of this disorder is type 2 diabetes.

The signs and symptoms of diabetes can include frequent urination, excessive thirst, extreme hunger, unusual weight loss, increased fatigue, irritability, and blurred vision. When these symptoms occur, it is imperative to seek medical advice, as early detection and treatment of diabetes can improve the chance of avoiding dangerous complications. (See the inset on page 257 for common complications.)

The causes of type 1 diabetes are not known, but many scientists are now viewing type 1 diabetes as a possible autoimmune disease. Although the precise causes of type 2 diabetes are also not known, we have learned that the risk factors for type 2 include obesity, high blood pressure (hypertension), high cholesterol, a family history of diabetes, a sedentary lifestyle, and stress.

It is vital to follow your doctor's recommendations concerning the treatment of diabetes, including the use of medications that lower blood sugar levels. In addition, it is important to choose foods that are low on the glycemic index, and therefore break down slowly during digestion, increasing blood glucose levels very gradually. A careful supplement plan can further improve treatment by resolving common deficiencies and enhancing the body's processing of glucose.

The following supplements can help keep diabetes mellitus under control. They affect your blood sugar level, so you may need less medication—or you may be able to stop taking your medication altogether. However, this is a decision that must be made with your healthcare provider. Regardless, continue to monitor your blood sugar closely so that it does not fall too low, which can cause hypoglycemia.

You may wish to try a product that contains several of the nutrients listed here. There are several great products that I recommend to my patients. An anti-aging fellowship physician can help you decide on a product, or you can visit a compounding pharmacist. (See Resource section for information on finding a compounding pharmacist in your area.)

SUPPLEMENTS TO TREAT DIABETES MELLITUS TYPE 2		
Supplements	Dosage	Considerations
Alpha-lipoic acid	100 to 300 mg daily	Consult your healthcare provider before taking.
Arginine	1,000 to 5,000 mg once a day	If you have kidney disease, liver disease, or herpes, consult your doctor before taking.
B-complex vitamins	50 mg twice a day	I suggest taking a multi-vitamin.
Biotin	8 to 16 mg once a day	
Bitter melon	2 oz of fresh juice or 100 ml of decoction once a day	
Carnitine	2,000 to 3,000 mg once a day	
Carnosine	2,000 mg once a day	
Chromium picolinate	300 to 1,000 mcg once a day	Some contain more chromium than necessary. Ask your healthcare provider for a recommendation on chromium consumption.
Coenzyme Q_{10}	30 to 200 mg daily	May reduce the effects of blood thinners. May cause diarrhea in dosages above 100 mg once a day.
Copper	2 to 3 mg once a day	Your copper-to-zinc ratio is very important for your health. Also, do not take copper supplement cupric oxide, which has a very low bioavailability.
EPA/DHA (fish oil)	1,000 to 2,000 mg once a day	Choose a source that contains vitamin E to prevent oxidation.
Fenugreek	Seed powder 50 mg twice a day or 2 to 4.5 ml of 1:2 liquid extract twice a day	
Fiber, soluble		Choose a fiber supplement with no added sugar. Supplement with several glasses of water.
Gamma-linolenic acid (GLA)	240 to 480 mg once a day	It is important to maintain the proper ratio of omega-6 fatty acids to omega-3 fatty acids. (See page 110.)

Ginkgo biloba	120 mg once daily	Do not use if taking a blood thinner.
Inositol	2,000 to 4,000 mg once a day	May stimulate uterine contractions. Women who wish to become pregnant should consult their doctor regarding its use.
Magnesium	400 to 800 mg once a day	Consult healthcare provider for dosage if you have kidney disease. Discontinue use and see your doctor if you experience abdominal pain. Take a lower dose if it causes diarrhea.
Manganese	2 to 5 mg once a day	
N-acetylcysteine (NAC)	500 mg once a day	When taking NAC supplements, also take extra vitamin C, copper, and zinc.
Quercetin	300 to 900 mg once a day	
Selenium	200 mcg once a day	
Taurine	1,000 to 1,500 mg once a day	Take between meals. Discontinue use if you suddenly have feelings of chest or throat tightness or if you break out in hives. Do not take with aspirin.
Vanadium	50 mg once a day	Do not take more than 50 mg a day.
Vitamin B_6 (pyridoxine)	75 mg twice a day	Do not take more than 500 mg a day. If you are taking L-dopa for Parkinson's disease, do not take B_6 without first consulting your doctor.
Vitamin B_{12} (cobalamin)	500 to 1,500 mcg twice a day	High doses can deplete your body of other vitamins in the B complex.
Vitamin C	500 to 1,500 mg twice a day	Do not take high dosages if you are prone to kidney stones or gout.
Vitamin D	Have your blood levels measured by your health-care provider, who will then determine proper dosage.	
Vitamin E	400 to 800 IU once a day	Take mixed tocopherols, the more active type of vitamin E. Consult healthcare provider first if you are taking a blood thinner.
Zinc	20 to 50 mg once a day	The best zinc supplements are zinc picolinate and zinc citrate. If you are taking zinc and iron supplements, take one in the morning and one in the evening. (Taking them together reduces the efficiency of both.)

Complications of Diabetes

When you have diabetes, it is vitally important to take good care of yourself. When diabetes is not carefully managed, the resulting complications can be serious, as shown by the following list.

- **Diabetic neuropathy.** This is one of the most common complications of diabetes. It involves damage to the nerves that run throughout the body, connecting the spinal cord to the skin, muscles, blood vessels, and other organs.

- **Eye problems.** People with diabetes have a higher risk of blindness than the rest of the population. Early detection and treatment of any eye problem is essential.

- **Kidney disease.** Diabetes can damage the kidneys, making them lose their ability to filter out waste products.

- **Heart disease and stroke.** Diabetes involves an increased risk for heart attack, stroke, and complications of the circulatory system.

- **Foot problems.** Because of poor circulation and/or nerve damage, diabetes can lead to many foot problems.

- **Skin complications.** About a third of those with diabetes have a related skin complication at some time in their lives. Fortunately, when caught early, these problems can usually be resolved.

- **Gastroparesis.** This condition, which involves extremely slow emptying of the stomach, affects people with both type 1 and type 2 diabetes.

- **Depression.** Depression has been associated with diabetes for almost three hundred years. In one out of every four patients, symptoms are severe enough to warrant treatment.

Insulin Resistance and Hyperinsulinism (High Insulin)

Insulin resistance and hyperinsulinism are conditions in which the body's insulin levels are too high. Both conditions can lead to the development of type 2 diabetes. The nutrients listed in the table "Supplements to Treat Insulin Resistance and Hyperinsulinism" can help control these two disorders and lower insulin levels, which can help decrease your risk of developing diabetes.

SUPPLEMENTS TO TREAT INSULIN RESISTANCE AND HYPERINSULINISM		
Supplements	**Dosage**	**Considerations**
Alpha-lipoic acid	200 to 600 mg once a day	Consult your healthcare provider before taking.
B-complex vitamins	25 mg twice a day	I recommend taking a multi-vitamin.
Chromium	400 to 1,200 mcg once a day	Combining with the protein picolinate allows your body to absorb chromium more efficiently. However, some chromium picolinate supplements contain more chromium than necessary. Ask your health-care provider for a recommendation on chromium consumption.
Coenzyme Q_{10}	30 to 200 mg once a day	May reduce the effects of blood thinners. May cause diarrhea in dosages above 100 mg once a day.
Conjugated linoleic acid (CLA)	1,000 to 3,000 mcg once a day	
EPA/DHA (fish oil)	2,000 mg once a day	Choose a source that contains vitamin E to prevent oxidation.
Fiber, soluble		Choose a fiber supplement with no added sugar. Supplement with several glasses of water.
Insinase	Used as directed.	Metagenics product. (See Resources.)
Magnesium	400 to 800 mg once a day	Consult healthcare provider for dosage if you have kidney disease. Discontinue use and see your doctor if you experience abdominal pain. Take a lower dose if it causes diarrhea.
Manganese	5 to 10 mg once a day	
Taurine	1,000 to 3,000 mg once a day	Take between meals. Discontinue use if you suddenly have feelings of chest or throat tightness or if you break out in hives. Do not take with aspirin.
Vanadium	50 mg once a day	Do not take more than 50 mg a day.
Vitamin B_7 (biotin)	2 to 4 mg twice a day	High doses can deplete your body of other vitamins in the B complex.
Vitamin C	500 to 1,500 mg twice a day	Do not take high dosages if you are prone to kidney stones or gout.

Vitamin D	Have your blood levels measured by your health-care provider, who will then determine proper dosage.	
Vitamin E	400 to 800 IU once a day	Take mixed tocopherols, the more active type of vitamin E. Consult healthcare provider first if you are taking a blood thinner.
Zinc	25 to 50 mg once a day	The best zinc supplements are zinc picolinate and zinc citrate. If you are taking zinc and iron supplements, take one in the morning and one in the evening. (Taking them together reduces the efficiency of both.)

Supplements to Treat Diabetic Neuropathy

Diabetic neuropathy is a progressive disorder that affects around 20 percent of diabetics. The body's nerves become damaged, and it can lead to a host of other neuropathic disorders. The following nutrients can slow the progression of diabetic neuropathy.

SUPPLEMENTS TO TREAT DIABETIC NEUROPATHY		
Supplements	Dosage	Considerations
Alpha-lipoic acid	300 to 1,500 mg once a day	Consult your healthcare provider before taking dosages larger than 600 mg.
Biotin	5 to 10 mg once a day	
Carnitine	2,000 mg once a day	
Carnosine	1,000 to 2,000 mg once a day	
EPA/DHA (fish oil)	1,000 to 2,000 mg once a day	Choose a source that contains vitamin E to prevent oxidation.
Gamma-linolenic acid (GLA)	1,000 mg once a day	It is important to maintain the proper ratio of omega-6 fatty acids to omega-3 fatty acids. (See page 110.)
Vitamin B_{12} (cobalamin)	1,000 to 2,500 mcg twice a day	High doses can deplete your body of other vitamins in the B complex.
Vitamin E	400 to 800 IU once a day	Take mixed tocopherols, the more active type of vitamin E. Consult healthcare provider first if you are taking a blood thinner.

DRY EYES

Dry eyes, also known as *keratoconjunctivitis sicca* (KCS), is an eye disorder that is most often caused by decreased tear production, but may also result from increased evaporation of the tear film due to abnormal tear composition. Symptoms can include dryness, burning, the sensation of having sand or grit in the eye, itching, stinging, tired eyes, redness, a pulling sensation, or a sensation of pressure behind the eye. Generally, both eyes are affected.

Dry eyes are usually age-related. This is especially true when there is an inadequate production of tears. Other causes include the use of contact lenses; eye surgery, including LASIK surgery; health conditions such as diabetes, menopause, rheumatoid arthritis, and lupus; the use of certain medications, such as sedatives, diuretics, tricyclic antidepressants, oral contraceptives, nasal decongestants, and antihistamines; and eye injuries, including thermal and chemical burns.

Most people suffer no long-term effects from dry eyes. But because the condition is uncomfortable, and because it can lead to eye damage if it is left untreated or becomes severe, it is important to identify and eliminate the cause of the condition, and to do what you can to relieve the symptoms. For many people, especially women, appropriate supplementation has been associated with a decreased incidence of dry eyes. *See also* Sjögren's Syndrome.

SUPPLEMENTS TO TREAT DIABETIC NEUROPATHY		
Supplements	Dosage	Considerations
Carnosine eye drops	Use as directed.	
EPA/DHA (fish oil)	2,000 to 3,000 mg once a day	Choose a source that contains vitamin E to prevent oxidation.

EATING DISORDER

See Anorexia Nervosa.

ECZEMA

Eczema is a noncontagious, inflammatory skin condition that is characterized by patches of dry, flaking skin that can become cracked and leathery, or blistered and oozing. Severe itching can occur in the affected areas. Eczema most frequently appears on the face and scalp, behind the ears, on the elbows, and in the creases behind the knees.

The two major types of eczema—*atopic dermatitis* and *contact dermatitis*—are both considered allergic responses. Those with atopic dermatitis often have a family history of eczema or allergic conditions like asthma and hay fever. Contact dermatitis, the more common form of the condition, is often an allergic response to an irritant that has come into contact with the skin. Soaps, wool and synthetic fabrics, dyes, latex, and certain cosmetic products are common culprits. Stressful or emotionally charged situations are also believed to trigger eczema flare-ups.

Cases of eczema can range from very mild to severe and, therefore, will require various treatment protocols. Proper skin care is often sufficient for treating mild cases, while more serious cases may require medication. For this reason, it is important to consult your health care provider for the best treatment options for your particular situation.

SUPPLEMENTS TO TREAT ECZEMA

Supplements	Dosage	Considerations
B-complex vitamins	25 to 50 mg twice a day	I suggest taking a multi-vitamin.
Copper	2 to 3 mg once a day	Your copper-to-zinc ratio is very important for your health. Also, do not take copper supplement cupric oxide, which has a very low bioavailability.
Dandelion	100 mg once a day	If you have gallstones or obstructed bile ducts, consult your healthcare practitioner before taking.
EPA/DHA (fish oil)	1,000 to 3,000 mg once a day	Choose a source that contains vitamin E to prevent oxidation.
Evening primrose oil	500 to 1,000 mg once a day	
Glucosamine	1,000 mg once a day	Don't take if you are allergic to shellfish. Consult use with your healthcare provider if you have diabetes because glucosamine can alter blood sugar levels.

Methylsulfonyl-methane (MSM)	3,000 to 10,000 mg once a day	When beginning supplementation, ingest with meals to avoid possible heartburn. May cause stomach upset in dosages larger than 6,000 mg.
Milk thistle	200 mg once a day	Reduces efficiency of certain blood pressure medication.
Probiotics	20 billion units once a day	If taking an antibiotic, wait three hours before taking probiotics.
Taurine	2,000 mg once a day	Take between meals. Discontinue use if you suddenly have feelings of chest or throat tightness or if you break out in hives. Do not take with aspirin.
Tea tree oil	Apply directly to skin once or twice a day.	Do not ingest or use in ears, eyes, or other mucous membranes.
Vitamin A and mixed carotenoids	20,000 to 50,000 IU— half vitamin A and half mixed carotenoids— once a day	Only take these dosages of vitamin A under the supervision of a healthcare provider. Do not take for extended periods of time. Do not take more than 8,000 IU a day if you have liver disease, are a smoker, or are exposed to asbestos.
Vitamin C	500 to 1,500 mg twice a day	Do not take high dosages if you are prone to kidney stones or gout.
Vitamin D	Have your blood levels measured by your health-care provider, who will then determine proper dosage.	
Vitamin E	400 IU once a day	Take mixed tocopherols, the more active type of vitamin E. Consult healthcare provider first if you are taking a blood thinner.
Zinc	25 to 75 mg once a day	The best zinc supplements are zinc picolinate and zinc citrate. If you are taking zinc and iron supplements, take one in the morning and one in the evening. (Taking them together reduces the efficiency of both.)

ENLARGED PROSTATE

See Benign Prostatic Hypertrophy.

ESTROGEN-RELATED PROBLEMS

Although estrogen is primarily thought of as a "women's hormone," it is actually present—and necessary—in the bodies of both sexes. It has many vital responsibilities, including proper brain function and the development of nerve cells. The proper use of estrogen by the body relies on its ratio of estrogen to progesterone. Although the actual ratio is different in men and women, it is equally important for good health in both sexes.

ESTROGEN DOMINANCE IN WOMEN

In women, estrogen has other functions as well. It forms the female body and reproductive organs, including the breasts, ovaries, and uterus, during puberty. It is also involved—along with the hormones progesterone and testosterone—with the menstrual cycle. Estrogen is clearly vital to many life functions. As mentioned above, however, the level of estrogen in the body is not nearly as important as the ratio of estrogen to progesterone.

As women age, their bodies release progessively less estrogen and progesterone. During perimenopause (the period of transition before menopause) and menopause, however, the decrease in the body's hormones becomes drastic. Progesterone levels usually decrease by as much as 75 percent—while estrogen levels tend to decrease by only 35 percent. Although the presence of both hormones has been reduced, the significantly greater drop in progesterone levels can cause *estrogen dominance.* Unfortunately, estrogen dominance—which occurs in many women at some point in their lives—can result in a host of different illnesses, such as osteoporosis, fibroids, fibrocystic breast disease, and breast cancer. The following supplements can help treat this common yet potentially serious problem.

SUPPLEMENTS TO TREAT ESTROGEN DOMINANCE IN WOMEN		
Supplements	Dosage	Considerations
Flaxseed	1,000 mg once a day	May interfere with anticoagulants, work as a laxative, or affect blood sugar levels.
Indole-3-carbinol (I-3-C)	300 to 500 mg once a day	
Progesterone, natural		As prescribed by your doctor.

ESTROGEN DOMINANCE IN MEN

Men make estrogen out of testosterone, with the help of an enzyme called aromatase. They require estrogen—although in smaller amounts than women—in large part because it helps the brain function properly. Yet an elevated level of this hormone can be very dangerous. It increases the risk of both prostate cancer and heart disease. The following list explains the reasons because of which a man's estrogen levels can become dangerously high. Then, the succeeding list provides various nutrients that can help lower these levels.

■ Causes of Estrogen Elevation in Men

- Alcohol abuse

- Consumption of grapefruit

- Drug abuse (amphetamines, marijuana, cocaine)

- General dietary deficiencies and malnutrition

- High doses of vitamin E

- Increase in aromatase activity

- Ingestion of estrogen-enhancing food or environmental substances

- Medications including pain relievers and anti-inflammatories (ibuprofen, acetaminophen, aspirin, propoxyphene), antibiotics (sulfas, tetracyclines, penicillins, cefazoline, erythromycins, floxacins, isoniazid), antifungal drugs (miconazole, itraconazole, fluconazole, ketoconazole), statin drugs, antidepressants (fluoxetine, fluvoxamine, paroxetine, sertraline), antipsychotic medicines (thorazine, haloperidol), heart and blood pressure medicine (propranolol, quinidine, amiodarone, coumadin, methyldopa), and calcium channel blockers (antacids, omeprazole, cimetidine)

- Obesity

- Poor liver function

- Stress

- Zinc deficiency

■ Causes of Decreased Estrogen Levels in Men

Consumption of the following has been found to lower estrogen levels in men.

- Cruciferous vegetables (broccoli, Brussels sprouts, cauliflower, kale)
- High-dose vitamin C
- Niacin
- Resveratrol (grape skin compound)
- Shellfish (oysters)
- Soy products
- Vegetarian diet

EXHAUSTION

See Adrenal Fatigue and Exhaustion.

EYE HEALTH

See Cataracts; Dry Eyes; Macular Degeneration.

FATIGUE

See Chronic Fatigue Syndrome.

FIBROIDS

Fibroids, which are also known as *leiomyomata*, are benign (non-cancerous) growths on or within the walls of the uterus. These tumors can be a variety of different sizes and quantities. The resulting symptoms depend upon these factors. If the fibroids are small and do not cause any symptoms, a doctor may recommend that no course of action be taken. However, larger—or multiple—fibroids can cause pain, excessive bleeding, and problems urinating, as well as infertility and premature labor. When fibroids cause serious problems such as these, treatment options include surgery (hysterectomy or myomectomy), medications (such as oral contraceptives), and procedures such as the high intensity focused ultrasound (which uses ultrasound waves to destroy the fibroid tissue). Although no substitute for necessary surgery or other medical action, the nutrients in the following table may allow these procedures to be avoided by shrinking the uterine fibroids naturally. You should also avoid drinking coffee.

Fibroids have estrogen receptors, and are thus responsive to the body's level of estrogen. During periods of pregnancy, when estrogen levels increase, fibroids tend to grow in size. After menopause, on the other hand, when estrogen levels drop significantly, fibroids usually become smaller. For this reason, doctors will often recommend a medication with an estrogen-lowering effect, which will artificially create this situation. Similarly, you may find it effective to take natural progesterone, which directly affects the estrogen in your body. Your doctor will be able to prescribe a specific daily dosage.

SUPPLEMENTS TO TREAT FIBROIDS

Supplements	Dosage	Considerations
Alpha-lipoic acid	300 mg once a day	Improves blood sugar levels so diabetics may be able to take less medication.
Carnitine	1,500 mg once a day	
Coenzyme Q_{10}	100 mg once a day	May reduce the effects of blood thinners. Dosages over 100 mg may cause diarrhea.
Gamma-linolenic acid (GLA)	240 to 720 mg once a day	It is important to maintain the proper ratio of omega-6 fatty acids to omega-3 fatty acids. (See page 110.)
Inositol	500 mg twice a day	May stimulate uterine contractions. Women who wish to become pregnant should consult their doctor regarding its use.
Magnesium	400 mg once a day	Consult healthcare provider for dosage if you have kidney disease. Discontinue use and see your doctor if you experience abdominal pain. Take a lower dose if it causes diarrhea.
Milk thistle	100 to 200 mg once a day	Reduces efficiency of certain blood pressure medication.
Phosphatidyl-choline (Lecithin)	2,000 mg once a day	Use with caution if you have malabsorption problems, as this could exacerbate them.

FOOD ALLERGIES

Scientists estimate that 60 percent of the US population suffers from food allergies. There are many different foods to which people are allergic, with the eight most common being eggs, fish, milk, peanuts, shell fish, soy, tree nuts, and wheat. Some reactions occur within three hours of eating the offending food, while others may not occur for several days. As you can see on the list below, there are also a large variety of reactions that can occur. They can range from mild to life threatening.

A doctor can help you determine the foods to which you are allergic. Although you may find that you crave these foods, you must eliminate the allergy-creating items from your diet. Then, begin supplementation with the nutrients listed in "Supplements to Treat Food Allergies." They will help lessen the severity of your allergy attacks.

■ Symptoms of Food Allergies

- ☐ Anal itching
- ☐ Anemia
- ☐ Anxiety, fear
- ☐ Backaches
- ☐ Belching
- ☐ Cracks at corners of mouth
- ☐ Dark circles under eyes
- ☐ Depression
- ☐ Destructive behavior
- ☐ Diarrhea
- ☐ Eczema
- ☐ Emotional outbursts
- ☐ Fluid behind eardrum

- ☐ Frequent urination
- ☐ Heartburn
- ☐ Hearing loss
- ☐ Heart palpitations
- ☐ Hives
- ☐ Hoarseness
- ☐ Inability to concentrate
- ☐ Indigestion
- ☐ Irritable behavior after meals
- ☐ Itchy, watery eyes
- ☐ Memory loss
- ☐ Muscle cramps

- ☐ Nervousness
- ☐ Panic attacks
- ☐ Rapid heart beat
- ☐ Red earlobes
- ☐ Red eyeballs
- ☐ Red rosy cheeks
- ☐ Restlessness
- ☐ Ringing in ears
- ☐ Sluggishness
- ☐ Spacey feeling
- ☐ Spastic colon
- ☐ Stomach aches
- ☐ Tension headaches
- ☐ Tremors
- ☐ Wrinkles under eyes

SUPPLEMENTS TO TREAT FOOD ALLERGIES

Supplements	Dosage	Considerations
Alpha-lipoic acid	200 to 300 mg once a day	Improves blood sugar levels so diabetics may be able to take less medication.
B-vitamin complex	25 mg twice a day	I suggest taking a multi-vitamin.
Curcumin	100 to 1,000 mg	
EPA/DHA (fish oil)	1,000 to 2,000 mg once a day	Choose a source that contains vitamin E to prevent oxidation.
Gamma-linolenic acid (GLA)	240 mg one to three times a day	It is important to maintain the proper ratio of omega-6 fatty acids to omega-3 fatty acids. (See page 110.)
Glutamine	1 to 6 g once a day	If you have a sensitivity to monosodium glutamate (MSG), use glutamine with caution. If you are taking medications for seizures, only take glutamine under the direction of your doctor.
Magnesium	400 to 600 mg once a day	Consult healthcare provider for dosage if you have kidney disease. Discontinue use and see your doctor if you experience abdominal pain. Take a lower dose if it causes diarrhea.
Perilla seed extract	5 to 10 g once a day	Use with caution if taking aspirin, nonsteroidal anti-inflammatory drugs (NSAIDs), ginkgo, or garlic.
Probiotics	20 billion units once a day	If taking an antibiotic, wait three hours before taking probiotics.
Quercetin	500 to 1,000 mg once a day	
Selenium	200 to 400 mcg once a day	
Vitamin C	500 to 1,000 mg twice a day	Do not take high dosages if you are prone to kidney stones or gout.
Vitamin E	400 to 800 IU once a day	Consult healthcare provider first if you are taking a blood thinner.
Zinc	25 mg once a day	The best zinc supplements are zinc picolinate and zinc citrate. If you are taking zinc and iron supplements, take one in the morning and one in the evening. (Taking them together reduces the efficiency of both.)

GALL BLADDER DISORDERS

The gall bladder is a small pear-shaped sac, located under the liver, that acts as a reservoir by storing bile made by the liver. This bile is then released by the gall bladder as needed, and used in the digestion of fats.

Although the gall bladder is not essential to life, it can be the site of much dysfunction and distress. *Gallstones* can form within the gall bladder, potentially obstructing the ducts, and causing pain and other symptoms as they pass. Inflammation of the gall bladder, called *cholecystitis*, can also occur. This condition—which can cause fever, nausea, and vomiting—must be treated immediately, as it can be life-threatening.

If gallstones or cholecystitis is suspected, a doctor should be contacted immediately. Once the problem has been professionally treated, the following supplements will allow you to maintain gallbladder health.

Supplements to Treat Gall Bladder Disorders

The following nutrients can both treat your gall bladder disorder and maintain your gall bladder's health. You should take 500 milligrams of taurine twice a day. Then, consume the following herbs. (See Chapter 5 for instructions on utilizing herbs.) These herbs can be used to make excellent *bitters*—alcohol in which herbs have been dissolved—which are very efficient for maintaining the health of your gall bladder.

- Chelidonium (greater celandine)
- Cynara (artichoke leaf)
- Humulus (hops)
- Mentha (peppermint)
- Rosmarinus (rosemary)
- Taraxacum (dandelion root)

GALLSTONES

See Gall Bladder Disorders.

GINGIVITIS

See Periodontal Disease.

GOUT

Uric acid, a byproduct of your metabolism, is usually oxidized by the enzyme uricase. But some people do not produce enough of this digestive enzyme, so the uric acid begins to first collect, and then crystallize, in their blood and tissues. When crystallizes, it becomes sharp and pokes into joints, causing severe pain and inflammation. Gout, also called *metabolic arthritis*, is one of the most painful forms of arthritis, but it is also one of the most treatable. Although it can occur to any joint in the body, it happens most often in the big toe.

The first stage of gout is symptomless. During this time, the uric acid level in your body rises. The second stage occurs when the uric acid begins to crystallize and causes pain in your joints. The attack may or may not be severe, and usually recedes afterwards for at least a few months and possibly even several years. However, in the third stage of gout, attacks occur with much greater frequency and severity. The gout can even begin to affect your vital organs.

To test for gout, a doctor will extract fluid from your inflamed joint. If you test positive, avoid niacin (vitamin B_3), which competes with uric acid for excretion and will make attacks worse. Avoid alcohol, anchovies, baker's and brewer's yeast, game meat, herring, high doses (1,000 micrograms a day or more) of molybdenum, high fructose corn syrup, mackerel, offal (organ meats), red meat, sardines, shellfish, and vitamin A.

You must see a doctor if you have gout. It is treatable—although not curable—but can be dangerous if not treated before the problem becomes serious. The following supplements will help until you can see a doctor. During gout attacks, eat only nuts, raw fruits and vegetables (particularly cherries and strawberries), and seeds.

SUPPLEMENTS TO TREAT GOUT

Supplements	Dosage	Considerations
Alpha-lipoic acid	200 mg once a day	Improves blood sugar levels so diabetics may be able to take less medication.
Baikal skullcap	3 capsules once a day	May cause low blood sugar levels.
Bilberry	60 mg once a day	
Carnitine	1,000 mg once a day	

Celery seed extract	450 mg once a day	
Chamomile	3 capsules or 3 cups of tea daily	Consult healthcare practitioner before taking if you are on a blood thinner. Do not take if you are allergic to other plants of the Asteraceae family (such as ragweed, aster, and chrysanthemums).
Chromium	400 to 1,000 mcg once a day	Combining with the protein picolinate allows your body to absorb chromium more efficiently. However, some chromium picolinate supplements contain more chromium than necessary. Ask your healthcare provider for a recommendation on chromium consumption.
Coenzyme Q_{10}	120 mg once a day	May reduce the effects of blood thinners. May cause diarrhea in dosages above 100 mg once a day.
EPA/DHA (fish oil)	2,000 mg once a day	Choose a source that contains vitamin E to prevent oxidation.
Grape seed extract	300 to 900 mg once a day	
Milk thistle	300 mg once a day	Reduces efficiency of certain blood pressure medication.
Quercetin	500 mg once a day	
Vitamin B_9 (folic acid)	5 to 10 mg twice a day	High doses can deplete your body of other vitamins in the B complex.
Vitamin C	500 to 1,500 mg twice a day	Do not take high dosages if you are prone to kidney stones or gout.
Vitamin E	400 IU once a day	Take mixed tocopherols, the more active type of vitamin E. Consult healthcare provider first if you are taking a blood thinner.
Yarrow	3 capsules daily	

HAIR LOSS

Hair loss, also called *alopecia,* is a common occurrence. Most often, it is the result of aging and genetics. Both men and women tend to lose hair thickness as they grow older. About 25 percent of men begin to bald by their thirties, with 66 percent either have a balding pattern or being completely bald by the age of sixty. However, there can be other causes of hair loss, including fungal infections of the scalp; high fever; cancer chemotherapy;

radiation therapy; hyperthyroidism (an overactive thyroid gland); autoimmune diseases such as lupus; nutritional deficiencies; emotional stress; and trichotillomania—a mental disorder that causes an individual to pull out his or her own hair. Even excessive shampooing and blow-drying can cause the hair to break and thin.

Clearly, it is important to know the cause of hair thinning and, if possible—as is the case with hyperthyroidism—to eliminate it. But it is also important to eat a well-balanced diet and take in adequate levels of hair-healthy nutrients. The following supplements have been found helpful in maintaining a thick head of hair and slowing hair loss.

- Biotin
- Indole-3-carbinol
- Nettles
- Rosemary
- Saw palmetto

HASHIMOTO'S THYROIDITIS

Hashimoto's thyroiditis, or *chronic lymphocytic thyroiditis,* is the most common type of *thyroiditis*—an inflammation of the thyroid gland. An autoimmune disease, Hashimoto's thyroiditis is genetic and much more prevalent in women than men.

The thyroid gland regulates growth and metabolism. When the immune system attacks the thyroid gland, as it does in Hashimoto's thyroiditis, growth and metabolism slow down. Weight gain is a common symptom, as are constipation, cramps, depression, fatigue, goiters, muscle weakness, and sensitivity to cold. *Hypothyroidism*—low levels of the thyroid hormones—often occurs. However, some people with Hashimoto's thyroiditis exhibit no symptoms.

See your doctor if you suspect you have Hashimoto's thyroiditis. He will perform a simple blood test to make this determination. If you do, he will probably prescribe thyroid hormone replacement to alleviate your hormone deficiency. However, the dosage of this pill is important. *Hyperthyroidism*—high levels of the thyroid hormones—can occur if you ingest too much thyroxine (one of the thyroid hormones). The symptoms of hyperthyroidism include insomnia, irritability, a racing heart, sensitivity to heat, and weight loss. You should, therefore, visit your doctor regularly to determine if you are ingesting the proper amount of thyroid hormone. You can also take the nutrients listed on page 273 to discourage the immune system from attacking the thyroid gland.

SUPPLEMENTS TO TREAT HASHIMOTO'S THYROIDITIS

Supplements	Dosage	Considerations
EPA/DHA (fish oil)	1,000 to 5,000 mg once a day	Choose a source that contains vitamin E to prevent oxidation.
Eleuthero	50 to 200 mg once a day	Do not use if you have a history of heart disease.
Flaxseed	1,000 mg once a day	May interfere with anticoagulants, work as a laxative, or affect blood sugar levels.
Gamma-linolenic acid (GLA)	1 to 5 mg once a day	It is important to maintain the proper ratio of omega-6 fatty acids to omega-3 fatty acids. (See page 110.)
Glucosamine	300 to 900 mg once a day	Don't take if you are allergic to shellfish. Consult use with your healthcare provider if you have diabetes because glucosamine can alter blood sugar levels.
Glutamine	1 to 5 g once a day	If you have a sensitivity to monosodium glutamate (MSG), use glutamine with caution. If you are taking medications f or seizures, only take glutamine under the direction of your doctor.
Kaprex AI	1 softgel capsule twice a day	Made by Metagenics. Do not use if taking an anticoagulant.
Magnesium	400 to 800 mg once a day	Consult healthcare provider for dosage if you have kidney disease. Discontinue use and see your doctor if you experience abdominal pain. Take a lower dose if it causes diarrhea.
Olive leaf extract	1 capsule one to three times daily	Take with food.
Probiotics	20 billion units once a day	If taking an antibiotic, wait three hours before taking probiotics.
Selenium	200 to 400 mcg once a day	
Vitamin C	500 to 1,500 mg twice a day	Do not take high dosages if you are prone to kidney stones or gout.
Vitamin E	400 IU once a day	Take mixed tocopherols, the more active type of vitamin E. Consult healthcare provider first if you are taking a blood thinner.

HEAD INJURY

See Closed Head Injury.

HEADACHES

See Migraine Headaches.

HEART FAILURE

See Congestive Heart Failure.

HEPATITIS C

Hepatitis C is a blood-borne infectious disease of the liver caused by the hepatitis C virus. It is the leading cause of liver transplants in the United States.

In the first six months of infection with the virus—the period referred to as *acute hepatitis C*—60 to 70 percent of the people infected have no symptoms at all, while others experience decreased appetite, fatigue, abdominal pain, jaundice, itching, or flu-like symptoms. When infection with the virus continues for more than six months—a condition called *chronic hepatitis C*—again, there may be no symptoms at all. Some patients, though, experience weight loss, flu-like symptoms, low-grade fever, muscle pain, joint pain, itching, abdominal pain, nausea, diarrhea, and more. If left untreated, this disorder can progress and cause inflammation of the liver, liver scarring, and cirrhosis. It should be noted, though, that the majority of those infected with hepatitis C experience either no symptoms or such mild symptoms that they do not seek treatment.

Hepatitis C is spread through contact with infected blood, and may be contracted through IV drug use; transfusions with unscreened blood; occupational exposure to blood; recreational exposure to drugs, as in sports; and even shared personal items such as razors. The condition has also been known to spread through sex with an infectious person, and from mother to infant during childbirth.

While prompt medical treatment of hepatitis C is important to avoid progression of the disease, a number of supplements can also be useful in the treatment of this disorder. At the same time, avoid high doses of vitamin A and beta carotene, and niacin supplementation greater than 100 milligrams.

SUPPLEMENTS TO TREAT HEPATITIS C		
Supplements	Dosage	Considerations
Alpha-lipoic acid	600 to 800 mg once a day	Consult healthcare practitioner before taking. High doses can cause hypothyroidism.
Astragalus	1 to 3 ml of tincture or capsule extract once a day	
B-complex vitamins	25 mg twice a day	I suggest taking a multi-vitamin.
Carnitine	500 to 3,000 mg once a day	The most effective form for this purpose is acetyl-L-carnitine (ALCAR).
Coenzyme Q_{10}	100 to 400 mg once a day	May reduce the effects of blood thinners. May cause diarrhea in dosages above 100 mg once a day.
Lysine	1,000 to 3,000 mg once a day	Taking for more than six months can cause an imbalance of arginine. Do not take if you have diabetes or are allergic to eggs, milk, or wheat.
N-acetylcysteine (NAC)	1,000 mg once a day	When taking NAC supplements, also take extra vitamin C, copper, and zinc.
Olive leaf extract	1 capsule one to three times daily	Take with food.
Phosphatidyl-choline (Lecithin)	2,000 to 10,000 mg once a day	Use with caution if you have malabsorption problems, as this could exacerbate them.
Probiotics	20 billion units once a day	If taking an antibiotic, wait three hours before taking probiotics.
Selenium	200 mcg once a day	
Silymarin	100 to 300 mg once a day	Found in milk thistle.
Taurine	1,000 to 3,000 mg once a day	Take between meals. Discontinue use if you suddenly have feelings of chest or throat tightness or if you break out in hives. Do not take with aspirin.

Vitamin B$_9$ (folic acid)	500 mcg twice a day	High doses can deplete your body of other vitamins in the B complex.
Vitamin B$_{12}$ (cobalamin)	5,00 to 1,000 mcg twice a day	High doses can deplete your body of other vitamins in the B complex.
Vitamin C	500 to 2,500 mg twice a day	Do not take high dosages if you are prone to kidney stones or gout.
Vitamin E	400 IU once a day	Take mixed tocopherols, the more active type of vitamin E. Consult healthcare provider first if you are taking a blood thinner.

HIGH BLOOD PRESSURE (HYPERTENSION)

Blood pressure is the measurement of the blood's force in the arteries as the heart pushes the blood through the body. High blood pressure, also called *hypertension,* occurs when too much pressure is exerted on the artery walls by the blood.

While researchers don't fully understand the cause of high blood pressure, they have identified several factors that contribute to the disorder. These factors include arteriosclerosis (hardening of the arteries), thickening of the artery walls, and excessive contraction of the small arteries. Researchers have also identified a number of risk factors for high blood pressure. (See the inset on page 277.)

While some people with early-stage hypertension experience dull headaches, dizziness, or nosebleeds, most sufferers have no symptoms whatsoever. Nevertheless, when untreated, high blood pressure increases the risk of serious health problems, including heart attack and stroke. This is why it is sometimes referred to as the "silent killer."

Although medications can reduce blood pressure to normal levels, they can also have a range of side effects, including depression; constipation; dizziness; deficiencies of potassium, magnesium, and other nutrients; kidney damage; impaired sexual function; and decreased alertness and memory. Fortunately, certain supplements can help you lower your blood pressure without the use of drugs. (These are listed in the table "Supplements that Can Lower Blood Pressure.") Other supplements can be used *with* drugs to augment their effects. Just keep in mind that hypertension is a serious disorder, so whether you are using these supplements to minimize or eventually discontinue your use of antihypertensive drugs, you must work with a physician to make sure that your blood pressure is being properly controlled. If you are currently taking blood pressure medication, *do not* stop taking it without the approval of your doctor. It is also important to realize that a good diet and regular exercise are extremely important in lowering and then maintaining your blood pressure.

SUPPLEMENTS THAT CAN LOWER BLOOD PRESSURE		
Supplements	Dosage	Considerations
Alpha-lipoic acid	200 mg once a day	Improves blood sugar levels so diabetics may be able to take less medication.
Arginine	5,000 mg once a day	If you have kidney disease, liver disease, or herpes, only take under a doctor's supervision.
B-complex vitamins	50 to 70 mg twice a day	I suggest taking a multi-vitamin.
Calcium	500 mg twice a day	Although most people are deficient in calcium, there is a danger in taking too much calcium. Do not ingest more than 1,000 to 1,200 mg of calcium a day.
Carnitine	1,000 to 2,000 mg once a day	The most effective form is acetyl-L-carnitine (ALCAR).
Celery seed powder	500 mg once a day	

Risk Factors for High Blood Pressure

Although scientists don't know exactly why some people have high blood pressure and some do not, they have identified a number of risk factors for high blood pressure. The following are some of the factors associated with hypertension.

- Age (being over 55).
- Excess weight.
- Genetics.

- Lack of exercise.
- Smoking.
- Alcohol abuse.

- The use of certain drugs, including amphetamine-like medications; cocaine; steroids; cyclosporine; decongestants; ephedra; erthropoietin; certain antidepressants; nonsteroidal anti-inflammatory drugs (NSAIDs), such as aspirin; COX inhibitors; and birth control and estrogen replacement pills.
- A poor diet—especially one that is high in sodium, saturated fat, trans fatty acids, sugar, refined carbohydrates, and caffeine.
- Stress.

Coenzyme Q$_{10}$	60 to 120 mg once a day	May reduce the effects of blood thinners. May cause diarrhea in dosages above 100 mg once a day.
EPA/DHA (fish oil)	3,000 to 4,000 mg once a day	Choose a source that contains vitamin E to prevent oxidation.
Garlic	10,000 mcg once a day	
Hawthorn berry	160 to 900 mg once a day	
Lycopene	10 to 20 mg once a day	
Magnesium	600 to 800 mg once a day	Consult healthcare provider for dosage if you have kidney disease. Discontinue use and see your doctor if you experience abdominal pain. Take a lower dose if it causes diarrhea.
N-acetylcysteine (NAC)	1,000 mg once a day	When taking NAC supplements, also take extra vitamin C, copper, and zinc.
Taurine	1,000 to 1,500 mg once a day	Take between meals. Discontinue use if you suddenly have feelings of chest or throat tightness or if you break out in hives. Do not take with aspirin.
Vitamin C	500 mg twice a day	Do not take high dosages if you are prone to kidney stones or gout.
Vitamin D	Have your blood levels measured by your health-care provider, who will then determine proper dosage.	
Vitamin E	400 to 800 IU once a day	Take mixed tocopherols, the more active type of vitamin E. Consult healthcare provider first if you are taking a blood thinner.
Zinc	25 mg once a day	The best zinc supplements are zinc picolinate and zinc citrate. If you are taking zinc and iron supplements, take one in the morning and one in the evening. (Taking them together reduces the efficiency of both.)

Medications that Can Lower Blood Pressure

Your doctor may feel that it is necessary for you to take one of the following types of medications. Yet, as stated above, many blood pressure medications cause a wide range of side effects. There are often nutrients that can be taken to augment the effects of the medication, so that a lower dosage can be used. This often causes many of the negative effects to subside. Sometimes you will even find that the nutrient can actually replace the medication. Before taking any nutrients on the following lists, however, discuss your options with your healthcare provider.

Diuretics

Diuretics can lower your blood pressure quite effectively. Unfortunately, they can also increase your risk of other health problems. The following nutrients will allow you to decrease—and possibly eliminate—your dosage of diuretics while continuing to lower your blood pressure. However, you should never stop taking your blood pressure medication without your doctor's approval.

- Calcium
- Carnitine
- Celery
- Coenzyme Q_{10}
- Fiber
- Gamma-linolenic acid (GLA)
- Hawthorn berry
- Magnesium
- Potassium
- Protein
- Taurine
- Vitamin B_6 (pyridoxine)
- Vitamin C

Direct Vasodilators

Direct vasodilators are drugs that decrease blood pressure by widening blood vessels. Yet they can cause serious side effects, including headaches, dizziness, upset stomach, and joint pain. Although these side effects may subside when the vasodilator is combined with a beta blocker medication, beta blockers can cause other problems, including worsened asthma and severe depression. Instead of taking a beta blocker with your direct vasodilator medication, try adding any of the following nutrients to your regimen. You may even find that taking the vasodilator is no longer necessary—but do not stop taking it without the approval of your doctor.

- Alpha-lipoic acid
- Angiotensin II Receptor Blockers (see list on page 280)
- Angiotensin-Converting Enzyme Inhibitors (see list on page 280)
- Arginine
- Calcium
- Celery
- Coenzyme Q_{10}
- Fiber
- Flavonoids
- Garlic
- Magnesium
- Omega-3 fatty acids
- Omega-9 fatty acids
- Potassium
- Soy
- Taurine
- Vitamin C
- Vitamin E

Angiotensin-Converting Enzyme Inhibitors

Angiotensin-Converting Enzyme Inibitors—or ACE Inhibitors—are vasodilators that act by restricting the production of the enzyme angiotensin II. This enzyme causes blood vessels to constrict, which results in their becoming more narrow. Restricting this enzyme allows the blood more room to move through the blood vessels, decreasing pressure. However, ACE Inhibitors can also decrease your body's store of important trace minerals such as copper, selenium, and zinc while increasing your potassium levels. The following supplements can limit these side effects and increase the effectiveness of your ACE Inhibitor. You may also find success when taking a multi-vitamin.

- Casein (a phosphoprotein found in milk and cheese)
- Egg yolks
- Garlic
- Gelatin
- Hawthorn berry
- Hydrolyzed wheat germ isolate
- Hydrolyzed whey protein
- Omega-3 fatty acids
- Pycnogenol
- Sake
- Sardine
- Seaweed
- Tuna
- Zinc

Angiotensin II Receptor Blockers

Angiotensin II Receptor Blockers (ARBs) are vasodilators that can help lower your blood pressure. They block the effects of the enzyme angiotensin II. ARBs are often effective for people for whom ACE Inihibitors have failed. The most common side effect is dizziness, but some people also experience fever, nasal congestion, back pain, dizziness, and more. The nutrients on the following list can help you avoid these possible side effects while allowing you to continue your medication. You may even find that you are able to decrease your dosage. Do not change your dosage without first consulting your healthcare provider.

- Celery
- Coenzyme Q_{10}
- Fiber
- Gamma-linolenic acid (GLA)
- Garlic
- Potassium
- Vitamin B_6 (pyridoxine)
- Vitamin C

Central Alpha Agonist

Central alpha agonists are medications that lower blood pressure. By stimulating alpha-receptors in the brain, central alpha agonists widen the peripheral arteries, releasing the pressure on the blood flow. However, these medications can cause dizziness, dry mouth, sedation, and rebound hypertension, so they are usually reserved as a last resort. The following nutrients can be taken with central alpha agonists to improve their function and reduce side effects.

- Celery
- Coenzyme Q_{10}
- Docosahexaenoic acid (DHA)
- Fiber
- Garlic

- Gamma-linolenic acid (GLA)
- Potassium
- Protein
- Sodium restriction

- Taurine
- Zinc
- Vitamin B_6 (pyridoxine)
- Vitamin C

Calcium Channel Blockers

Calcium channel blockers decrease blood pressure by limiting the movement of calcium into the blood vessels. The negative effect of these medications is that they can affect the strength of the heart muscle's contractions. The following nutrients can help counter this effect as well as lower blood pressure.

- Alpha-lipoic acid
- Calcium
- Celery
- Garlic

- Hawthorn berry
- Magnesium
- NAC
- Omega-3 fatty acids

- Vitamin B_6 (pyridoxine)
- Vitamin C
- Vitamin E

HIGH CHOLESTEROL

Cholesterol is a wax-like fatty substance (lipid) found in the cell membranes of all body tissues. About 75 percent of it is synthesized by the body, with the rest being of dietary origin. Despite cholesterol's bad reputation, it is actually necessary for proper body function, and plays a central role in many biochemical processes including production of sex hormones. But at the same time, excessively high levels of cholesterol—referred to as *hypercholesterolemia*—pose a threat to good health.

There are two major forms of cholesterol. *High-density lipoproteins (HDLs)*, which are often referred to as "good cholesterol," carry cholesterol from the blood to the liver for elimination from the body. *Low-density lipoproteins (LDLs)*, or "bad cholesterol," carry cholesterol from the liver to the rest of the body. Your *total cholesterol* considers both LDL and HDL levels, because they are both important for good health. When there are high levels of LDLs in the blood—and especially when this is accompanied by low levels of HDLs—cholesterol can be deposited on the walls of the arteries, causing atherosclerosis (hardening of the arteries). This condition, in turn, is the underlying cause of strokes, heart attacks, and most cardiovascular disease in general.

These disorders are also linked to high *triglyceride* levels. This refers to the form that fat takes when it is being stored for energy in your body. Triglycerides, like cholesterol, are vital for human life but unhealthy if at too high a level. Your doctor will be able to test your HDL, LDL, and triglyceride levels by taking a simple blood test. (You may need to fast the day of the test. Your doctor will provide you with details.)

Dietary changes are key to lowering both cholesterol and triglycerides. Red meat and other foods high in saturated fats should eaten sparingly (or, preferably, eliminated), while heart-healthy fish, vegetables, fruits, grains, and nuts should be included in greater amounts. Exercise is also very important for achieving and maintaining healthy cholesterol levels. Additionally, certain nutrients—such as those listed in the table "Supplements that Decrease Cholesterol Levels"—can help lower bad cholesterol, raise good cholesterol, and restore heart health. To specifically lower your triglycerides, see the nutrients listed in the table "Supplements that Decrease Triglycerides." Causes of high triglyceride levels can be found on page 286.

■ Causes of High Cholesterol

- Alcoholism

- Amino acid deficiency

- Biotin deficiency

- Carnitine deficiency

- Deficiency of hormones such as DHEA, estrogen, or testosterone

- Deficiency of natural antioxidants such as beta-carotene or selenium

- Essential fatty acid deficiency

- Excess dietary starch

- Excess dietary sugar

- Fiber deficiency

- Food allergies

- Hydrogenated, partially hydrogenated, or processed fats (lard, margarine, palm oil, shortening)

- Increased tissue damage due to infection, radiation, or oxidative activity (free radical production)

- Liver dysfunction

- Vitamin C deficiency

■ Causes of Low Cholesterol

- Adrenal stress

- Cancer

- Cholesterol-lowering drugs

- Chronic hepatitis

- Essential fatty acid deficiency

- Excessive exercise

- Immune decline

- Liver infection or disease

- Low-fat diets

- Manganese deficiency

- Psychological stress

- Recreational drugs such as marijuana or cocaine

SUPPLEMENTS THAT DECREASE CHOLESTEROL LEVELS		
Supplements	Dosage	Considerations
Carnitine	1,000 to 2,000 mg once a day	L-carnitine is most effective.
Chromium	200 to 300 mcg once a day	Decreases total cholesterol and LDL (bad) cholesterol.
Coenzyme Q_{10}	60 to 120 mg once a day	Increases HDL (good) cholesterol and decreases platelet stickiness. May reduce the effects of blood thinners.

Fiber, soluble	20 to 30 g once a day	Decreases total cholesterol and LDL (bad) cholesterol. Choose a fiber supplement with no added sugar. Supplement with several glasses of water.
Garlic (supplements or cloves)		Decreases triglycerides and decreases total cholesterol.
Gugulipid	50 mg twice a day	Decreases LDL (bad) cholesterol, increases HDL (good) cholesterol, and decreases platelet stickiness. I suggest either Lipotain by Metagenics or Policosanol + Gugulipid by Designs for Health. Consult a doctor before combining with any medication.
Magnesium	600 mg once a day	Decreases total cholesterol, decreases LDL (bad) cholesterol, increases HDL (good) cholesterol, decreases triglycerides, and decreases platelet stickiness. Do not take if you have problems with your kidneys. Discontinue use if you experience diarrhea or abdominal pain.
Niacin, non-extended release	100 to 500 mg once a day	Decreases total cholesterol, decreases LDL (bad) cholesterol, increases HDL (good) cholesterol, and decreases triglycerides. Do not drink alcohol or hot drinks within one hour of taking niacin. See page 36 for side effects of niacin.
Pantethine	900 mg once a day	Decreases total cholesterol, decreases LDL (bad) cholesterol, increases HDL (good) cholesterol, decreases triglycerides.
Policosanol	20 mg once a day	Increases HDL (good) cholesterol, lowers LDL (bad) cholesterol, and decreases platelet stickiness. Discuss use with doctor if taking an anticoagulant. I recommend Policosanol Extra Strength capsules from Vital Life Nutritionals.
Red yeast rice	600 mg twice a day	Take 200 mg of Coenzyme Q_{10} with red yeast rice, which lowers total cholesterol. Use with caution if you have liver disease because it may elevate liver enzymes.
Soy		Decreases total cholesterol, decreases LDL (bad) cholesterol, and decreases triglycerides. Consuming too much soy may be unhealthy, so I suggest eating soy foods rather than taking soy supplements.

| Tocotrienols | 400 IU once a day | Modifies HMG-CoA reductase, an enzyme that can decrease the rate at which your body makes cholesterol; decreases plaque formation in arteries; and reduces lipoprotein plasma levels. Consult health-care provider first if you are taking a blood thinner. I suggest UltraTrienols from Designs for Health. |

SUPPLEMENTS THAT DECREASE TRIGLYCERIDES

Supplements	Dosage	Considerations
Alpha-ketoglutarate	500 to 1,000 mg once a day	Use with caution if you get cold sores.
Arginine	2 to 4 g once a day	If you have kidney disease, liver disease, or herpes, only take under a doctor's supervision.
Carnitine	2,000 mg once a day	The most effective form is L-carnitine.
Chromium	300 mcg once a day	Combining with the protein picolinate allows your body to absorb chromium more efficiently. However, some chromium picolinate supplements contain more chromium than necessary. Ask your health-care provider for a recommendation on chromium consumption.
Coenzyme Q_{10}	60 to 120 mg once a day	May reduce the effects of blood thinners. May cause diarrhea in dosages above 100 mg once a day.
EPA/DHA (fish oil)	2,000 to 4,000 mg once a day	Choose a source that contains vitamin E to prevent oxidation.
Gugulipid	500 to 1,000 mg once a day	
Lysine	1,000 to 3,000 mg once a day	Taking for more than six months can cause an imbalance of arginine. Do not take if you have diabetes or are allergic to eggs, milk, or wheat.
Magnesium	600 mg once a day	Consult healthcare provider for dosage if you have kidney disease. Discontinue use and see your doctor if you experience abdominal pain. Take a lower dose if it causes diarrhea.
Methionine	250 to 500 mg once a day	Take with vitamins B_6 and B_9 to prevent a build-up of homocysteine. May counter the effects of levodopa (a drug used to treat Parkinson's disease).

Niacin	1 to 2 g once a day	Do not take the suggested dosage without first consulting your doctor. Large dosages can cause a "flush" feeling, which can be eliminated by taking an aspirin one hour before the niacin. Do not drink alcohol or hot drinks within one hour of taking niacin.
Policosanol	10 to 20 mg once a day	
Vitamin B$_5$ (pantothenic acid)	100 mg once a day	High doses can deplete your body of other vitamins in the B complex.
Vitamin B$_9$ (folic acid)	1 mg twice a day	High doses can deplete your body of other vitamins in the B complex.
Vitamin E	400 IU once a day	Take tocotrienols, the most active type of vitamin E.
Zinc	25 mg once a day	The best zinc supplements are zinc picolinate and zinc citrate. If you are taking zinc and iron supplements, take one in the morning and one in the evening. (Taking them together reduces the efficiency of both.)

Causes of High Triglyceride Levels

Triglycerides are fat cells that are stored in your body and later transferred into energy. Yet high levels of triglycerides have been strongly linked to coronary heart disease. The supplements in the table beginning on page 285 may help lower triglyceride levels and increase your heart health. The list below, on the other hand, describes factors and foods that can cause your triglyceride levels to rise.

- Alcohol
- Birth control pills or any other progestin-containing drug
- Caffeine
- Cakes, cookies, and candies
- Diuretics
- Fruit juice
- Genetics
- High fat diet
- Lack of physical activity
- Nicotine
- Skipping an early meal and compensating in the evening
- Soft drinks
- Stress
- Too many carbohydrates
- Too much fruit
- White bread
- White flour
- White sugar

HOMOCYSTEINE

Homocysteine is an amino acid that promotes free radical production (which was discussed on page 4). It also elevates triglycerides and cholesterol levels. Studies have indicated that high homocysteine levels are directly related to strokes, peripheral vascular disease, and cardiovascular disease.

■ Reasons that Homocysteine Levels May Be Elevated

• Coronary artery disease

• Dementia

• Diabetes

• Drugs

• Elevated testosterone levels in women

• Hereditary predisposition

• Hypothyroidism

• Menopause

• Osteoarthritis

• Renal failure

• Rheumatoid arthritis

• Smoking

• Toxins

Eliminating alcohol, birth control pills, caffeine, diuretics, niacin, and tobacco can help decrease homocysteine. The following nutrients can also be effective.

SUPPLEMENTS TO LOWER HOMOCYSTEINE LEVELS		
Supplements	Dosage	Considerations
Betaine (trimethylglycine)	500 to 1,000 mg once a day	
N-acetylcysteine (NAC)	500 to 1,000 mg once a day	When taking NAC supplements, also take extra vitamin C, copper, and zinc.
Phosphatidylcholine (Lecithin)	2,000 to 4,000 mg once a day	Use with caution if you have malabsorption problems, as this could exacerbate them.

Taurine	2,000 to 4,000 mg once a day	Take between meals. Discontinue use if you suddenly have feelings of chest or throat tightness or if you break out in hives. Do not take with aspirin.
Vitamin B_6 (pyridoxine)	50 mg twice a day	Do not take more than 500 mg a day. If you are taking L-dopa for Parkinson's disease, do not take B6 without first consulting your doctor.
Vitamin B_9 (folic acid)	800 mcg once a day	High doses can deplete your body of other vitamins in the B complex.
Vitamin B_{12} (cobalamin)	1,000 mcg once a day	High doses can deplete your body of other vitamins in the B complex.

FIBRINOGEN

Fibrinogen is a clot-promoting substance in your blood. Elevated levels of fibrinogen can cause a heart attack.

■ Ways to Lower Fibrinogen Levels

• Bromelain

• EPA/DHA (fish oil)

• Estrogen hormone replacement

• Garlic

• Ginger

• Ginkgo

• Stop smoking

• Vitamin E

LIPOPROTEIN(A)

Lipoprotein(a) is a small cholesterol particle that can cause inflammation and clog blood vessels when present in the body in elevated levels. High lipoprotein(a) levels can also greatly increase a person's risk of developing heart disease. Along with diabetes and menopause, taking statin medications and eating soy has been shown to increase this particle's presense in the body.

SUPPLEMENTS TO LOWER LIPOPROTEIN (A) LEVELS

Supplements	Dosage	Considerations
Coenzyme Q_{10}	100 to 300 mg once a day	May reduce the effects of blood thinners. May cause diarrhea in dosages above 100 mg once a day.
EPA/DHA (fish oil)	1,000 to 2,000 mg once a day	Choose a source that contains vitamin E to prevent oxidation.
L-carnatine	1,000 to 2,000 mg once a day	
L-proline	5000 to 1,000 mg once a day	
Lysine	5000 to 1,000 mg once a day	Taking for more than six months can cause an imbalance of arginine. Do not take if you have diabetes or are allergic to eggs, milk, or wheat.
N-acetylcysteine (NAC)	500 mg once a day	When taking NAC supplements, also take extra copper, vitamin C, and zinc.
Niacin	1,000 to 2,000 mg once a day	Discuss use and dose with doctor prior to taking. Do not drink alcohol or hot drinks within one hour of taking niacin.
Vitamin E	See healthcare provider for dosage recommendation	Take mixed tocopherols, the more active type of vitamin E. Consult healthcare provider first if you are taking a blood thinner.
Vitamin C	2,000 to 4,000 mg twice a day	Do not take high dosages if you are prone to kidney stones or gout.

C-REACTIVE PROTEIN

C-reactive protein is a protein found in the blood. Its levels become elevated when the body detects an infection or need for inflammation. C-reactive protein levels can also rise due to a previous infection, obesity, depression, or diabetes mellitus. In addition, raised levels may be indicative of future problems including cardiovascular disease and atherosclerosis.

Besides the supplements listed in the table on page 290, exercise and the Metagenics product UltraInflamX can help lower elevated c-reactive proteins levels. One baby aspirin a day may also be effective, but check with your healthcare provider regarding usage before starting this regimen.

■ Causes of Increased C-Reactive Protein Levels

• Depression

• Diabetes mellitus

• Inflammation

• Obesity

• Previous infection

SUPPLEMENTS TO LOWER C-REACTIVE PROTEIN LEVELS		
Supplements	Dosage	Considerations
Coenzyme Q$_{10}$	200 to 300 mg once a day	May reduce the effects of blood thinners. May cause diarrhea in dosages above 100 mg once a day.
Curcumin	300 to 600 mg once a day	
EPA/DHA (fish oil)	2,000 to 3,000 mg once a day	Choose a source that contains vitamin E to prevent oxidation.
Grapeseed extract	100 to 200 mg once a day	
Green tea	3 cups or 3 capsules daily	
Quercetin	500 mg once a day	
Rosemary		
Vitamin E	800 IU once a day	Take mixed tocopherols, the more active type of vitamin E. Consult healthcare provider first if you are taking a blood thinner.

HPV INFECTION

See Cervical Cancer.

HYPERCHOLESTEROLEMIA

See High Cholesterol.

HYPERTENSION

See High Blood Pressure.

HYPERTHYROIDISM

The thyroid gland is the body's internal thermostat. It regulates temperature by secreting hormones that control how quickly the body burns calories and uses energy. Hypothyroidism occurs when there is an excess of thyroid hormones. As a result, body processes, including metabolism, occur quicker than they should. Dramatic weight loss, fast heart rate, nervousness, fatigue, weakness, depression, and a host of other symptoms can result.

There are many different forms of treatment for hyperthyroidism, including hormone-suppressing medication, antithyroid medications, radioactive iodine, and surgery. Based on the cause of the problem and the patient's age and overall health, the healthcare provider will determine which treatment route is most appropriate. The following nutrient list can help ease the problem but *always* see your physician for ongoing care if you have hyperthyroidism.

SUPPLEMENTS TO TREAT HYPERTHYROIDISM		
Supplements	Dosage	Considerations
Carnitine	3,000 to 4,000 mg once a day	

HYPOTHYROIDISM

The thyroid gland is the body's internal thermostat. It regulates temperature by secreting hormones that control how quickly the body burns calories and uses energy. Hypothyroidism develops due to an underactive thyroid gland that does not produce enough hormones. Common symptoms include fatigue, intolerance to cold, slowed heart rate, unexplained weight gain, muscle weakness, hair loss (including the eyebrows), dry skin, and heavy menstrual periods. Severity of symptoms depends on the degree of the hormone deficiency. In a large number of cases, this disorder comes on so gradually, the person is unaware that he or she has a problem. If you suspect you may have this condition, check your thyroid function by following the directions in the inset below.

Hypothyroidism affects about 5 million people in the United States, and five to eight times more women than men. Many cases are the result of an autoimmune disorder known as *Hashimoto's thyroiditis* (see page 272) in which the body develops antibodies that attack the thyroid gland. Other common causes of this disorder include surgical removal of the thyroid and radioactive iodine therapy. Less common causes or contributors include infections of the thyroid, too much or too little dietary iodine, an excess of calcium and copper, and deficiencies of iron, selenium, zinc, and vitamins A, B_2, B_3, B_6, and C. Medications, including beta blockers, lithium, certain oral contraceptives, and chemotherapy drugs, are also possible contributors.

Certain foods—especially seafood, sea vegetables, and other rich sources of iodine—are recommended for those with an underactive thyroid gland. And be aware that, when eaten raw, cabbage, Brussels sprouts, broccoli, turnips, cauliflower, mustard greens, and spinach can contribute to a low-functioning thyroid. These foods should be eaten in moderation and only when cooked. Other foods that should be eaten only in moderate amounts include almonds, walnuts, peanuts, pine nuts, millet, tapioca, and soy products.

Self-Test for an Underactive Thyroid

The following self-test can give you a good indication of whether or not you have an underactive thyroid.

Keep a thermometer next to your bed. As soon as you awake in the morning, before getting out of bed, tuck the basal body thermometer under your armpit and keep it there for fifteen minutes while lying very still. (Any motion can affect the reading.) Write down the temperature, which is called a basal body temperature. Do this for three days in a row.* Determine your average temperature by adding up the three readings and dividing by three. If it is below 97.2°F, there is a good chance you may have a low-functioning thyroid. Contact your doctor to discuss your findings.

* Because hormonal shifts affect body temperature, women should not take this test during the middle of a menstrual cycle, when ovulation usually occurs.

SUPPLEMENTS TO TREAT HYPOTHYROIDISM

Supplements	Dosage	Considerations
Ashwagandha root	500 to 1,000 mg once a day	
B-complex vitamins	100 mg once a day	I suggest taking a multi-vitamin.
Carnitine	1,000 to 4,000 mg once a day	I suggest taking L-carnitine.
Chromium	200 mcg once a day	Combining with the protein picolinate allows your body to absorb chromium more efficiently. However, some chromium picolinate supplements contain more chromium than necessary. Ask your health-care provider for a recommendation on chromium consumption.
Coenzyme Q_{10}	30 to 120 mg once a day	May reduce the effects of blood thinners. May cause diarrhea in dosages above 100 mg once a day.
Copper	1 to 3 mg once a day	Your copper-to-zinc ratio is very important for your health. Also, do not take copper supplement cupric oxide, which has a very low bioavailability.
EPA/DHA (fish oil)	500 to 2,000 mg once a day	Choose a source that contains vitamin E to prevent oxidation.
Gamma-linolenic acid (GLA)	240 mg once a day	It is important to maintain the proper ratio of omega-6 fatty acids to omega-3 fatty acids. (See page 110.)
Iodine	100 to 300 mcg once a day	Most table salts contain iodine, but sea salts do not.
Magnesium	400 to 600 mg once a day	Consult healthcare provider for dosage if you have kidney disease. Discontinue use and see your doctor if you experience abdominal pain. Take a lower dose if it causes diarrhea.
Milk thistle	200 to 300 mg once a day	Reduces efficiency of certain blood pressure medication.
Myrrh	20 to 60 mg once a day	
Sage	40 to 60 mg once a day	
Selenium	200 mcg once a day	
Tyrosine	1,000 mg once a day	Do not take if you are taking an MAO inhibitor medication.

Vitamin A and mixed carotenoids	5,000 to 10,000 IU— half vitamin A and half mixed carotenoids— once a day	Use caution when taking vitamin A supplements because they have the potential to be toxic. Do not take for extended periods of time. Do not take high dosages if you have liver disease, are a smoker, or are exposed to asbestos.
Vitamin B$_3$ (niacin)	500 mg twice a day	Use with caution if you have kidney disease, liver disease, or an ulcer. High doses can deplete your body of other vitamins in the B complex.
Vitamin B$_6$ (pyridoxine)	50 mg twice a day	Do not take more than 500 mg a day. If you are taking L-dopa for Parkinson's disease, do not take B$_6$ without first consulting your doctor.
Vitamin B$_{12}$ (cobalamin)	500 mcg twice a day	High doses can deplete your body of other vitamins in the B complex.
Vitamin C	500 to 1,500 mg twice a day	Do not take high dosages if you are prone to kidney stones or gout.
Vitamin D	Have your blood levels measured by your health-care provider, who will then determine proper dosage.	
Vitamin E	400 IU once a day	Take mixed tocopherols, the more active type of vitamin E. Consult healthcare provider first if you are taking a blood thinner.
Zinc	25 to 50 mg once a day	The best zinc supplements are zinc picolinate and zinc citrate. If you are taking zinc and iron supplements, take one in the morning and one in the evening. (Taking them together reduces the efficiency of both.)

IBS

See Irritable Bowel Syndrome.

INFLAMMATION

Acute inflammation, characterized by redness, swelling, pain, and heat, is a localized reaction to an injury, infection, or other irritation. It can occur to any organ or tissue, and protects the body from the affected area by allowing the stimuli to be removed and the healing to begin. Sometimes, unfortunately, the immune system may not perform this process properly. Chronic inflammation occurs when the body's reaction does not lead to healing within a reasonable amount of time. It can last indefinitely and lead to disease and discomfort.

There are many different causes of inflammation, as well as many different diseases to which it can lead. The following nutrients help reduce the length of both acute and chronic inflammation, and can alleviate some uncomfortable symptoms. You should also avoid eating soda, sugar, and white flour products. *See also* Asthma; Atherosclerosis; Autoimmune Diseases; Crohn's Disease; Gout; Hashimoto's Thyroiditis; Lupus; Myasthenia Gravis; Rheumatoid Arthritis; Ulcerative Colitis; Wound Healing.

SUPPLEMENTS TO TREAT INFLAMMATION		
Supplements	**Dosage**	**Considerations**
Bromelain	250 to 750 mg three times a day	Bromelain is a protease, an enzyme that dissolves protein.
Essential fatty acids such as eicosapenta-enoic acid (EPA) and gamma-linolenic acid (GLA)	2,000 to 10,000 mg once a day	In dosages above 4,000 mg, may cause the blood to thin. It is important to maintain the proper ratio of omega-6 fatty acids to omega-3 fatty acids. (See page 110.)
Gamma-tocopherol	800 IU once a day	Form of Vitamin E. Consult healthcare provider first if you are taking a blood thinner.
Glucosamine	500 to 1,000 mg three times a day	Don't take if you are allergic to shellfish. Consult use with your healthcare provider if you have diabetes because glucosamine can alter blood sugar levels.
Methylsulfonyl-methane (MSM)	3,000 to 10,000 mg once a day	Use with caution if you have kidney disease, liver disease, or an ulcer. High doses can deplete your body of other vitamins in the B complex.
Vitamin B_3 (niacinamide)	100 mg twice a day	Use with caution if you have kidney disease, liver disease, or an ulcer. High doses can deplete your body of other vitamins in the B complex.
Vitamin B_5 (pantothenic acid)	100 mg twice a day	High doses can deplete your body of other vitamins in the B complex.

INFLAMMATORY BOWEL DISEASE

See Crohn's Disease; Ulcerative Colitis.

INSOMNIA

Insomnia is a sleep disorder characterized by an inability to sleep and/or an inability to remain asleep for a reasonable period of time. People with this problem have difficulty falling asleep, staying asleep, or sleeping

Factors That Can Contribute to Insomnia

As explained on page 297, insomnia can exist on its own, without outside causes, or can be brought about by a variety of activities, lifestyle choices, disorders, and substances. Some people may find that the following factors can cause or contribute to insomnia.

- **Diet:** Caffeinated beverages, food additives, and allergen-containing foods. Eating sugary foods right before bed.

- **Illnesses:** Urinary disorders, nasal and sinus problems, reflux esophagitis, asthma, gall bladder disease, chronic pain, and emotional disorders such as anxiety and depression.

- **Hormonal problems:** Thyroid dysfunction, growth hormone loss, progesterone loss, testosterone loss, estrogen loss, and elevated cortisol.

- **Medications:** Asthma medications, blood pressure medications, and synthetic progestins.

- **Lack of exercise.**

- **Sleep apnea.**

- **Light.**

- **Night work.**

- **Nutritional deficiencies:** Deficiencies of niacin, magnesium, copper, iron, tryptophan, and vitamin B_6.

- **Chemical exposure:** Over a hundred chemicals are known to interfere with sleep.

soundly. As a result, they often suffer from daytime fatigue, lack of energy, poor concentration, and irritability. Insomnia is estimated to affect at least half of the adults in the United States.

Insomnia is often categorized in terms of its duration. *Transient insomnia* lasts less than a week; *short-term insomnia* lasts a week to a month; and *chronic insomnia* lasts more than a month. Moreover, insomnia may be considered *primary*, meaning that it exists on its own; or *secondary*, meaning that it has other causes. Secondary insomnias include sleep problems caused by stress; lack of an enforced bedtime during childhood; an underlying psychiatric disorder, such as anxiety or depression; a medical condition, such as restless legs syndrome; or consumption of or withdrawal from alcohol, caffeine, or another substance. (See the inset on page 296 for more factors that can contribute to insomnia.)

When a specific cause for insomnia can be found, the elimination of the causative factor can often end the sleep problem. Healthy habits, such as limited caffeine consumption, a consistent bedtime routine, and exercise, can also end or minimize insomnia. Moreover, a sound supplement program can relieve sleep problems by eliminating nutritional deficiencies; inducing relaxation; and helping to restore the body's normal rhythms.

SUPPLEMENTS TO TREAT INSOMNIA		
Supplements	Dosage	Considerations
Astragalus	4.5 to 8.5 ml of 1:2 liquid extract once a day or 1 to 4 g of dried root three times a day	Do not use after organ transplant, if you have a gum allergy, or for an extended period of time.
Chamomile	3 to 6 ml of 1:2 high grade liquid extract once a day or 300 to 400 mg of extract three times a day	Consult healthcare practitioner before taking if you are on a blood thinner. Do not take if you are allergic to other plants of the Asteraceae family (such as ragweed, aster, and chrysanthemums).
5-Hydroxy-tryptophan (5-HTP)	100 to 200 mg once a day	Do not take with vitamin B_6. Consult your healthcare provider regarding use if you are taking antidepressants. Do not take at the same time as antidepressants or any serotonin-affecting drugs.
Gamma-amino-butyric acid (GABA) plus	300 to 900 mg once a day	May make you drowsy, so you may want to take before going to bed.

Inositol	1,000 mg once a day	May stimulate uterine contractions. Women who wish to become pregnant should consult their doctor regarding its use.
Jujube	6 to 11.5 ml of 1:2 liquid extract once a day	
Lemon balm	3 to 6 ml of 1:2 liquid extract or 80 to 100 mg of dry extract once a day	Do not use if you have glaucoma.
Magnesium	600 mg once a day	Consult healthcare provider for dosage if you have kidney disease. Discontinue use and see your doctor if you experience abdominal pain. Take a lower dose if it causes diarrhea.
Melatonin	1 to 6 mg once a day	Take directly before bedtime and while in the dark.
Passion flower	1 to 2 g of either dried plant or tea, 4 to 6 ml of 1:5 tincture, 1 to 2 ml of 1:1 fluid extract, or 200 to 400 mg of solid extract once a day	Do not take if on MAO inhibitor.

INSULIN-DEPENDENT DIABETES

See Diabetes Mellitus.

IRRITABLE BOWEL SYNDROME (IBS)

Irritable bowel syndrome, or IBS, is a "functional" disorder of the lower intestinal tract. This means that although no structural abnormalities can be found, the body's function in terms of the movement of the intestines is impaired. IBS is believed to affect up to 20 percent of the US population—about one person in every five. It occurs more often in women than in men.

Bloating and abdominal pain and cramping are the major symptoms of IBS. Other symptoms vary from person to person, and may include constipation, diarrhea, or alternating constipation and diarrhea; nausea; and vomiting. Both emotional stress and the consumption of certain foods tend to exacerbate symptoms. No one knows what causes IBS, and it is usually a lifelong problem.

In most cases, IBS can be controlled through medication and a diet that avoids problem foods. These foods vary from person to person, but often include grains, breads, crackers, cakes, cookies, potatoes, beans, and other carbohydrates that increase the formation of gas. You can also take certain nutrients to aid the digestive process, such as those in the table "Supplements to Treat Irritable Bowel Syndrome."

You may find it helpful to contact an anti-aging, fellowship-trained practitioner that has a 4R Program. At our office, the patient goes through a four-tier program to *remove* allergens, antigens, pathogens, and parasites; *reinoculate* with good bacteria; *replace* with symbiotic flora; and *repair* gut mucosal nutrients. This allows us to treat various gastrointestinal illnesses by both identifying the cause of the problem and detoxifying the body.

SUPPLEMENTS TO TREAT IRRITABLE BOWEL SYNDROME		
Supplements	Dosage	Considerations
Boswellia extract	1 to 2 capsules once or twice a day	Take with a meal.
Colostrum	1,000 to 4,000 mg once a day	Consult with your doctor regarding use. Do not use if you have dairy allergies or hyperthyroid disease.
Deglycyrrhizinated licorice (DGL)	1 to 4 tablets	Consult your healthcare practitioner before taking if you have hypertension, glaucoma, diabetes, kidney or liver disease, heart disease, or are on the medication digitalis.
EPA/DHA (fish oil)	1,000 to 2,000 mg once a day	Choose a source that contains vitamin E to prevent oxidation.
Fiber, soluble and insoluble	10 to 20 g of supplements in addition to a diet high in fiber	Choose a fiber supplement with no added sugar. Supplement with several glasses of water.
Gamma-linolenic acid (GLA)	240 to 720 mg once a day	It is important to maintain the proper ratio of omega-6 fatty acids to omega-3 fatty acids. (See page 110.)
Glutamine	6,000 mg once a day	If you have a sensitivity to monosodium glutamate (MSG), use glutamine with caution. If you are taking medications for seizures, only take glutamine under the direction of your doctor.

Inflamma-bLOX	Follow instructions on bottle.	Ortho Molecular product. (See Resources.)
Magnesium	400 to 800 mg once a day	Consult healthcare provider for dosage if you have kidney disease. Discontinue use and see your doctor if you experience abdominal pain. Take a lower dose if it causes diarrhea.
Olive leaf extract	1 capsule one to three times daily	Take with food.
Pancreatic enzymes	1 to 2 capsules either with meal or one hour after eating	Do not take if you have an ulcer.
Peppermint oil	1 capsule after meal or 1 drop of oil into water/tea after meal	Consult doctor regarding use if you have gall bladder problems, liver problems, or diabetes.
Probiotics	20 billion units once a day	If taking an antibiotic, wait three hours before taking probiotics.
Querectin	500 to 2,000 mg once a day	
UltraInflamX	Follow instructions on bottle.	Metagenics product. (See Resources.) Do not use if taking a diuretic.
Vitamin A and mixed carotenoids	5,000 to 10,000 IU— half vitamin A and half mixed carotenoids —once a day	Use caution when taking vitamin A supplements because they have the potential to be toxic. Do not take for extended periods of time. Do not take high dosages if you have liver disease, are a smoker, or are exposed to asbestos.
Vitamin B_9 (folic acid)	800 mcg once a day	High doses can deplete your body of other vitamins in the B complex.
Vitamin C	500 to 1,500 mg twice a day	Do not take high dosages if you are prone to kidney stones or gout.
Vitamin E	200 to 400 IU once a day	Consult healthcare provider first if you are taking a blood thinner.
Zinc	25 to 75 mg once a day	The best zinc supplements are zinc picolinate and zinc citrate. If you are taking zinc and iron supplements, take one in the morning and one in the evening. (Taking them together reduces the efficiency of both.)

LEAKY GUT SYNDROME

A common but poorly recognized problem, leaky gut syndrome occurs when spaces develop between the cells of the gut (the intestines), allowing bacteria, toxins, medications, and partially digested particles of food to leak into the body. This can lead to a host of problems, including poor absorption of nutrients, infection, food allergies, chemical sensitivities, and autoimmune disease.

The symptoms of leaky gut syndrome are wide in range, and include gastrointestinal complaints, such as abdominal pain, constipation, bloating, gas, and diarrhea; neurological problems, such as anxiety, confusion, mood swings, and poor memory; breathing problems, such as shortness of breath and asthma; and various other difficulties, including poor immunity, recurrent bladder infections, chronic joint pain, and fatigue.

Leaky gut syndrome can have a number of causes. These include heavy metal toxicity; environmental toxins; nutritional deficiencies; the use of certain medications, such as broad-spectrum antibiotics, birth control pills, prednisone, and non-steroidal anti-inflammatory drugs (NSAIDs); fungal infection; food allergies; excess consumption of refined sugar, caffeine, and alcohol; a deficiency of digestive enzymes or hydrochloric acid in the stomach; and even stress.

A healthy diet can help avoid leaky gut syndrome, and aid in repairing the gut when problems occur. A number of supplements can also improve gut health.

SUPPLEMENTS TO TREAT LEAKY GUT SYNDROME

Supplements	Dosage	Considerations
EPA/DHA (fish oil)	500 mg to 1,000 mg three times a day	Choose a source that contains vitamin E to prevent oxidation.
Fiber, soluble and insoluble	10 to 20 g of supplements in addition to a diet high in fiber	Choose a fiber supplement with no added sugar. Supplement with several glasses of water.
Gamma-linolenic acid (GLA)	500 mg three times a day	It is important to maintain the proper ratio of omega-6 fatty acids to omega-3 fatty acids. (See page 110.)

Glutamine	2,000 to 6,000 mg once a day	If you have a sensitivity to monosodium glutamate (MSG), use glutamine with caution. If you are taking medications for seizures, only take glutamine under the direction of your doctor.
Inflamma-bLOX	Follow instructions on bottle.	Ortho Molecular product. (See Resources.)
Methylsulfonyl-methane (MSM)	1,000 mg three times a day	When beginning supplementation, ingest with meals to avoid possible heartburn. May cause stomach upset in dosages larger than 6,000 mg.
N-acetylcysteine (NAC)	500 mg once a day	When taking NAC supplements, also take extra vitamin C, copper, and zinc.
Pancreatic enzymes	1 to 2 capsules with meal or one hour after eating	Do not use if you have an ulcer.
Probiotics	20 billion units once a day	If taking an antibiotic, wait three hours before taking probiotics.
Quercetin	500 mg three times a day	
UltraInflamX	Follow instructions on bottle.	Metagenics product. (See Resources.) Do not use if taking a diuretic.
Vitamin A and mixed carotenoids	5,000 to 15,000 IU—half vitamin A and half mixed carotenoids—once a day	Use caution because vitamin A supplements can be toxic. Do not take for extended periods of time. Do not take more than 8,000 IU a day if you have liver disease, are a smoker, or are exposed to asbestos.
Vitamin B_5 (pantothenic acid)	100 to 200 mg three times a day	High doses can deplete your body of other vitamins in the B complex.
Vitamin C	500 mg twice a day	Do not take high dosages if you are prone to kidney stones or gout.
Vitamin E	400 IU once a day	If you are taking a blood thinner, vitamin E may allow you to lower your dosage.
Zinc	10 to 20 mg three times a day	The best zinc supplements are zinc picolinate and zinc citrate. If you are taking zinc and iron supplements, take one in the morning and one in the evening. (Taking them together reduces the efficiency of both.)

LEG CRAMPS

A leg cramp is a painful, involuntary contraction of a single muscle or group of muscles in the leg. Most commonly, leg cramps occur in the calf muscles, but the thigh muscles can also be affected. Typically, these cramps take place at night, sometimes awakening the individual from sleep, and last anywhere from less than a minute to several minutes before subsiding. They are most often experienced by adolescents and the elderly.

The exact cause of leg cramps is not understood. However, the occurrence of these cramps has been linked to a number of risk factors, including muscle fatigue, heavy exercising, dehydration, excess weight, electrolyte imbalance, and the use of certain medications.

Gentle stretching of the muscles, a well-balanced diet, adequate rest, and warm baths or showers taken before retiring at night can all reduce the occurrence of leg cramps. By helping to ensure electrolyte balance, nutritional supplements can also normalize muscle function and prevent painful contractions.

SUPPLEMENTS TO TREAT LEG CRAMPS		
Supplements	Dosage	Considerations
Calcium	600 mg twice a day	Although most people are deficient in calcium, there is a danger in taking too much calcium. Do not ingest more than 1,000 to 1,200 mg of calcium a day.
EPA/DHA (fish oil)	1,000 mg once a day	Choose a source that contains vitamin E to prevent oxidation.
Magnesium	600 to 800 mg once a day	Consult healthcare provider for dosage if you have kidney disease. Discontinue use and see your doctor if you experience abdominal pain. Take a lower dose if it causes diarrhea.
Potassium	As prescribed by your doctor.	
Vitamin B$_3$ (niacin)	100 mg once a day	High doses can deplete your body of other vitamins in the B complex.
Vitamin E	400 to 800 IU daily	Consult healthcare provider first if you are taking a blood thinner.

LUPUS

The immune systems of people who have lupus, also known as *systemic lupus erythematosus,* are unable to distinguish between foreign antigens and the person's own body. As a result, the immune system creates antibodies that attack otherwise healthy tissues and organs. The resulting inflammation can cause permanent damage to almost any body part, including the blood, brain, heart, joints, kidneys, liver, lungs, and skin.

Lupus affects many more women than men. The most common symptoms are fever, joint and muscle pain, and rashes. However, because lupus can affect so many different body parts, there are many possible symptoms. There is also no simple, definitive test for diagnosis. Unfortunately, the disease can often be mistaken for other illnesses for months or even years.

Although there is no cure for this chronic autoimmune disease, treatment can make life much more comfortable for people with lupus. They are often prescribed an anti-inflammatory or immunosuppressive drug, which may help shorten or even prevent flair-ups. Steroids may be prescribed, but are usually avoided because of the extent of their side effects. Doctors also focus on treating the disease's symptoms.

SUPPLEMENTS TO TREAT LUPUS

Supplements	Dosage	Considerations
EPA/DHA (fish oil)	1,000 to 5,000 mg once a day	Dosages above 4,000 mg a day may act as a blood thinner. Choose a source that contains vitamin E to prevent oxidation.
Eleuthero	50 to 200 mg once a day	Do not use if you have a history of heart disease.
Flaxseed	1,000 mg once a day	May interfere with anticoagulants; work as a laxative; or affect blood sugar levels.
Gamma-linolenic acid (GLA)	240 to 720 mg once a day	It is important to maintain the proper ratio of omega-6 fatty acids to omega-3 fatty acids. (See page 110.)
Glucosamine	300 to 900 mg once a day	Don't take if you are allergic to shellfish. Consult use with your healthcare provider if you have diabetes because glucosamine can alter blood sugar levels.

Glutamine	1 to 5 g once a day	If you have a sensitivity to monosodium glutamate (MSG), use glutamine with caution. If you are taking medications for seizures, only take glutamine under the direction of your doctor.
Kaprex AI	1 softgel capsule twice a day	Made by Metagenics. (See Resources.) Do not use if taking an anticoagulant.
Magnesium	400 to 800 mg once a day	Consult healthcare provider for dosage if you have kidney disease. Discontinue use and see your doctor if you experience abdominal pain. Take a lower dose if it causes diarrhea.
Olive leaf extract	1 capsule one to three times daily	Take with food.
Probiotics	20 billion units once a day	If taking an antibiotic, wait three hours before taking probiotics.
Selenium	100 to 200 mcg once a day	
Vitamin C	500 to 1,500 mg twice a day	Do not take high dosages if you are prone to kidney stones or gout.
Vitamin E	400 IU once a day	Take mixed tocopherols, the more active type of vitamin E. Consult healthcare provider first if you are taking a blood thinner.

MACULAR DEGENERATION

Macular degeneration is the progressive destruction of the *macula,* an oval spot in the eye that is responsible for central vision and is specialized for fine detail. Because this condition usually affects the elderly, it is also referred to as *age-related macular degeneration,* or AMD. In the United States, macular degeneration is the leading cause of vision loss and blindness in those over sixty-five years of age.

There are two types of macular degeneration. *Dry (non-neovascular) macular degeneration* is an early stage of the disease, and is diagnosed when deteriorating tissue begins to accumulate as yellowish spots known as drusen. *Wet (neovascular) macular degeneration* occurs when new blood vessels grow beneath the retina, leaking blood and fluid, and permanently damaging retinal cells.

Macular degeneration usually results in a slow and painless loss of vision, although more rapid vision loss sometimes occurs. Early signs of AMD-related vision loss include shadowy areas in central vision, or unusually fuzzy or distorted vision. Even before symptoms appear, your healthcare provider may detect AMD through a retinal examination. A special graph pattern called an Amsler grid may then be used to help determine if AMD is the problem.

As already mentioned, macular degeneration is usually associated with aging and the related deterioration of eye tissues. Specific variants of one or more genes have also been linked to AMD. Other risk factors include smoking, high blood pressure, light eye color, not wearing sunglasses when exposed to sunlight, obesity, the use of certain drugs, and a poor diet—especially one that is high in fat. Many researchers believe that certain nutrients can help lower the risk for AMD.

SUPPLEMENTS TO TREAT MACULAR DEGENERATION

Supplements	Dosage	Considerations
Alpha-lipoic acid	300 to 400 mg once a day	Improves blood sugar levels so diabetics may be able to take less medication.
B-complex vitamins	50 mg twice a day	I suggest taking a multi-vitamin.
Bilberry	120 mg once a day	May cause low blood sugar levels.
Carnitine	200 mg once a day	
Coenzyme Q_{10}	100 mg once a day	May reduce the effects of blood thinners. May cause diarrhea in dosages above 100 mg once a day.
Copper	2 mg once a day	Your copper-to-zinc ratio is very important for your health. Also, do not take copper supplement cupric oxide, which has a very low bioavailability.
EPA/DHA (fish oil)	1,000 to 2,000 mg once a day	Choose a source that contains vitamin E to prevent oxidation.
Ginkgo biloba	120 mg once a day	Do not use if taking a blood thinner.
Lutein	12 mg once a day	Taking for more than six months can cause an imbalance of arginine. Do not take if you have diabetes or are allergic to eggs, milk, or wheat.
N-acetylcysteine (NAC)	1,000 to 3,000 mg once a day	When taking NAC supplements, also take extra vitamin C, copper, and zinc.
Selenium	200 to 400 mcg once a day	

Taurine	3,000 mg once a day	Take between meals. Discontinue use if you suddenly have feelings of chest or throat tightness or if you break out in hives. Do not take with aspirin.
Vitamin A and mixed carotenoids	5,000 to 20,000 IU— half vitamin A and half mixed carotenoids— once a day	Do not take more than 8,000 IU a day if you have liver disease, are a smoker, or are exposed to asbestos. Do not use large dosage of vitamin A long term.
Vitamin C	1,000 to 1,500 mg twice a day	Do not take high dosages if you are prone to kidney stones or gout. Higher dosages may cause diarrhea.
Vitamin E	400 to 800 IU once a day	Take mixed tocopherols, the more active type of vitamin E. Consult healthcare provider first if you are taking a blood thinner.
Zinc	25 to 80 mg once a day	The best zinc supplements are zinc picolinate and zinc citrate. If you are taking zinc and iron supplements, take one in the morning and one in the evening. (Taking them together reduces the efficiency of both.)

MENOPAUSE-RELATED PROBLEMS

Menopause occurs when a woman has permanently stopped menstruating. Prior to menopause, most women experience *perimenopause,* during which periods become progessively less frequent and regular. When the cycle has stopped for at least one full year, the woman has entered menopause. Women are usually between the ages of thirty-five and fifty-five when this occurs.

During menopause, the body experiences hormone changes. Hormones such as estrogen and progesterone—which were previously involved in regulating the menstrual cycle—are suddenly at much lower levels. Resulting symptoms can occur quickly or gradually, and at varying degrees of severity. (They often begin during perimenopause.) These include anxiety, mood swings, hot flashes, night sweats, headaches, and decreased bone density (which can lead to osteoporosis).

Some women claim that their only relief from menopause symptoms came from alternative medicine. Some of the more popular natural herbs for this purpose are listed on page 308. You may find that these nutrients, along with a healthy lifestyle and the implementation of relaxation techniques, successfully decrease your menopausal symptoms. (See also "Hormone Replacement Therapy" on page 371.)

■ Supplements to Ease Symptoms of Menopause

- Black cohash (should not be taken for extended periods of time)
- Chasteberry
- Dong Quai
- Soy

MIGRAINE HEADACHES

A migraine headache is a moderate to severe headache, usually occurring on one side of the head only. It can last from several hours to three days, and is often accompanied by gastrointestinal problems such as nausea and vomiting. Other symptoms characteristic of migraines include pain that has a pulsating or throbbing quality, pain that worsens with physical activity, and sensitivity to light and sound.

Fifteen to thirty minutes before the migraine begins, some people experience an *aura*—a "warning" that comes in the form of sparkling flashes of light, dazzling zigzag lines, slowly spreading blind spots, tingling sensations in an arm or leg, or even speech problems. Although auras typically occur before the onset of a migraine, they sometimes continue after the headache starts or even occur after it begins.

Experts are still debating the cause and mechanism of the migraine headache. What is known is that migraines can have various triggers, including hormonal changes; the consumption of certain foods, such as aged cheese, wine, chocolate, fermented and marinated foods, and monosodium glutamate; stress; sensory stimuli such as bright lights and sun glare; changes in the sleep-wake cycle; changes in the weather; and the use of certain medications.

If you suffer from migraine headaches, it makes sense to avoid potential triggers. In addition, certain nutrients are known to help prevent the occurrence of migraines.

SUPPLEMENTS TO TREAT MIGRAINE HEADACHES

Supplements	Dosage	Considerations
B-complex vitamins	50 mg twice a day	I suggest taking a multi-vitamin.
Calcium	500 mg once or twice a day	Although most people are deficient in calcium, there is a danger in taking too much calcium. Do not ingest more than 1,000 to 1,200 mg of calcium a day.
Carnitine	1,000 to 3,000 once a day	The most effective form for this purpose is acetyl-L-carnitine (ALCAR).
Coenzyme Q_{10}	100 mg twice a day	May reduce the effects of blood thinners. Dosages above 100 mg once a day may cause diarrhea.
Curcumin	100 to 1,000 mg once a day	
EPA/DHA (fish oil)	1,000 to 2,000 mg once a day	Choose a source that contains vitamin E to prevent oxidation.
Feverfew	100 mg once a day for at least one month	If you are allergic to plants in the daisy family (such as chamomile or ragweed), do not take feverfew. It also has the potential to interact with anticoagulant drugs such as coumadin.
Magnesium	600 to 800 mg once a day	Consult healthcare provider for dosage if you have kidney disease. Discontinue use and see your doctor if you experience abdominal pain. Take a lower dose if it causes diarrhea.
Probiotics	20 billion units once a day	If taking an antibiotic, wait three hours before taking probiotics.
Selenium	200 mcg once a day	
Vitamin B_2 (riboflavin)	100 to 200 mg twice a day	High doses can deplete your body of other vitamins in the B complex.
Vitamin C	500 to 1,500 mg twice a day	Higher dosages can cause diarrhea. Do not take high dosages if you are prone to kidney stones or gout.
Vitamin D	Have your blood levels measured by your health-care provider, who will then determine proper dosage.	
Vitamin E	400 to 800 IU once a day	Consult healthcare provider first if you are taking a blood thinner.

| Zinc | 25 mg once a day | The best zinc supplements are zinc picolinate and zinc citrate. If you are taking zinc and iron supplements, take one in the morning and one in the evening. (Taking them together reduces the efficiency of both.) |

MULTIPLE SCLEROSIS

Multiple sclerosis (MS) is a degenerative disease of the nervous system that affects the brain, spinal cord, and optic nerves. In this disorder, which is usually diagnosed in young adults between ages twenty and forty, the myelin sheaths that protect the nerve fibers degenerate, leaving the nerves vulnerable to damage. Areas of the body that are controlled by the damaged nerves become impaired. Symptoms will vary, depending on which nerves are involved, and commonly include visual disturbances, muscle fatigue, slurred speech, numbness, dizziness, thinking and memory problems, and impaired balance and coordination.

Although the exact cause of MS is not known, most researchers believe it that an unknown virus triggers the autoimmune process responsible for damaging the myelin sheaths. Heredity seems to play a role—15 percent of those with this disease have a close relative who is also affected. It is also much more prevalent in colder climates.

Currently, there is no cure for MS, although a number of promising treatments are being investigated. Nutritional supplements, moderate exercise, and the avoidance of stress have all shown to be helpful, especially during the early stages of the disease. Proper diet is also important. Several studies have shown that a low-fat, high-fiber diet can help decrease the number of new MS lesions. Saturated fats, especially those found in meat (red meat in particular) and dairy products, should be avoided, as well as hydrogenated and partially hydrogenated fats. Diet should include lots of fresh fruits and vegetables, especially leafy greens, and foods that contain beneficial omega-3 fatty acids.

SUPPLEMENTS TO TREAT MULTIPLE SCLEROSIS

Supplements	Dosage	Considerations
Alpha-lipoic acid	100 to 300 mg once a day	Improves blood sugar levels so diabetics may be able to take less medication.

Carnitine	500 to 3,000 mg once a day	
Coenzyme Q_{10}	100 to 300 mg once a day	May reduce the effects of blood thinners. May cause diarrhea in dosages above 100 mg once a day.
Copper	1 to 2 mg once a day	Your copper-to-zinc ratio is very important for your health. Also, do not take copper supplement cupric oxide, which has a very low bioavailability.
EPA/DHA (fish oil)	1,000 to 3,000 mg once a day	Choose a source that contains vitamin E to prevent oxidation.
Gamma-linolenic acid (GLA)	300 to 720 mg once a day	It is important to maintain the proper ratio of omega-6 fatty acids to omega-3 fatty acids. (See page 110.)
Ginkgo biloba	30 mg once a day	Do not use if taking a blood thinner.
Magnesium	400 to 600 mg once a day	Consult healthcare provider for dosage if you have kidney disease. Discontinue use and see your doctor if you experience abdominal pain. Take a lower dose if it causes diarrhea.
N-acetylcysteine (NAC)	200 mg once a day	When taking NAC supplements, also take extra vitamin C, copper, and zinc.
NADH	5 mg twice a day	Reduced and more active form of niacin.
Phosphatidylserine	200 to 300 mg once a day	
Selenium	200 mcg once a day	
Vitamin B_3 (niacin)	25 mg twice a day	High doses can deplete your body of other vitamins in the B complex.
Vitamin B_6 (pyridoxine)	25 mg twice a day	Do not take more than 500 mg a day. If you are taking L-dopa for Parkinson's disease, do not take B_6 without first consulting your doctor.
Vitamin B_9 (folic acid)	500 mcg once a day	High doses can deplete your body of other vitamins in the B complex.
Vitamin B_{12} (cobalamin)	1,000 mcg once a day	High doses can deplete your body of other vitamins in the B complex.
Vitamin C	500 mg twice a day	Do not take high dosages if you are prone to kidney stones or gout.
Vitamin D	Have your blood levels measured by your healthcare provider, who will then determine proper dosage.	

Vitamin E	400 IU once a day	Take mixed tocopherols, the more active type of vitamin E. Consult healthcare provider first if you are taking a blood thinner.
Zinc	10 to 15 mg once a day	The best zinc supplements are zinc picolinate and zinc citrate. If you are taking zinc and iron supplements, take one in the morning and one in the evening. (Taking them together reduces the efficiency of both.)

MUSCLE CRAMPS

See Leg Cramps.

MYASTHENIA GRAVIS

Myasthenia gravis is a chronic autoimmune disease in which the immune system attacks the body's own proteins as foreign antigens. Specifically, the immune system targets and interferes with acetylcholine, a neurotransmitter that transmits messages between the nerves and muscles. This results in moderate to severe muscle weakness that can occur throughout the body.

The muscle weakness is usually first seen in the eye. Often, other effects on the face—such as eye movement, facial expression, and swallowing—then become visible as well. A person with myasthenia gravis may have double vision or impaired speech. The disease can affect any voluntary muscle, including any limb and the lungs.

Myasthenia gravis can be medicated by either treating the symptom or trying to suppress the autoimmune disease. The symptom can be treated by increasing muscle strength through medication. To suppress the disease, doctors can prescribe immunosuppressant drugs, which would discourage the immune system from attacking acetylcholine. However, because immunosuppressant drugs can have dangerous side effects, they are usually only recommended for a short period of time and when found to be extremely necessary. Anticholinesterase agents, on the other hand, both treat the weakened muscles and suppress the immune system. A patient could also decide to have his thymus gland removed, a procedure that is often effective—but it can sometimes take years for the effects to be felt.

Because myasthenia gravis can restrict vitally important muscles, such as the lungs, patients can have life-threatening episodes. In these situations, immediate and professional medical help is critical.

SUPPLEMENTS TO TREAT MYASTHENIA GRAVIS		
Supplements	Dosage	Considerations
EPA/DHA (fish oil)	1,000 to 5,000 mg once a day	Choose a source that contains vitamin E to prevent oxidation.
Eleuthero	50 to 200 mg once a day	Do not use if you have a history of heart disease.
Flaxseed	1,000 mg once a day	May interfere with anticoagulants; work as a laxative; or affect blood sugar levels.
Gamma-linolenic acid (GLA)	240 to 720 mg once a day	It is important to maintain the proper ratio of omega-6 fatty acids to omega-3 fatty acids. (See page 110.)
Glucosamine	300 to 900 mg once a day	Don't take if you are allergic to shellfish. Consult use with your healthcare provider if you have diabetes because glucosamine can alter blood sugar levels.
Glutamine	1 to 5 g once a day	If you have a sensitivity to monosodium glutamate (MSG), use glutamine with caution. If you are taking medications for seizures, only take glutamine under the direction of your doctor.
Kaprex AI	1 softgel capsule twice a day	Made by Metagenics. (See Resources.) Do not use if taking an anticoagulant.
Magnesium	400 to 800 mg once a day	Consult healthcare provider for dosage if you have kidney disease. Discontinue use and see your doctor if you experience abdominal pain. Take a lower dose if it causes diarrhea.
Olive leaf extract	1 to 3 capsules once a day	Take with food.
Probiotics	20 billion units once a day	If taking an antibiotic, wait three hours before taking probiotics.
Selenium	200 to 300 mcg once a day	
Vitamin C	500 to 1,500 mg twice a day	Do not take high dosages if you are prone to kidney stones or gout.

| Vitamin E | 400 IU once a day | Take mixed tocopherols, the more active type of vitamin E. Consult healthcare provider first if you are taking a blood thinner. |

NON-INSULIN-DEPENDENT DIABETES

See Diabetes Mellitus.

OSTEOARTHRITIS

Also known as *osteoarthrosis, degenerative arthritis,* and *degenerative joint disease,* osteoarthritis is a gradual wearing down of *cartilage*—the firm, elastic tissue that connects bones with muscles and protects the joints. This can cause swelling and inflammation of the joints, reduced mobility, and muscle spasms. Simple movement often causes pain, which is usually characterized by either a sharp ache or burning sensation. Painful *bone spurs*—abnormal growths of bone—can form as well. It is most likely to occur to the hips, knees, spine, feet, and hands.

The most common type of arthritis, osteoarthritis affects more than 20 million people in the United States. It usually begins around middle age. Sufferers tend to feel best in the morning, with symptoms becoming progressively worse as the day continues. Osteoarthritis is irreversible, so treatment aims to reduce pain and improve mobility.

SUPPLEMENTS TO TREAT OSTEOARTHRITIS		
Supplements	**Dosage**	**Considerations**
B-complex vitamins	25 to 50 mg twice a day	I suggest a multi-vitamin.
Boron	1,000 mcg once a day	
Chondroitin sulfate	500 to 2,000 mg once a day	
EPA/DHA (fish oil)	1,000 to 2,000 mg once a day	Choose a source that contains vitamin E to prevent oxidation.
Gamma-linolenic acid (GLA)	240 to 720 mg once a day	It is important to maintain the proper ratio of omega-6 fatty acids to omega-3 fatty acids. (See page 110.)

Ginger	100 mg once a day	Do not take with coumadin or nonsteroidal anti-inflammatory pain medications (NSAIDs).
Glucosamine	1,000 mg three times a day	Don't take if you are allergic to shellfish. Consult use with your healthcare provider if you have diabetes because glucosamine can alter blood sugar levels.
Manganese	5 to 10 mg once a day	
Methylsulfonyl-methane (MSM)	1,000 to 10,000 mg once a day	When beginning supplementation, ingest with meals to avoid possible heartburn. May cause stomach upset when taken in large doses.
Quercetin	500 to 1,000 mg once a day	
UltraInflamX	Follow instructions on bottle.	Metagenics product. (See Resources.) Do not use if taking a diuretic.

OSTEOPOROSIS

Osteoporosis is a progressive disease in which the bones become porous and brittle, making them susceptible to fractures. It is the cause of approximately 1.2 million cases of broken bones each year in the United States. Although one-third of the cases involve men, osteoporosis occurs primarily in postmenopausal women. In most cases, the bone loss does not cause any symptoms, so the condition usually goes unnoticed until a break occurs.

Osteoporosis tends to occur more often in small, fine-boned individuals, rather than those with larger, denser bones. It is particularly threatening to women after menopause because that is when the ovaries stop producing estrogen, which helps maintain bone mass. Other causes of osteoporosis include calcium deficiency and a deficiency in vitamin D, which helps the body absorb calcium. If the body does not get a sufficient amount of calcium through foods and/or supplements, it will rob this essential mineral from the bones. Other dietary factors that increase the risk of osteoporosis include excessive intakes of protein, salt, sugar, caffeine, and carbonated soft drinks. Foods containing oxalic acid, such as spinach, Swiss chard, beet and dandelion greens, rhubarb, asparagus, and chocolate, which bind with calcium and decrease its absorption, should also be avoided. Smoking and alcohol consumption are additional risk factors, as are a number of medications, including certain blood thinners, steroids, seizure medications, chemotherapy drugs, lithium, and tetracycline. Abnormal cortisol (a stress hormone) levels can also lead to bone loss.

A diet high in calcium and vitamin D is suggested to help prevent bone loss. Also recommended is regular weight-bearing exercise, especially walking, which helps maintain strong bones.

SUPPLEMENTS TO TREAT OSTEOPOROSIS		
Supplements	**Dosage**	**Considerations**
Boron	1 to 5 mg once a day	
Calcium	500 to 1,200 mg daily, in dosages no larger than 500 mg.	Use calcium hydroxyapatite or calcium citrate. Do not use calcium carbonate. Although most people are deficient in calcium, there is a danger in taking too much calcium. Do not ingest more than 1,000 to 1,200 mg of calcium a day.
Copper	1 to 2 mg once a day	Your copper-to-zinc ratio is very important for your health. Also, do not take copper supplement cupric oxide, which has a very low bioavailability.
EPA/DHA (fish oil)	500 to 1,000 mg once a day	Choose a source that contains vitamin E to prevent oxidation.
Gamma-linolenic acid (GLA)	240 mg once a day	It is important to maintain the proper ratio of omega-6 fatty acids to omega-3 fatty acids. (See page 110.)
Ipriflavone	150 to 200 mg three times a day	
Potassium		Consume foods high in potassium, such as those listed on page 74.
Vitamin B_9 (folic acid)	500 mcg once a day	High doses can deplete your body of other vitamins in the B complex.
Vitamin B_{12} (cobalamin)	1,000 mcg once a day	High doses can deplete your body of other vitamins in the B complex.
Magnesium	400 to 800 mg once a day	Consult healthcare provider for dosage if you have kidney disease. Discontinue use and see your doctor if you experience abdominal pain. Take a lower dose if it causes diarrhea.
Manganese	5 to 10 mg once a day	
Vitamin C	500 mg twice a day	Do not take high dosages if you are prone to kidney stones or gout.

Vitamin D	Have your blood levels measured by your health-care provider, who will then determine proper dosage.	
Vitamin K	150 mcg once a day	High dosages can cause toxicity. Consult your healthcare provider before taking if you are on an anticoagulant. K_2 is particularly effective at maintaining bone structure.
Zinc	25 mg once a day	The best zinc supplements are zinc picolinate and zinc citrate. If you are taking zinc and iron supplements, take one in the morning and one in the evening. (Taking them together reduces the efficiency of both.)

OVARIAN CYSTS

See Polycystic Ovarian Syndrome.

PARKINSON'S DISEASE

Also known as *palsy* or *paralysis agitans*, Parkinson's disease is a degenerative condition that affects the nervous system. It is caused by a lack of the neurotransmitter *dopamine* in the brain. Normally, dopamine, together with the neurotransmitter *acetylcholine*, transmits messages between nerve cells that control muscle function. Acetylcholine sends the signal that causes muscles to contract, while dopamine keeps the contractions at manageable levels. In people with Parkinson's, the imbalance between these two chemicals causes involuntary tremors and muscle stiffness.

More common in men than women, and often occurring in those over sixty years old, Parkinson's disease usually starts with mild tremors in a hand or leg that worsens when it is resting. As the disease progresses, so does the trembling, which eventually affects both sides of the body. Later symptoms typically include stiffness, muscle weakness, a shaking head, and shuffling gait. A "pill-rolling" movement in which the thumb and forefinger rub together is another characteristic of the disease. Speech becomes impaired and everyday activities require assistance.

The cause of Parkinson's disease is not known. One popular theory suggests that an accumulation of environmental toxins may be a factor.

SUPPLEMENTS TO TREAT PARKINSON'S DISEASE

Supplements	Dosage	Considerations
Alpha-lipoic acid	100 to 600 mg once a day	Improves blood sugar levels so diabetics may be able to take less medication.
Bilberry	100 to 300 mg once a day	May cause low blood sugar levels.
Carnitine	1,500 to 3,000 mg once a day	
Coenzyme Q_{10}	100 to 1,200 mg once a day	May reduce the effects of blood thinners. May cause diarrhea in dosages above 100 mg once a day.
Gingko biloba	240 to 360 mg once a day	Do not use if taking a blood thinner.
Grape seed extract	50 to 200 mg once a day	
N-acetylcysteine (NAC)	500 to 2,000 mg once a day	When taking NAC supplements, also take extra vitamin C, copper, and zinc.
NADH	5 to 10 mg twice a day	Reduced and more active form of niacin.
Phosphatidylserine	300 to 500 mg once a day	
Probiotics	20 billion units once a day	If taking an antibiotic, wait three hours before taking probiotics.
Selenium	200 mcg once a day	
Silymarin	100 to 300 mg once a day	
Vitamin C	500 to 2,500 mg twice a day	Do not take high dosages if you are prone to kidney stones or gout.
Vitamin D	Have your blood levels measured by your health-care provider, who will then determine proper dosage.	
Vitamin E	800 to 1,200 IU once a day	Consult healthcare provider first if you are taking a blood thinner.

PCOS

See Polycystic Ovarian Syndrome.

PERIMENOPAUSE

See Menopause-Related Problems.

PERIODONTAL DISEASE

Periodontal disease refers to any infection of the tissues that support the teeth. It begins just below the gum line, where it causes the tooth attachment and the gums to break down. This type of disease is classified according to its severity, of which there are two major stages—gingivitis and periodontitis. Gingivitis, which affects only the gums, is a milder and reversible form of the disease. Left untreated, it can lead to periodontitis (also called *pyorrhea*), a more serious, destructive condition that erodes the underlying bone and leads to tooth loss. Periodontal disease is also a major risk factor for heart disease. In the United States, over 75 percent of adults over age thirty-five have some degree of periodontal disease.

Poor nutrition and inadequate oral hygiene are key factors in the development of periodontal disease. Other factors that can increase its risk include excessive alcohol and sugar consumption, tobacco chewing or smoking, and a number of medications, including certain cancer therapy drugs, steroids, and oral contraceptives. Individuals with systemic diseases such as diabetes are also at greater risk.

Although there are several signs that can signal a possible periodontal problem—gums that are red, swollen, and tender; persistent bad breath; gums that bleed easily; permanent teeth that begin to separate or loosen; and gums that have receded from the teeth—it is possible to experience no warning signs at all! This is one reason that regular dental checkups are so important. Of course good daily hygiene, which includes brushing and flossing, is essential as well.

SUPPLEMENTS TO TREAT PERIODONTAL DISEASE

Supplements	Dosage	Considerations
Calcium	500 mg once or twice a day	Although most people are deficient in calcium, there is a danger in taking too much calcium. Do not ingest more than 1,000 to 1,200 mg of calcium a day.

Carnitine	1,000 to 2,000 mg once a day	
Coenzyme Q_{10}	50 to 200 mg once a day	Available at compounding pharmacies as a prescription paste to brush on gums or can be swallowed as supplement.
Copper	2 mg once a day	Your copper-to-zinc ratio is very important for your health. Also, do not take copper supplement cupric oxide, which has a very low bioavailability.
EPA/DHA (fish oil)	2,000 mg once a day	Choose a source that contains vitamin E to prevent oxidation.
Probiotics	20 billion units once a day	If taking an antibiotic, wait three hours before taking probiotics.
Vitamin A and mixed carotenoids	20,000 IU—half vitamin A and half mixed carotenoids—once a day, short term only (one to two months)	Do not take for extended periods of time. Do not take more than 8,000 IU a day if you have liver disease, are a smoker, or are exposed to asbestos.
Vitamin B_6 (pyridoxine)	100 mg twice a day	Do not take more than 500 mg a day. If you are taking L-dopa for Parkinson's disease, do not take B_6 without first consulting your doctor.
Vitamin B_9 (folic acid)	500 to 1,000 mcg once a day	High doses can deplete your body of other vitamins in the B complex.
Vitamin C	1,000 mg twice a day	Do not take high dosages if you are prone to kidney stones or gout.
Vitamin E	400 IU once a day	Consult healthcare provider first if you are taking a blood thinner.
Zinc	25 mg once a day	The best zinc supplements are zinc picolinate and zinc citrate. If you are taking zinc and iron supplements, take one in the morning and one in the evening. (Taking them together reduces the efficiency of both.)

PERIODONTITIS

See Periodontal Disease.

PIMPLES

See Acne.

PMS

See Premenstrual Syndrome.

POLYCYSTIC OVARIAN SYNDROME (PCOS)

Polycystic Ovarian Syndrome (PCOS), also known as *Stein-Leventhal syndrome,* is an endocrine disorder in which multiple cysts may develop in the ovaries. Affecting 5 to 7 percent of women, PCOS can have very serious health consequences, including type 2 diabetes, uterine cancer, high cholesterol, high blood pressure, heart disease, and infertility.

A woman with PCOS may have any number of the following symptoms and signs: irregular menstruation and/or menstruation cycles; lack of ovulation; elevated levels of male hormones, specifically testosterone, androstenedione, and dehydroepiandrosterone sulfate (DHEAS); obesity, usually particularly concentrated at the torso; pain during sexual intercourse; larger than normal ovaries; excess hair on face or body; acne; sleep apnea; and insulin resistance.

There are a variety of medication options for women with PCOS. Doctors also recommend regular exercise and a change in diet, to one that is either low in carbohydrates or low according to the glycemic index. The addition of the following nutrients will add to the likelihood of success of most treatments.

SUPPLEMENTS TO TREAT POLYCYSTIC OVARIAN SYNDROME

Supplements	Dosage	Considerations
Alpha-lipoic acid	100 to 300 mg once a day	Improves blood sugar levels so diabetics may be able to take less medication.
B-complex vitamins	25 mg twice a day	I suggest taking a multi-vitamin.
Carnitine	1,000 to 3,000 mg once a day	

Chromium	600 to 1,000 mcg once a day	Combining with the protein picolinate allows your body to absorb chromium more efficiently. However, some chromium picolinate supplements contain more chromium than necessary. Ask your health-care provider for a recommendation.
Copper	1 to 3 mg once a day	Your copper-to-zinc ratio is very important for your health. Also, do not take copper supplement cupric oxide, which has a very low bioavailability.
EPA/DHA (fish oil)	500 to 1,000 mg once a day	Choose a source that contains vitamin E to prevent oxidation.
Gamma-linolenic acid (GLA)	240 to 480 mg once a day	It is important to maintain the proper ratio of omega-6 fatty acids to omega-3 fatty acids. (See page 110.)
Inositol	6,000 mg twice a day	Only take this dosage under the direction of a physician. May stimulate uterine contractions. Women who wish to become pregnant should consult their doctor regarding its use.
Magnesium	400 to 800 mg once a day	Consult healthcare provider for dosage if you have kidney disease. Discontinue use and see your doctor if you experience abdominal pain. Take a lower dose if it causes diarrhea.
Taurine	500 to 2,000 mg once a day	Take between meals. Discontinue use if you suddenly have feelings of chest or throat tightness or if you break out in hives. Do not take with aspirin.
Vanadium	50 mg once a day	Do not take more than 50 mg a day.
Vitamin C	1,000 to 3,000 mg once a day	Do not take high dosages if you are prone to kidney stones or gout.
Vitamin D	Have your blood levels measured by your health-care provider, who will then determine proper dosage.	
Vitamin E	400 to 800 IU once a day	Take mixed tocopherols, the more active type of vitamin E. Consult healthcare provider first if you are taking a blood thinner.
Zinc	25 to 50 mg once a day	The best zinc supplements are zinc picolinate and zinc citrate. If you are taking zinc and iron supplements, take one in the morning and one in the evening. (Taking them together reduces the efficiency of both.)

PREMENSTRUAL SYNDROME (PMS)

Premenstrual syndrome (PMS) occurs to some women in the week before they begin menstruating each month and continues until menstruation begins. It may even last one or two days after the period begins. Emotional symptoms include tension, anxiety, irritability, mood swings, and depression. Physical symptoms include weight gain from water retention, backache, sensitivity of breasts, swelling of feet or ankles, acne, headache, and joint or muscle pain. Many women experience some of these symptoms during menstruation, but for women with PMS, the severity of these symptoms is disabling and interferes with their regular lives.

The cause of PMS is unknown and debated, although many people believe hormones to be at the root of the problem. Treatment—such as anti-inflammatories, diuretics, anti-anxiety medication, antidepressants, and medications that fluctuate hormones—tend to deal with different causes and different symptoms. Every woman is unique, and may find success with a different method. However, before beginning one of the aforementioned treatments, some people find that a simple change to a more healthy, well-balanced diet with less sugar, salt, and candy in the week before menstruation can help immensely. Other women find that their symptoms are sufficiently improved after implementing a healthier diet with the addition of the nutrients in the following table.

There are also some women who experience symptoms that are even more severe and last for as long as two weeks. These women have premenstrual dysphoric disorder (PMDD). Sufferers of PMDD should see their healthcare provider.

SUPPLEMENTS TO TREAT PREMENSTRUAL SYNDROME

Supplements	Dosage	Considerations
B-complex vitamins	50 mg mg once a day	I suggest taking a multi-vitamin.
Calcium	500 mg twice daily	Although most people are deficient in calcium, there is a danger in taking too much calcium. Do not ingest more than 1,000 to 1,200 mg of calcium a day.
Carnitine	500 mg once a day	
Chasteberry	50 mg once a day	

Chromium	400 mcg once a day	Combining with the protein picolinate allows your body to absorb chromium more efficiently. However, some chromium picolinate supplements contain more chromium than necessary. Ask your healthcare provider for a recommendation.
Copper	1 to 2 mg once a day	Your copper-to-zinc ratio is very important for your health. Also, do not take copper supplement cupric oxide, which has a very low bioavailability.
Gamma-linolenic acid (GLA)	240 mg once a day	It is important to maintain the proper ratio of omega-6 fatty acids to omega-3 fatty acids. (See page 110.)
Inositol	500 to 1,000 mg twice a day	May stimulate uterine contractions. Women who wish to become pregnant should consult their doctor regarding its use.
Magnesium	400 to 800 mg once a day	Consult healthcare provider for dosage if you have kidney disease. Discontinue use and see your doctor if you experience abdominal pain. Take a lower dose if it causes diarrhea.
Manganese	2 to 5 mg once a day	
Vitamin A and mixed carotenoids	10,000 to 20,000 IU— half vitamin A and half mixed carotenoids— once a day	Use caution when taking vitamin A supplements because they have the potential to be toxic. Do not take for extended periods of time. Do not take more than 5,000 IU a day if you have liver disease, are a smoker, or are exposed to asbestos.
Vitamin C	1,000 mg once a day	Do not take high dosages if you are prone to kidney stones or gout.
Vitamin E	400 IU once a day	Take mixed tocopherols, the more active type of vitamin E. Consult healthcare provider first if you are taking a blood thinner.
Zinc	25 to 50 mg once a day	The best zinc supplements are zinc picolinate and zinc citrate. If you are taking zinc and iron supplements, take one in the morning and one in the evening. (Taking them together reduces the efficiency of both.)

SUPPLEMENTS TO TREAT PAINFUL MENSTRUAL CYCLES

Supplements	Dosage	Considerations
EPA/DHA (fish oil)	2,000 to 3,000 mg once a day	Choose a source that contains vitamin E to prevent oxidation.
Gamma-linolenic acid (GLA)	500 to 1,000 mg once a day	It is important to maintain the proper ratio of omega-6 fatty acids to omega-3 fatty acids. (See page 110.)
Vitamin B_{12} (cobalamin)	1,000 mcg once a day	High doses can deplete your body of other vitamins in the B complex.

PROSTATE DISORDER

See Benign Prostatic Hypertrophy.

PSORIASIS

A common skin disorder that affects 2 percent of the population, psoriasis is characterized by thick patches of raised, reddish skin that is covered by what looks like silvery-white scales. In this condition, the body produces new skin cells at a much faster rate than normal; however, the old skin cells on the surface are shed at a slower, more normal rate. Because of this, the cells beneath the surface of the skin accumulate and form thick patches, while the "scales" on top are actually unshed dead skin cells. These patches, which typically appear on the scalp, elbows, knees, and lower back, often itch and may crack and bleed.

Although psoriasis is not contagious, it generally occurs in members of the same family. Flare-ups are followed by periods of healing, although the condition never disappears. The duration and severity of the cases range—some are so mild that people don't even realize they have the condition, while others are so severe the patches may cover large areas of the body. The cause of psoriasis is not known, although breakouts can be triggered by stress, infections, overexposure to the sun, and alcohol abuse. Medications, including beta blockers and nonsteroidal anti-inflammatory drugs (NSAIDS), are other possible triggers.

Psoriasis is not curable, but it is treatable. Keeping this condition under control requires lifelong therapy. Treatments, which can be recommended by a healthcare professional, will vary depending on the severity of the condition.

SUPPLEMENTS TO TREAT PSORIASIS		
Supplements	Dosage	Considerations
B-complex vitamins	25 to 50 mg twice a day	I suggest taking a multi-vitamin.
Copper	2 to 3 mg once a day	Your copper-to-zinc ratio is very important for your health. Also, do not take copper supplement cupric oxide, which has a very low bioavailability.
Dandelion	100 mg once a day	If you have gallstones or obstructed bile ducts, consult your healthcare practitioner before taking.
EPA/DHA (fish oil)	1,000 to 3,000 mg once a day	Choose a source that contains vitamin E to prevent oxidation.
Evening primrose oil	500 to 1,000 mg once a day	
Glucosamine	1,000 mg once a day	Don't take if you are allergic to shellfish. Consult use with your healthcare provider if you have diabetes because glucosamine can alter blood sugar levels.
Methylsulfonyl-methane (MSM)	3,000 to 10,000 mg once a day	When beginning supplementation, ingest with meals to avoid possible heartburn. May cause stomach upset in dosages larger than 6,000 mg.
Milk thistle	200 mg once a day	Reduces efficiency of certain blood pressure medication.
Probiotics	20 billion units once a day	If taking an antibiotic, wait three hours before taking probiotics.
Taurine	2,000 mg once a day	Take between meals. Discontinue use if you suddenly have feelings of chest or throat tightness or if you break out in hives. Do not take with aspirin.
Tea tree oil	Apply directly to skin once or twice a day.	Do not ingest or use in ears, eyes, or other mucous membranes.
Vitamin A and mixed carotenoids	10,000 to 20,000 IU—half vitamin A and half mixed carotenoids—once a day for one month.	Your physician may recommend higher dosages, but only take these dosages under the supervision of your healthcare provider.
Vitamin C	500 to 1,500 mg twice a day	Do not take high dosages if you are prone to kidney stones or gout.
Vitamin D	Have your blood levels measured by your health-care provider, who will then determine proper dosage.	

Vitamin E	400 IU once a day	Take mixed tocopherols, the more active type of vitamin E. Consult healthcare provider first if you are taking a blood thinner.
Zinc	25 to 75 mg once a day	The best zinc supplements are zinc picolinate and zinc citrate. If you are taking zinc and iron supplements, take one in the morning and one in the evening. (Taking them together reduces the efficiency of both.)

PYORRHEA

See Periodontal Disease.

RHEUMATOID ARTHRITIS

Rheumatoid arthritis is an autoimmune disease in which the body's immune system mistakenly attacks healthy tissue and joints, resulting in chronic inflammation. It is a debilitating disease because it can create a severe lack of mobility. Rheumatoid arthritis causes pain, stiffness, swelling, and even destruction of the joints during periods of inflammation, which are followed by periods of remission. This chronic illness can affect any joint in the body. For most people, the effects are worst upon wakening and gradually subside as the day progresses.

Although there is no known cause, many people hypothesize that rheumatoid arthritis is related to a prior infection from a bacteria, fungus, or virus. Other people believe that the disease is genetic. Still others believe it to be a result of lifestyle choices, such as smoking tobacco. Scientists are currently studying rheumatoid arthritis in an effort to pinpoint its cause.

Treatment for rheumatoid arthritis addresses the inflammatory component of the disease while also attempting to stabilize the immune system. Patients with rheumatoid arthritis should decrease their intake of foods from the nightshade group, such as eggplants, peppers, potatoes, and tomatoes.

SUPPLEMENTS TO TREAT RHEUMATOID ARTHRITIS

Supplements	Dosage	Considerations
Alpha-lipoic acid	300 to 400 mg once a day	Improves blood sugar levels so diabetics may be able to take less medication.
Arginine	2,000 mg once a day	If you have kidney disease, liver disease, or herpes, only take under a doctor's supervision.
B-complex vitamins	50 mg once a day	I suggest a multi-vitamin.
Boswellia resin	400 mg once a day	
Carnitine	500 to 1,000 mg once a day	Doses above 100 mg can cause diarrhea.
Coenzyme Q_{10}	60 to 120 mg once a day	May reduce the effects of blood thinners. May cause diarrhea in dosages above 100 mg once a day.
Copper	2 mg once a day	Your copper-to-zinc ratio is very important for your health. Also, do not take copper supplement cupric oxide, which has a very low bioavailability.
Curcumin	100 to 1,000 mg once a day	
EPA/DHA (fish oil)	1,500 to 2,000 mg once a day	Choose a source that contains vitamin E to prevent oxidation.
Gamma-linolenic acid (GLA)	900 mg once a day	It is important to maintain the proper ratio of omega-6 fatty acids to omega-3 fatty acids. (See page 110.)
Ginger	100 mg once a day	Do not take with coumadin or nonsteroidal anti-inflammatory pain medications (NSAIDs).
Glutamine	1,500 mg once a day	If you have a sensitivity to monosodium glutamate (MSG), use glutamine with caution. If you are taking medications for seizures, only take glutamine under the direction of your doctor.
Grape seed extract	300 to 600 mg once a day	
Magnesium	600 mg once a day	Consult healthcare provider for dosage if you have kidney disease. Discontinue use and see your doctor if you experience abdominal pain. Take a lower dose if it causes diarrhea.

Methylsulfonyl-methane (MSM)	3,000 to 10,000 mg once a day	When beginning supplementation, ingest with meals to avoid possible heartburn. May cause stomach upset in dosages larger than 6,000 mg.
N-acetylcysteine (NAC)	500 to 1,000 mg once a day	When taking NAC supplements, also take extra vitamin C, copper, and zinc.
Quercetin	500 mg once a day	
Selenium	100 to 200 mcg once a day	
Vitamin C	500 to 1,000 mg twice a day	Do not take high dosages if you are prone to kidney stones or gout.
Zinc	25 mg once a day	The best zinc supplements are zinc picolinate and zinc citrate. If you are taking zinc and iron supplements, take one in the morning and one in the evening. (Taking them together reduces the efficiency of both.)

SCLERODERMA (SYSTEMIC SCLEROSIS)

Scleroderma is a chronic, degenerative disease that causes excess buildup of *collagen*—a protein chemical that strengthens connective tissue. It is then deposited throughout the skin or other organs. The collagen buildup usually appears as small white lumps under the skin that burst and become white fluid.

There are three types of scleroderma. *Limited scleroderma* is a localized disorder. The skin, particularly of the extremities, becomes hard and thick, and may also appear red and scaly. Although it can affect the muscles as well as the skin, the disease travels slowly and does not usually spread to the organs. *Diffuse scleroderma,* (also called *systemic sclerosis* and *CREST syndrome,*) a generalized disorder, spreads quickly through the body and can affect many of the body's organs. It is the most serious and potentially fatal type of scleroderma. *Morphea scleroderma,* or *linear scleroderma,* can affect different parts of the skin but does not interfere with the body's other organs.

People with scleroderma may experience a wide array of symptoms. Their skin may appear shiny, discolored, or hard, and may be itchy. They may feel fatigued, short of breath, pain in their joints, or numbness in their toes or fingers. They may also lose weight or experience damage to the affected organs. There is no cure for scleroderma, but there is much that can be done to alleviate many of the symptoms. Your doctor can suggest therapy for your specific ailments. You should also moisturize your skin, refrain from smoking, get good sleep, avoid strong detergents, and reduce as much stress from your life as you can. These safeguards, as well as the following list of nutrients, will help reduce the effects of scleroderma.

SUPPLEMENTS TO TREAT SCLERODERMA		
Supplements	**Dosage**	**Considerations**
Carnitine	1,000 to 2,000 mg once a day	
EPA/DHA (fish oil)	1,000 to 4,000 mg once a day	Choose a source that contains vitamin E to prevent oxidation.
Flaxseed oil	1 to 3 tbsp once a day	May interfere with anticoagulants, work as a laxative, or affect blood sugar levels.
Gamma-linolenic acid (GLA)	240 to 720 mg once a day	It is important to maintain the proper ratio of omega-6 fatty acids to omega-3 fatty acids. (See page 110.)
Glucosamine	300 to 900 mg once a day	Don't take if you are allergic to shellfish. Consult use with your healthcare provider if you have diabetes because glucosamine can alter blood sugar levels.
Glutamine	1,000 to 6,000 mg once a day	If you have a sensitivity to monosodium glutamate (MSG), use glutamine with caution. If you are taking medications for seizures, only take glutamine under the direction of your doctor.
Probiotics	20 billion units once a day	If taking an antibiotic, wait three hours before taking probiotics.
Selenium	200 mcg once a day	
Vitamin B$_{10}$ (para-aminobenzoic acid)	2 to 6 g twice a day	Use with caution if you have renal disease. Stop taking immediately if anorexia results from usage.
Vitamin C	500 to 2,500 mg twice a day	Do not take high dosages if you are prone to kidney stones or gout.
Vitamin E	400 to 800 IU once a day	Consult healthcare provider first if you are taking a blood thinner.

SJÖGREN'S SYNDROME

Sjögren's syndrome is a common autoimmune disease which affects several million people in the United States. It occurs when the body's white blood cells attack the exocrine glands that produce moisture. The eyes, mouth, nose, skin, and vagina can become dry, the voice can become hoarse, and major organs can be damaged. Some people experience mild symptoms, while others become severely ill from the disease. Like many other autoimmune diseases, Sjögren's syndrome can be difficult to diagnose because of the wide range of symptoms as well as the similarity of these symptoms to those of other disorders.

A large majority of people with this illness are women. In 50 percent of cases, Sjögren's syndrome occurs alone. The other 50 percent of cases affect people who also have one of the following autoimmune diseases: rheumatoid arthritis, lupus, diffuse scleroderma, or dermatomyositis.

There is no cure for Sjögren's syndrome. Care focuses on treating the symptoms. There are various moisture replacement therapies that are quite effective. Your doctor will be able to recommend the appropriate course of action for your treatment. There are also immunosuppressive medications that hinder the immune system's function.

SUPPLEMENTS TO TREAT SJÖGREN'S SYNDROME

Supplements	Dosage	Considerations
EPA/DHA (fish oil)	1,000 to 5,000 mg once a day	Your healthcare provider may recommend a higher dosage. More than 4,000 mg a day can act as a blood thinner. Choose a source that contains vitamin E to prevent oxidation.
Eleuthero	50 to 200 mg once a day	Do not use if you have a history of heart disease.
Flaxseed	1,000 mg once a day	May interfere with anticoagulants; work as a laxative; or affect blood sugar levels.
Gamma-linolenic acid (GLA)	240 to 720 mg once a day	It is important to maintain the proper ratio of omega-6 fatty acids to omega-3 fatty acids. (See page 110.)
Glucosamine	300 to 900 mg once a day	Don't take if you are allergic to shellfish. Consult use with your healthcare provider if you have diabetes because glucosamine can alter blood sugar levels.

Glutamine	1 to 5 g once a day	If you have a sensitivity to monosodium glutamate (MSG), use glutamine with caution. If you are taking medications for seizures, only take glutamine under the direction of your doctor.
Kaprex AI	1 softgel capsule twice a day	Made by Metagenics. (See Appendix.) Do not use if taking an anticoagulant.
Magnesium	400 to 800 mg once a day	Consult healthcare provider for dosage if you have kidney disease. Discontinue use and see your doctor if you experience abdominal pain. Take a lower dose if it causes diarrhea.
Olive leaf extract	1 to 3 capsules once a day	Take with food.
Probiotics	20 billion units once a day	If taking an antibiotic, wait three hours before taking probiotics.
Selenium	200 mcg once a day	
Vitamin C	500 to 1,500 mg twice a day	Do not take high dosages if you are prone to kidney stones or gout.
Vitamin E	400 IU once a day	Take mixed tocopherols, the more active type of vitamin E. Consult healthcare provider first if you are taking a blood thinner.

SKIN DISORDERS

See Acne; Eczema; Psoriasis.

SLEEP DISORDERS

See Insomnia.

STRESS

See Adrenal Fatigue and Exhaustion; Anxiety.

STROKE

Also called a *cerebrovascular accident*, a stroke occurs when the blood supply to the brain is interrupted, and the brain is deprived of the oxygen it needs to function. An *ischemic* stroke, the most common type, is caused by a blocked blood vessel in the brain. A *hemorrhagic* stroke develops when an artery in the brain leaks or bursts. Brain damage can begin within minutes, so it is important to recognize stroke symptoms and act fast. Quick treatment can help limit damage to the brain and increase the chance of a full recovery.

Symptoms of a stroke, which happen quickly, typically include numbness or paralysis on one side of the body (usually the face, arm, or leg); dim, blurry, or double vision; difficulty speaking and understanding; dizziness; unsteadiness when walking; and severe headache. (See the "Warning" below.) About 80 percent of strokes are caused by atherosclerosis, which results from a gradual buildup of plaque on artery walls, eventually causing them to close. High blood pressure is another major risk factor.

After experiencing a stroke, following your doctor's orders is crucial for stabilizing your condition and reducing the risk of having another one. In addition to any prescribed medications and therapies, eating a well-balanced diet that includes lots of fresh vegetables, whole grains, and lean protein is recommended. This type of diet will help protect blood vessels, oxygenate tissues, and fight damaging free radicals. The following nutritional supplement program is designed to further support stroke recovery. However, if your stroke was hemorrhagic, do not take these nutrients until your physician confirms that there is no further risk of bleeding.

WARNING

If you experience any symptoms of a stroke, immediately call 911 or another emergency service. If the symptoms occur, but go away quickly, be sure to contact your doctor immediately. You may have had a *transient ischemic attack (TIA)*. Also known as a *mini-stroke*, a TIA is often a warning that a stroke may occur soon. Seeking immediate treatment can help prevent it.

SUPPLEMENTS FOR STROKE RECOVERY		
Supplements	**Dosage**	**Considerations**
Carnitine	400 mg once a day	
Coenzyme Q_{10}	150 to 200 mg once a day	May reduce the effects of blood thinners. May cause diarrhea in dosages above 100 mg once a day.
EPA/DHA (fish oil)	1,000 to 2,000 mg once a day	Choose a source that contains vitamin E to prevent oxidation.
Glycerophospho-choline (GPC)	300 to 1,200 mg once a day	
NADH	5 mg twice a day	Reduced and more active form of niacin.
Phosphatidylserine	100 to 300 mg once a day	
Vinpocetine	10 mg once a day	Do not take if you are taking a blood thinner.
Vitamin B_3 (niacin)	100 mg twice a day	High doses can deplete your body of other vitamins in the B complex.
Vitamin B_6 (pyridoxine)	100 mg twice a day	Do not take more than 500 mg a day. If you are taking L-dopa for Parkinson's disease, do not take B_6 without first consulting your doctor.
Vitamin B_9 (folic acid)	800 mcg once a day	High doses can deplete your body of other vitamins in the B complex.
Vitamin B_{12} (cobalamin)	200 mcg once a day	High doses can deplete your body of other vitamins in the B complex.

SYSTEMIC SCLEROSIS

See Scleroderma.

THYROID DISORDERS

See Hyperthyroidism; Hypothyroidism.

TYPE 1 DIABETES

See Diabetes Mellitus.

TYPE 2 DIABETES

See Diabetes Mellitus.

ULCERATIVE COLITIS

Ulcerative colitis is a disorder that causes inflammation of the inner lining of the digestive tract, along with sores (*ulcers*). This disorder is referred to as an inflammatory bowel disease (IBD), which is a general term for conditions that cause inflammation of the small intestine and colon. More than 500,000 Americans have ulcerative colitis.

There are several types of this disorder, with each form occurring in a specific location. The different forms include *ulcerative prostates,* in which inflammation is confined to the rectum, causing rectal bleeding and/or pain; *left-sided colitis,* which extends from the rectum to the left side of the colon, resulting in bloody diarrhea, abdominal cramping and pain, and weight loss; *pan colitis,* which affects the entire colon, causing bloody diarrhea, abdominal cramping, weight loss, fatigue, and night sweats; and *fulminant colitis,* a rare form that affects the entire colon and causes severe pain, diarrhea, and sometimes dehydration.

No one knows exactly what causes ulcerative colitis, but researchers are exploring possible connections to viral or bacterial infection, poor diet, heredity, and use of antibiotics. Until the cause is found, treatments aim at reducing inflammation. Medications, including anti-inflammatory drugs, are often prescribed, and surgery is sometimes needed. Supplements can play an important role in relieving inflammation and helping the digestive tract to heal.

SUPPLEMENTS TO TREAT ULCERATIVE COLITIS

Supplements	Dosage	Considerations
EPA/DHA (fish oil)	500 to 1,000 mg three times a day	Choose a source that contains vitamin E to prevent oxidation.
Fiber, soluble		Choose a fiber supplement with no added sugar. Supplement with several glasses of water.

Gamma-linolenic acid (GLA)	500 mg three times a day	It is important to maintain the proper ratio of omega-6 fatty acids to omega-3 fatty acids. (See page 110.)
Glutamine	2,000 to 6,000 mg daily	If you have a sensitivity to monosodium glutamate (MSG), use glutamine with caution. If you are taking medications for seizures, only take glutamine under the direction of your doctor.
Methylsulfonyl-methane (MSM)	1,000 mg three times a day	When beginning supplementation, ingest with meals to avoid possible heartburn. May cause stomach upset in dosages larger than 6,000 mg.
N-acetylcysteine (NAC)	500 mg once a day	When taking NAC supplements, also take extra vitamin C, copper, and zinc.
Pancreatic enzymes	1 to 2 capsules with meal or one hour after eating	Use with caution if you have a severe ulcer.
Probiotics	20 billion units once a day	If taking an antibiotic, wait three hours before taking probiotics.
Quercitin	500 mg three times a day	
UltraInflamX	Follow instructions on bottle.	Metagenics product. (See Resources.) Do not use if taking a diuretic.
Vitamin A and mixed carotenoids	5,000 to 20,000 IU— half vitamin A and half mixed carotenoids— once a day	Use caution when taking vitamin A supplements because they have the potential to be toxic. Do not take for extended periods of time. Do not take more than 8,000 IU a day if you have liver disease, are a smoker, or are exposed to asbestos.
Vitamin B_5 (pantothenic acid)	100 mg to 200 mg three a day	High doses can deplete your body of other vitamins in the B complex.
Vitamin C	500 mg twice a day	Do not take high dosages if you are prone to kidney stones or gout.
Vitamin E	400 IU once a day	Take mixed tocopherols, the more active type of vitamin E. Consult healthcare provider first if you are taking a blood thinner.
Zinc	10 to 20 mg three times a day	The best zinc supplements are zinc picolinate and zinc citrate. If you are taking zinc and iron supplements, take one in the morning and one in the evening. (Taking them together reduces the efficiency of both.)

UTERINE FIBROIDS

See Fibroids.

VARICOSE VEINS

Dark blue or purple in color, varicose veins are veins that are swollen, bulging, and often appear twisted—like cords. They are unsightly and can form anywhere from the groin to the ankles, although they usually appear on the back of the calves or the inner legs. Usually accompanied by dull aches and a heavy feeling in the legs, varicose veins can also cause swollen feet and ankles, as well as severe pain.

To understand how varicose veins are formed, it's important to first be aware of how veins are designed, as well as their purpose. This is explained in "Circulation 101" in the inset below. If a vein's one-way valves, which keep the blood flowing back to the heart, fail to work properly, the blood will back up and overfill the vein. Eventually, the blood-clogged vein will begin to bulge. Varicose veins occur in the legs because the blood coursing through the leg veins has to work against gravity to get back to the heart.

Although varicose veins seem to run in families, the exact reason for their development is not known. Certain contributing factors can include lack of regular exercise, standing or sitting for extended periods, heavy lifting, chronic constipation, obesity, and pregnancy. Generally, varicose veins

Circulation 101

The job of the circulatory system—the heart, lungs, and blood vessels—is to keep blood continually traveling through the body. Basically, the heart pumps fresh nutrient-rich, oxygenated blood through the arteries to various parts of the body. When the blood makes the return trip to the heart, it does so through the veins. On this return trip, the blood is no longer powered by the pumping heart—instead, the muscles surrounding the veins expand and contract, squeezing the veins and pushing the blood along. The veins themselves are designed with one-way valves that keep the blood flowing in the right direction.

do not cause serious health problems. In some cases, however, they can cause complications such as bleeding under the skin or blood clot formation. It is important to speak with your doctor for treatment recommendations.

SUPPLEMENTS TO TREAT VARICOSE VEINS		
Supplements	Dosage	Considerations
EPA/DHA (fish oil)	2,000 mg once a day	Choose a source that contains vitamin E to prevent oxidation.
Gotu kola	200 to 400 mg of a 40-percent extract once a day	
Grape seed extract	100 to 200 mg once a day	
Horse chestnut	300 to 600 mg once a day	
Pine bark extract	50 to 100 mg once a day	
Vessel Max	Use as directed.	Ortho Molecular product (See Resources.)
Vitamin C	500 mg twice a day	Do not take high dosages if you are prone to kidney stones or gout.
Vitamin E	400 IU once a day	Take mixed tocopherols, the more active type of vitamin E. Consult healthcare provider first if you are taking a blood thinner.

WOUND HEALING

Wound healing is the body's natural process of regenerating dermal and epidermal tissue—in other words, the skin—when physical injury occurs. The events that constitute the wound-healing process overlap in time, but include blood clotting, platelet aggregation, inflammation, the formation of new capillaries and collagen, contraction of the wound edges, and formation of scar tissue. This process begins at the moment of injury, and can continue for months or years.

The ability of wounds to heal properly is determined by adequate blood supply, appropriate wound-care techniques, and control of any existing medical problems. For healthy people, wound healing usually progresses well. People who are vulnerable to problems with wound healing include the elderly, diabetics, those with congestive heart failure, and those with suppressed immune systems.

The most important aspect of wound care is constant attention to the wound with frequent cleansing and changing of dressings. It has also been found that a supplement program which combines antioxidant nutrients can speed wound healing by 20 percent.

SUPPLEMENTS TO ENCOURAGE WOUND HEALING

Supplements	Dosage	Considerations
Arginine	1,000 to 3,000 mg once a day	If you have kidney disease, liver disease or herpes, only take under a doctor's supervision.
Carnosine	1,000 to 2,000 mg once a day	
Grape seed extract	50 to 200 mg once a day	
Vitamin B_5 (pantothenic acid)	50 mg twice a day	High doses can deplete your body of other vitamins in the B complex.
Vitamin C	1,000 mg twice a day	Do not take high dosages if you are prone to kidney stones or gout.

YEAST INFECTIONS

See Candidiasis.

PART 3

Maintaining Well-Being

After reading Part 2, you know how to treat and manage a variety of different conditions. Yet it is preferable to implement good nutrition before the development of a problem. This section explains how people with various schedules and goals can maintain good health, while improving their lives and futures by strengthening their immune systems and increasing their energy levels.

Please note the following precautions, along with the considerations given throughout this section. The dosages given are intended for adults without kidney or liver disease. If you have kidney or liver disease, you may need to take lower dosages of most supplements, and should consult your doctor before embarking upon any nutritional program. Similarly, if you are pregnant or nursing, consult your doctor before following any of these protocols.

If you are taking coumadin or any other blood thinner, your dosage of garlic, ginkgo, and vitamin E must be lower than what is suggested. Please ask your physician to help you determine the appropriate dosage. If you are having surgery, do not take any nutrients (except for the surgery pre- and post-operative protocol that your doctor gives you) for two weeks before and one week after your surgery date.

You should never take any supplement with which you are unfamiliar. The nutrients found throughout Part 3 were described in Part 1. All supplements should be taken with a full glass of water, which will allow the nutrients to be properly dispersed throughout your body.

BIRTH CONTROL PILLS AND NUTRITION

Hormones are very much involved in pregnancy, from conception through labor. Birth control pills, or *oral contraceptives,* can prevent pregnancy by adjusting certain hormone levels. They are among the most popular and effective means of birth control. There are many different kinds to choose from, and your doctor can recommend which one is right for you.

However, these pills can also deplete your body of other nutrients, including zinc and vitamins B_{12}, B_6, and B_9, and elevate levels of nutrients such as copper. The following list of nutrients can be extremely helpful for anyone taking birth control.

SUPPLEMENTS TO TAKE WHILE TAKING BIRTH CONTROL PILLS		
Supplements	Dosage	Considerations
Alpha-lipoic acid	200 mg once a day	Improves blood sugar levels so diabetics may be able to take less medication.
B-complex vitamins	50 mg twice a day	I suggest taking a multi-vitamin.
Carnitine	1,000 mg once a day	
Gamma-linolenic acid (GLA)	240 mg once a day	It is important to maintain the proper ratio of omega-6 fatty acids to omega-3 fatty acids. (See page 110.)
Inositol	500 mg twice a day	May stimulate uterine contractions. Women who wish to become pregnant should consult their doctor regarding its use.
Magnesium	400 mg once a day	Consult healthcare provider for dosage if you have kidney disease. Discontinue use and see your doctor if you experience abdominal pain. Take a lower dose if it causes diarrhea.
Phosphatidylcholine (Lecithin)	2,000 mg once a day	Use with caution if you have malabsorption problems, as this could exacerbate them.
Zinc	25 mg once a day	The best zinc supplements are zinc picolinate and zinc citrate. If you are taking zinc and iron supplements, take one in the morning and one in the evening. (Taking them together reduces the efficiency of both.)

BODYBUILDER'S NUTRITION

Some 650 muscles make up approximately 43 percent of an average man's body weight and 34 percent of a woman's. Along with the support of the skeletal system, about 620 of these muscles work together to create movement. The remaining muscles, which include the cardiac and smooth muscles, perform a number of vital bodily functions that include pumping blood and assisting in the operation of various internal organs. During bodybuilding, focus is on the skeletal muscles.

Skeletal muscles are composed of two types of muscle fibers—fast-twitch and slow-twitch. When heavy work is called for, fast-twitch muscles are used. They contract quickly and provide short bursts of energy, making them useful for high-intensity, low-endurance activities, such as weightlifting, sprinting, and swinging a baseball bat. Fast-twitch muscle fibers tire quickly; they can also become painful due to the buildup of lactic acid. On the other hand, slow-twitch muscle fibers produce slow, steady contractions; they are used for low-intensity, high-endurance activities like long-distance running and other aerobic-type exercises. These activities produce very little lactic acid. Endurance athletes tend to develop more slow-twitch muscle fibers, while power athletes develop more fast-twitch.

Proper nutrition combined with an effective weight-training program is integral for building muscles. In addition, dietary supplements are recommended to maintain a strong, healthy body and to replace any nutrients that are lost through sweating or training activities. The following list of nutrients includes supplements that should be taken after every workout.

SUPPLEMENTS TO RELIEVE SORE MUSCLES AFTER EXERCISE		
Supplements	Dosage	Considerations
Carnitine	1,000 to 2,000 mg once a day	
Coenzyme Q_{10}	100 to 200 mg once a day	May reduce the effects of blood thinners. Dosages over 100 mg may cause diarrhea.
Methylsulfonyl-methane (MSM)	1,000 three times a day	When beginning supplementation, ingest with meals to avoid possible heartburn. May cause stomach upset in dosages larger than 6,000 mg.
Zinc	25 to 50 mg once a day	The best zinc supplements are zinc picolinate and zinc citrate. If you are taking zinc and iron supplements, take one in the morning and one in the evening. (Taking them together reduces the efficiency of both.)

DIETER'S NUTRITION

Every year, more and more Americans become overweight—even obese. This unfortunate trend has been linked to a growing number of health issues, including potentially fatal cardiovascular diseases and weakness of limbs and organs. Many people have a difficult time losing weight and then keeping it off—but with the right diet and exercise program, you truly have the ability to make your body significantly healthier.

There are many popular diets. There are diets that recommend decreasing consumption of fats, diets that restrict eating carbohydrates while increasing protein consumption, and diets that carefully balance intake of the different food groups. Interestingly, different people find success with different diets. It is important to find a diet that works for you. Yet the most reliable way to lose weight is the tried-and-true method of decreasing total calorie consumption while increasing the number of calories burned, through exercise and other physical activity. (If you find that your diet-and-exercise plan has no effect after a month of true, prevailing effort, see a fellowship-trained anti-aging practitioner who can look at other possible issues, such as thyroid dysfunction, allergies, gut health, and insulin resistance. You may also wish to read my book *Demystifying Weight Loss*.)

However, good nutrition is as key an aspect of losing weight as cutting calories and intensifying exercise sessions. Being overweight can be dangerous to your health and well-being, but dropping pounds without continued consumption of the proper nutrients can be just as unhealthy. At the same time, these supplements will provide you with the energy you need to successfully continue your diet.

SUPPLEMENTS TO TAKE WHILE DIETING		
Supplements	Dosage	Considerations
Alpha-lipoic acid	100 to 600 mg once a day	Improves blood sugar levels so diabetics may be able to take less medication.
Ashwagandha root	200 to 400 mg twice a day	
Carnitine	3,000 to 4,000 mg once a day	

Chromium	200 to 600 mcg once a day	Combining with the protein picolinate allows your body to absorb chromium more efficiently. However, some chromium picolinate supplements contain more chromium than necessary. Ask your healthcare provider for a recommendation on chromium consumption.
Coenzyme Q$_{10}$	60 to 200 mg once a day	May reduce the effects of blood thinners. Dosages over 100 mg may cause diarrhea.
Conjugated linoleic acid (CLA)	3,000 to 4,000 mg once a day	Do not take for longer than 6 months at a time.
Eleuthero	100 to 200 mg once a day	Do not use if you have a history of heart disease.
Flaxseed oil	1 tbsp once a day	May interfere with anticoagulants, work as a laxative, or affect blood sugar levels.
Gamma-linolenic acid (GLA)	240 to 480 mg once a day	It is important to maintain the proper ratio of omega-6 fatty acids to omega-3 fatty acids. (See page 110.)
Green tea extract	1,000 mg once a day	Use with caution if you have intestinal problems, such as an ulcer, or kidney disease.
Multi-vitamin	1 tablet once a day or as directed	
N-acetylcysteine (NAC)	500 to 1,000 mg once a day	When taking NAC supplements, also take extra vitamin C, copper, and zinc.
Selenium	100 to 200 mcg once a day	
Vitamin E	400 IU once a day	Take mixed tocopherols, the more active type of vitamin E. Consult healthcare provider first if you are taking a blood thinner.
Zinc	25 mg once a day	The best zinc supplements are zinc picolinate and zinc citrate. If you are taking zinc and iron supplements, take one in the morning and one in the evening. (Taking them together reduces the efficiency of both.)

ENHANCING DETOXIFICATION

Detoxification is the process through which toxic substances—environmental pollutants, medications, byproducts of metabolism, and more—are removed from the body. This process is one of the major functions of the liver, lower gastrointestinal tract, kidneys, and skin, with the liver being the most important organ of detoxification. Studies have shown that each individual has a different ability to break down toxins.

Detoxification in the liver is largely accomplished in two phases. In Phase I, enzymes change toxins into intermediate compounds. In Phase II, the intermediate compounds are neutralized through the addition of a water-soluble molecule. The body is then able to eliminate the transformed toxins through the urine or feces.

When the body is unable to properly detoxify, the resulting toxic accumulations can, at a low level, cause chronic fatigue, loss of concentration, and poor memory. When toxic accumulations reach higher levels, more serious problems can result. Because the detoxification process is very nutrient dependent, a number of vitamins, minerals, and other supplements can help ensure that toxins are quickly removed from the body. In our office, we also use UltraClear Plus by Metagenics and 200 milligrams of milk thistle twice a day.

Activities and Habits
That Increase Exposure to Toxins

Although the human body has the ability to neutralize and eliminate many toxins, an overload of toxic substances can overwhelm the organs of detoxification. One way to prevent this overload is to avoid or minimize the following practices.

- Drinking tap water.
- Excessive consumption of processed foods and fats.
- Excessive consumption of caffeine.
- Excessive consumption of alcohol.
- Tobacco use.
- Recreational drug use.
- Chronic use of medication(s).
- Lack of exercise.
- Occupational or other exposure to pesticides, paints, and other toxic substances without adequate protective equipment.
- Living or working near areas of high traffic or industrial plants.

■ Supplements for Phase I Detoxification

- Bioflavonoids
- Copper
- Folic acid
- Magnesium

- Vitamin B_2 (riboflavin)
- Vitamin B_3 (niacin)
- Vitamin B_6 (pyridoxine)

- Vitamin B_{12} (cobalamin)
- Vitamin C
- Zinc

ENHANCING ENERGY

Every cell in the body is packed with small organelles called mitochondria. Referred to as "intracellular powerhouses," these cell components produce most of the energy used by the body. Cells with a high metabolic rate, like those in the heart muscles, can contain thousands of mitochondria. Other cells may contain only a few dozen.

Energy production via the mitochondria is absolutely essential for physical strength, stamina, and life itself. When production drops even slightly, fatigue, weakness, and reduced cognitive ability can result. Many researchers believe that mitochondrial dysfunction, which is age-related, is linked to heart disease, fatigue syndromes, Parkinson's disease, and Alzheimer's disease.

There is no nutritional "magic bullet" that can restore compromised mitochondrial function. But it has been found that a combination of nutrients can normalize the function of the mitochondria, increase energy production, and delay age-related decline.

SUPPLEMENTS FOR ENERGY ENHANCEMENT		
Supplements	Dosage	Considerations
Alpha-lipoic acid	100 to 300 mg once a day	Improves blood sugar levels so diabetics may be able to take less medication.
B-complex vitamins	50 mg twice a day	I suggest taking a multi-vitamin.
Carnitine	1,000 to 2,000 mg once a day	
Coenzyme Q_{10}	100 to 200 mg once a day	May reduce the effects of blood thinners. Dosages over 100 mg may cause diarrhea.
Magnesium	600 mg once a day	Consult healthcare provider for dosage if you have kidney disease. Discontinue use and see your doctor if you experience abdominal pain. Take a lower dose if it causes diarrhea.

Manganese	2.5 to 5 mg once a day	
N-acetylcysteine (NAC)	500 to 1,000 mg once a day	When taking NAC supplements, also take extra vitamin C, copper, and zinc.
NADH (reduced form of niacin)	5 mg twice a day	
Ribose	5 g three times a day	D-ribose is the most effective form.
Vitamin C	500 to 1,000 mg twice a day	Do not take high dosages if you are prone to kidney stones or gout.
Vitamin E	400 to 800 IU once a day	
Zinc	25 mg once a day	The best zinc supplements are zinc picolinate and zinc citrate. If you are taking zinc and iron supplements, take one in the morning and one in the evening. (Taking them together reduces the efficiency of both.)

ENHANCING IMMUNITY

The immune system is comprised of several mechanisms that protect the body against infection by identifying and killing *pathogens*—harmful bacteria, viruses, protozoa, fungi, and parasites. In simplest terms, the immune system discriminates between those things that are "self" (belong in the body), and those things that are "nonself" (foreign to the body). It then neutralizes and/or eliminates all that is nonself.

The immune system is composed of many different structures and substances, including various proteins, cells, organs, tissues, and even healthful bacteria. These structures and substances form an elaborate and dynamic network that is constantly acting to protect and defend the body. When the immune system is working well, the body remains healthy and does not easily succumb to the threats posed by cuts, scrapes, bacteria, viruses, and other potential dangers. But when the efficiency of the immune system is compromised—as it can be by lack of sleep, toxic exposure, serious infection, stress, poor diet, the overuse of antibiotics, and other factors—the body becomes vulnerable to many threats. Fortunately, a healthy lifestyle coupled with a good supplement plan can strengthen the immune system, enabling the body to better protect itself.

SUPPLEMENTS THAT ENHANCE IMMUNITY

Supplements	Dosage	Considerations
Astragalus	1,000 to 2,000 mg (or 1 to 4 droppers full of tincture) once a day	
B-complex vitamins	25 mg twice a day	I suggest taking a multi-vitamin.
Carnitine	1,000 to 3,000 mg once a day	
Chlorella/spirulina	1 to 2 tbsp once a day	Stop taking if experience nausea or gastrointestinal distress. Use with caution if you have allergic tendencies.
Coenzyme Q_{10}	50 to 300 mg once a day	May reduce the effects of blood thinners. Dosages over 100 mg may cause diarrhea.
Colostrum		Consult with your doctor regarding use. Do not use if you have dairy allergies or hyperthyroid disease.
Curcuminoids	100 to 1,500 mg once a day	
Echinacea	2 tablets once a day	Short-term use only.
Gamma-linolenic acid (GLA)	240 to 480 mg once a day	It is important to maintain the proper ratio of omega-6 fatty acids to omega-3 fatty acids. (See page 110.)
Garlic	300 to 900 mg once a day	
Glutamine	1,000 to 6,000 mg once a day	If you have a sensitivity to monosodium glutamate (MSG), use glutamine with caution. If you are taking medications for seizures, only take glutamine under the direction of your doctor.
Green tea extract	1,000 mg once a day	Use with caution if you have intestinal problems, such as an ulcer, or kidney disease.
Magnesium	400 to 600 mg once a day	Consult healthcare provider for dosage if you have kidney disease. Discontinue use and see your doctor if you experience abdominal pain. Take a lower dose if it causes diarrhea.
N-acetylcysteine (NAC)	500 to 2,000 mg once a day	When taking NAC supplements, also take extra vitamin C, copper, and zinc.
Probiotics	20 billion units once a day	If taking an antibiotic, wait three hours before taking probiotics.

Selenium	400 mcg once a day	
Taurine	1,000 to 3,000 mg once a day	L-taurine is most effective. Take between meals. Discontinue use if you suddenly have feelings of chest or throat tightness or if you break out in hives. Do not take with aspirin.
Vitamin A and mixed carotenoids	5,000 to 25,000 IU— half vitamin A and half mixed carotenoids— once a day	Do not take over 10,000 IU daily for more than three months. Do not take more than 5,000 IU daily if you have liver disease, are a smoker, or are exposed to asbestos.
Vitamin C	500 to 5,000 mg twice a day	Do not take high dosages if you are prone to kidney stones or gout. May cause diarrhea in dosages about 2,000 mg a day.
Vitamin E	400 to 800 IU once a day	Take mixed tocopherols, the more active type of vitamin E. Consult healthcare provider first if you are taking a blood thinner.
Zinc	15 to 50 mg once a day	The best zinc supplements are zinc picolinate and zinc citrate. If you are taking zinc and iron supplements, take one in the morning and one in the evening. (Taking them together reduces the efficiency of both.)

LIVER HEALTH

The largest gland in the human body, the liver lies below the diaphragm, in the thoracic region of the abdomen. The liver has a number of important functions, including storage of glycogen, the body's primary source of short-term energy; synthesis of plasma protein; detoxification; and production of bile, a compound that aids in the digestion of lipids. The inset on page 352 lists more functions of the liver.

The human body cannot live without the liver, and currently, there is no artificial device capable of performing the many functions of this vital organ. Thus, it is important to maintain liver health and prevent the development of diseases such as hepatitis and cirrhosis. Both a sound diet and a wise program of nutritional supplements can protect the liver from harm and help maintain liver health.

Functions of the Liver

Although most people don't give the liver much thought, the fact is that without the liver, human life cannot continue. In fact, the liver performs so many important tasks that so far, no artificial device has been able to replace it. The liver:

- Produces and excretes bile.
- Aids in carbohydrate metabolism.
- Synthesizes cholesterol and triglycerides.
- Stores glycogen, vitamin B_{12}, iron, and copper.
- Produces proteins that maintain blood pressure.
- Produces coagulation factors.
- Breaks down hemoglobin.
- Breaks down toxic substances.
- Converts ammonia to urea.

SUPPLEMENTS FOR LIVER HEALTH

Supplements	Dosage	Considerations
Alpha-lipoic acid	100 to 600 mg once a day	Improves blood sugar levels so diabetics may be able to take less medication.
Artichoke		Consult healthcare practitioner for dosage.
B-complex vitamins	25 mg twice a day	I suggest a multi-vitamin.
Carnitine	500 to 3,000 mg once a day	
Coenzyme Q_{10}	100 to 400 mg once a day	May reduce the effects of blood thinners. Dosages over 100 mg may cause diarrhea.
Curcuminoids	100 to 1,500 mg once a day	
Dandelion	100 mg once a day	
Inositol	500 mg twice a day	May stimulate uterine contractions so women who wish to become pregnant should consult their doctor regarding its use.
Isothiocyanates		Phytochemicals found in cruciferous vegetables. I suggest eating these vegetables rather than taking supplements.

Limonene		A hydrocarbon found in lemon oil that promotes liver health.
Magnesium	400 to 600 mg once a day	Consult healthcare provider for dosage if you have kidney disease. Discontinue use and see your doctor if you experience abdominal pain. Take a lower dose if it causes diarrhea.
Milk thistle	100 to 300 mg once a day	Reduces efficiency of certain blood pressure medication.
N-acetylcysteine (NAC)	1,000 mg once a day	When taking NAC supplements, also take extra vitamin C, copper, and zinc.
Perillyl alcohol		Found in cherries.
Phosphatidylcholine (Lecithin)	1,000 to 3,000 mg once a day	Use with caution if you have malabsorption problems, as this could exacerbate them.
Quercetin	500 mg once a day	
Rosemary	2 to 4.5 ml of 1:2 liquid extract once a day	Contains carnosol, an effective antioxidant that also helps reduce liver toxicity.
Selenium	200 to 400 mcg once a day	
Taurine	1,000 to 3,000 mg once a day	Take between meals. Discontinue use if you suddenly have feelings of chest or throat tightness or if you break out in hives. Do not take with aspirin.
Vitamin B_9 (folic acid)	500 mcg twice a day	High doses can deplete your body of other vitamins in the B complex.
Vitamin B_{12} (cobalamin)	500 to 1,000 mcg twice a day	High doses can deplete your body of other vitamins in the B complex.
Vitamin C	500 to 2,500 mg twice a day	Do not take high dosages if you are prone to kidney stones or gout.
Vitamin E	400 IU once a day	Take mixed tocopherols, the more active type of vitamin E. Consult healthcare provider first if you are taking a blood thinner.
Zinc	25 mg once a day	The best zinc supplements are zinc picolinate and zinc citrate. If you are taking zinc and iron supplements, take one in the morning and one in the evening. (Taking them together reduces the efficiency of both.)

MEMORY ENHANCEMENT

Memory loss—the failure to retrieve stored mental information—can be caused by a variety of factors. Mental and physical stress, lack of sleep, hormonal imbalance, recreational drug use, and alcoholism, as well as medical conditions such as thyroid disorders, allergies, head injury, candidiasis, depression, and hypoglycemia, are all possible contributors. Various drugs, including certain painkillers, antihistamines and decongestants, steroids, statin drugs, and blood-pressure medications, are other possible contributors.

The aging process is another factor that can affect memory. Brain cells communicate with each other through special chemicals called neurotransmitters, which are necessary for learning, concentration, and recall. As the body ages, it produces fewer neurotransmitters. If, however, the brain receives an increased supply of the nutrients needed to produce neurotransmitters, it can slow down memory loss. Other possible causes of memory impairment include free-radical damage and cholesterol-clogged blood, which can restrict the necessary supply of nutrients to the brain.

The following suggested protocols were developed by Dr. Robert Goldman, cofounder of the American Academy of Anti-Aging Medicine and founder and president of the National Academy of Sports Medicine. I personally follow this program and have found it very useful in my patients. *See also* Alzheimer's Disease.

MEMORY-ENHANCING BRAIN-NUTRIENT PROGRAM

Supplements	Dosage	Considerations
Alpha-lipoic acid	100 mg once a day	Improves blood sugar levels so diabetics may be able to take less medication.
B-complex vitamins	50 mg twice a day	I suggest taking a multi-vitamin.
Choline	25 to 50 mg twice a day	
Coenzyme Q$_{10}$	60 to 100 mg once a day	May reduce the effects of blood thinners. Dosages over 100 mg may cause diarrhea.
Eicosapentaenoic acid EPA/DHA (fish oil)	1,000 mg once a day	Choose a source that contains vitamin E to prevent oxidation.
Gingko biloba	50 to 150 mg once a day	Do not use if taking a blood thinner.

Magnesium	600 to 800 mg once a day	Consult healthcare provider for dosage if you have kidney disease. Discontinue use and see your doctor if you experience abdominal pain. Take a lower dose if it causes diarrhea.
Phosphatidylcholine (Lecithin)	200 to 500 mg once a day	Use with caution if you have malabsorption problems, as this could exacerbate them.
Phosphatidylserine	300 to 500 mg once a day	
Vitamin B_9 (folic acid)	250 to 400 mcg twice a day	High doses can deplete your body of other vitamins in the B complex.
Vitamin B_{12} (cobalamin)	500 mcg twice a day	High doses can deplete your body of other vitamins in the B complex.
Vitamin C	500 to 1,000 mg twice a day	Do not take high dosages if you are prone to kidney stones or gout.
Zinc	30 to 50 mg once a day	The best zinc supplements are zinc picolinate and zinc citrate. If you are taking zinc and iron supplements, take one in the morning and one in the evening. (Taking them together reduces the efficiency of both.)

SUPPLEMENTS FOR ENHANCING MENTAL ALERTNESS

Supplements	Dosage	Considerations
B-complex vitamins	25 to 50 mg twice a day	I suggest taking a multi-vitamin.
Carnitine	500 to 1,000 mg once a day	
Coenzyme Q_{10}	60 mg once a day	May reduce the effects of blood thinners. Dosages over 100 mg may cause diarrhea.
EPA/DHA (fish oil)	1,000 mg once a day	Choose a source that contains vitamin E to prevent oxidation.
Gingko biloba	50 to 100 mg once a day	Do not use if taking a blood thinner.
Ginseng	200 to 500 mg once a day	
Glutamine	1,000 to 2,000 mg once a day	If you have a sensitivity to monosodium glutamate (MSG), use glutamine with caution. If you are taking medications for seizures, only take glutamine under the direction of your doctor.
Magnesium	600 mg once a day	Consult healthcare provider for dosage if you have kidney disease. Discontinue use and see your doctor if you experience abdominal pain. Take a lower dose if it causes diarrhea.

Phosphatidylcholine (Lecithin)	1,000 to 4,000 mg once a day	Use with caution if you have malabsorption problems, as this could exacerbate them.
Phosphatidylserine	300 to 500 mg once a day	
Tyrosine	1,000 to 2,000 mg once a day	Do not take if you are taking an MAO inhibitor medication.
Vitamin B$_5$ (pantothenic acid)	25 to 50 mg twice a day	High doses can deplete your body of other vitamins in the B complex.
Vitamin C	1,500 mg twice a day	Do not take high dosages if you are prone to kidney stones or gout.
Zinc	30 mg once a day	The best zinc supplements are zinc picolinate and zinc citrate. If you are taking zinc and iron supplements, take one in the morning and one in the evening. (Taking them together reduces the efficiency of both.)

MEN'S HEALTH

There are many health problems (discussed in Part 2) facing men today, but there are also many men who have yet to experience any of these disorders. The following table includes nutrition recommendations for healthy men who wish to maintain their well-being. To encourage good health, men should also limit their stress levels, improve their diets, and make sure they get enough exercise.

At the same time, it is critically important that all men have regular physicals, as well as the good sense to see a doctor when curious symptoms arise. One of the biggest obstacles standing in the way of men's health is the hurdle of simply going to the doctor to get something checked out. People should be familiar with their bodies so that they notice if something out of the ordinary happens or appears. Unfortunately, many men allow symptoms to persist until they become intolerable and do not take proper care of themselves. Yet, because early detection is crucial to the treatment of so many conditions, problems should not be put off or ignored.

SUPPLEMENTS FOR MEN UNDER THE AGE OF FIFTY

Supplements	Dosage	Considerations
B-complex vitamins	50 mg twice a day	I suggest taking a multi-vitamin.
Calcium	500 mg once a day	Although most people are deficient in calcium, there is a danger in taking too much calcium. Do not ingest more than 1,000 to 1,200 mg of calcium a day.

Chromium	200 mcg once a day	Combining with the protein picolinate allows your body to absorb chromium more efficiently. However, some chromium picolinate supplements contain more chromium than necessary. Ask your healthcare provider for a recommendation.
Copper	2 to 3 mg once a day	Your copper-to-zinc ratio is very important for your health. Also, do not take copper supplement cupric oxide, which has a very low bioavailability.
EPA/DHA (fish oil)	1,000 mg once a day	Choose a source that contains vitamin E to prevent oxidation.
Magnesium	250 mg once a day	Consult healthcare provider for dosage if you have kidney disease. Discontinue use and see your doctor if you experience abdominal pain. Take a lower dose if it causes diarrhea.
Manganese	2 mg once a day	
Selenium	100 mcg daily	
Vitamin A and mixed carotenoids	5,000 to 10,000 IU— half vitamin A and half mixed carotenoids— once a day	Use caution when taking vitamin A supplements because they have the potential to be toxic. Do not take for extended periods of time. Do not take more than 8,000 IU a day if you have liver disease, are a smoker, or are exposed to asbestos.
Vitamin C	250 to 500 mg twice a day	Do not take high dosages if you are prone to kidney stones or gout.
Vitamin D		Have your blood levels measured by your healthcare provider to determine proper dosage.
Vitamin E	400 IU once a day	Take mixed tocopherols, the more active type of vitamin E. Consult healthcare provider first if you are taking a blood thinner.
Zinc	25 mg once a day	The best zinc supplements are zinc picolinate and zinc citrate. If you are taking zinc and iron supplements, take one in the morning and one in the evening. (Taking them together reduces the efficiency of both.)

SUPPLEMENTS FOR MEN OVER THE AGE OF FIFTY

Supplements	Dosage	Considerations
Alpha-lipoic acid	100 mg once a day	Improves blood sugar levels so diabetics may be able to take less medication.
B-complex vitamins	50 mg twice a day	I suggest taking a multi-vitamin.
Bilberry	60 to 120 mg once a day	May cause low blood sugar levels.
Calcium	500 mg once a day	Although most people are deficient in calcium, there is a danger in taking too much calcium. Do not ingest more than 1,000 to 1,200 mg of calcium a day.
Chromium	200 to 600 mcg once a day	Combining with the protein picolinate allows your body to absorb chromium more efficiently. However, some chromium picolinate supplements contain more chromium than necessary. Ask your health-care provider for a recommendation.
Coenzyme Q_{10}	100 mg once a day	May reduce the effects of blood thinners. May cause diarrhea in dosages above 100 mg once a day.
Copper	3 to 4 mg once a day	Your copper-to-zinc ratio is very important for your health. Also, do not take copper supplement cupric oxide, which has a very low bioavailability.
EPA/DHA (fish oil)	2,000 mg once a day	Choose a source that contains vitamin E to prevent oxidation.
Gamma-linolenic acid (GLA)	500 mg once a day	It is important to maintain the proper ratio of omega-6 fatty acids to omega-3 fatty acids. (See page 110.)
Lutien	6 mg once a day	Do not take for extended periods of time. Do not take high dosages if you have liver disease, are a smoker, are exposed to asbestos, or are pregnant.
Lycopene	10 to 20 mg once a day	
Magnesium	250 mg once a day	Consult healthcare provider for dosage if you have kidney disease. Discontinue use and see your doctor if you experience abdominal pain. Take a lower dose if it causes diarrhea.
Manganese	2 mg once a day	
Phosphatidylserine	300 mg once a day	
Saw palmetto	320 mg once a day	

Selenium	100 to 200 mcg once a day	
Soy isoflavones	50 to 300 mg once a day	
Vitamin A and mixed carotenoids	5,000 IU—half vitamin A and half mixed carotenoids—once a day	Use caution when taking vitamin A supplements because they have the potential to be toxic. Do not take for extended periods of time. Do not take more than 8,000 IU a day if you have liver disease, are a smoker, or are exposed to asbestos.
Vitamin B$_9$ (folate)	400 mcg twice a day	High doses can deplete your body of other vitamins in the B complex.
Vitamin B$_{12}$ (cobalamin)	1,000 mcg once a day	High doses can deplete your body of other vitamins in the B complex.
Vitamin C	1,000 to 2,000 mg once a day	Do not take high dosages if you are prone to kidney stones or gout.
Vitamin D		Have your blood levels measured by your healthcare provider to determine proper dosage.
Vitamin E	400 to 800 IU once a day	Take mixed tocopherols, the more active type of vitamin E. Consult healthcare provider first if you are taking a blood thinner.
Zinc	50 mg once a day	The best zinc supplements are zinc picolinate and zinc citrate. If you are taking zinc and iron supplements, take one in the morning and one in the evening. (Taking them together reduces the efficiency of both.)

ORAL CONTRACEPTIVES AND NUTRITION

See Birth Control Pills and Nutrition.

SMOKER'S NUTRITION

Containing over 4,000 chemicals, including more than sixty known carcinogenic (cancer-causing) substances, tobacco smoke has an obvious negative impact on health. People who smoke cigarettes or any other form of tobacco are at greater risk for such serious respiratory illnesses as lung cancer, emphysema, and chronic bronchitis, as well as coronary heart disease, stroke, circulatory problems, periodontal disease, and osteoporosis.

Smoking robs the body of a number of important vitamins and minerals, and it also affects the body's ability to absorb these essential nutrients. The primary nutrient affected by cigarette smoke is vitamin C, which helps boost the immune system, is needed for maintaining healthy bones and teeth, and is essential for healing wounds. It is also necessary to form collagen, a protein that is required to make blood vessels, skin, scar tissue, and ligaments. As one of the body's many antioxidants, vitamin C helps block some of the damage caused by free radicals.

To help counteract the damage caused by cigarette smoke, your body needs increased nutrient levels, especially vitamin C. Following the supplement program below and eating vitamin-rich foods can help protect against the damage caused by smoking, but make no mistake—these steps will not offer full protection. The best alternative, of course, is to quit smoking altogether.

SUPPLEMENTS FOR SMOKERS		
Supplements	Dosage	Considerations
Alpha-lipoic acid	100 mg once a day	Improves blood sugar levels so diabetics may be able to take less medication.
Carnitine	1,000 mg once a day	
Coenzyme Q_{10}	100 mg once a day	May reduce the effects of blood thinners. Dosages over 100 mg may cause diarrhea.
N-acetylcysteine (NAC)	1,000 mg once a day	When taking NAC supplements, also take extra vitamin C, copper, and zinc.
Selenium	100 mcg once a day	
Vitamin C	1,500 to 2,500 mg twice a day	Do not take high dosages if you are prone to kidney stones or gout.
Vitamin E	400 to 800 IU once a day	Take mixed tocopherols, the more active type of vitamin E. Consult your health-care provider first if you are taking a blood thinner.

Warning

You already know that very high dosages of vitamin A and beta-carotene can cause certain health risks. However, recent studies have shown that smokers who intake high dosages of vitamin A and/or beta-carotene may have an increased risk of developing lung cancer. Consequently, do not take more than 8,000 IU a day of vitamin A or beta-carotene—especially if you are a smoker.

SPORTS NUTRITION

Sound sports nutrition gives any athlete the winning edge by allowing the body to efficiently make energy, fuel performance, build muscle, and repair injury. The best nutrition for each individual depends on that person's age, size, physical condition, and specific type of exercise or sport. However, some general guidelines hold true for everyone.

Water is perhaps the most important aspect of sports nutrition. Water is involved in almost every bodily process, and because it is sweated out during physical exercise, it is especially important for the athlete. Dehydration can cause muscle cramping, fatigue, and other problems that can impair physical performance, and can even lead to permanent harm.

All athletes must also be certain to fuel themselves with a balanced diet of carbohydrates, proteins, and fats. During exercise, the body first draws its energy from carbohydrates, then from proteins, and finally, from fats. Emphasis should be placed on fruits, vegetables, whole grains, and whole-grain breads and pastas; lean proteins such as fish, poultry, eggs, beans, nuts, and low-fat dairy products; and relatively small amounts of heart-healthy fats. Foods to be avoided include high-sugar products, which can lead to exhaustion during endurance sports; high-fat foods, which can slow digestion; and foods high in caffeine, which can cause dehydration. In addition, a good program of nutritional supplements can help boost the body's immune system, provide optimal energy during workout and performance, and repair any injuries experienced during sports activities.

ENDURANCE TRAINING NUTRITION

Supplements	Dosage	Considerations
Alpha-lipoic acid	100 to 200 mg once a day	Take 600 mg if you are preparing for a marathon. Improves blood sugar levels so diabetics may be able to take less medication.
Beta-carotene	5,000 IU once a day	
Calcium	500 mg once or twice a day	Although most people are deficient in calcium, there is a danger in taking too much calcium. Do not ingest more than 1,000 to 1,200 mg of calcium a day.
Carnitine	3,000 to 10,000 mg once a day	

Chromium	200 to 1,200 mcg once a day	Combining with the protein picolinate allows your body to absorb chromium more efficiently. However, some chromium picolinate supplements contain more chromium than necessary. Ask your healthcare provider for a recommendation on chromium consumption
Coenzyme Q$_{10}$	100 to 200 mg once a day	May reduce the effects of blood thinners. Dosages over 100 mg may cause diarrhea.
Dimethylglycine (DMG)	125 to 250 mg once a day	
EPA/DHA (fish oil)	1,000 to 2,000 mg once a day	Choose a source that contains vitamin E to prevent oxidation.
Eleuthero	1,000 mg once a day	Do not use if you have a history of heart disease.
Flaxseed oil	1 tbsp once a day	May interfere with anticoagulants, work as a laxative, or affect blood sugar levels.
Gingko biloba	40 to 60 mg once a day	Do not use if taking a blood thinner.
Glutamine	1,000 to 3,000 mg once a day	If you have a sensitivity to monosodium glutamate (MSG), use glutamine with caution. If you are taking medications for seizures, only take glutamine under the direction of your doctor.
Glycine	1,000 mg once a day	Do not take with clozapine or other atypical antipsychotic medications.
Magnesium	400 to 600 mg once a day	Consult healthcare provider for dosage if you have kidney disease. Discontinue use and see your doctor if you experience abdominal pain. Take a lower dose if it causes diarrhea.
Multi-vitamin	1 tablet once a day or as directed	
N-acetylcysteine (NAC)	100 to 2,000 mg once a day	When taking NAC supplements, also take extra vitamin C, copper, and zinc.
Phosphatidylserine	100 to 300 mg once a day	
Reishi mushroom	1,000 mg once a day	
Selenium	200 mcg once a day	

Taurine	1,000 mg once a day	Take between meals. Discontinue use if you suddenly have feelings of chest or throat tightness or if you break out in hives. Do not take with aspirin.
Vitamin A and mixed carotenoids	5,000 IU—half vitamin A and half mixed carotenoids—once a day	Use caution when taking vitamin A supplements because they have the potential to be toxic. Do not take for extended periods of time.
Vitamin C	1,000 to 5,000 mg twice a day	Do not take high dosages if you are prone to kidney stones or gout.
Vitamin E	400 to 800 IU once a day	Take mixed tocopherols, the more active type of vitamin E. Consult healthcare provider first if you are taking a blood thinner.
Zinc	10 to 60 mg once a day	The best zinc supplements are zinc picolinate and zinc citrate. If you are taking zinc and iron supplements, take one in the morning and one in the evening. (Taking them together reduces the efficiency of both.)

The Warning Signs of Overtraining

Every athlete must keep fit and adequately train for competitions. But it is possible for athletes to overtrain, destroying the delicate balance between overload and recovery, and actually impairing performance. The following are possible signs of overtraining.

- Sudden drop in performance
- Muscle soreness, joint pain, and/or general achiness
- Increased incidence of injuries
- Slow recovery from injuries
- Fatigue during both exercise and rest
- Excessive sweating
- Increased susceptibility to infection
- Insomnia
- Headaches
- Decreased appetite
- Loss of purpose, energy, competitive drive, and enthusiasm
- Feeling trapped in a routine
- Anxiety, irritability, and moodiness
- Depression
- Loss of libido

STRENGTH TRAINING NUTRITION		
Supplements	**Dosage**	**Considerations**
Arginine	2,000 to 10,000 mg once a day	If you have kidney disease, liver disease, or herpes, only take under a doctor's supervision. For long-term use must balance with lysine.
Carnitine	3,000 to 10,000 mg once a day	
Chromium	400 to 1,200 mcg once a day	Combining with the protein picolinate allows your body to absorb chromium more efficiently. However, some chromium picolinate supplements contain more chromium than necessary. Ask your healthcare provider for a recommendation on chromium consumption.
Magnesium	400 to 600 mg once a day	Consult healthcare provider for dosage if you have kidney disease. Discontinue use and see your doctor if you experience abdominal pain. Take a lower dose if it causes diarrhea.
N-acetylcysteine (NAC)	500 to 1,000 mg once a day	When taking NAC supplements, also take extra vitamin C, copper, and zinc.
Glutamine	4,000 to 6,000 mg once a day	If you have a sensitivity to monosodium glutamate (MSG), use glutamine with caution. If you are taking medications for seizures, only take glutamine under the direction of your doctor.
Taurine	1,000 mg once a day	Take between meals. Discontinue use if you suddenly have feelings of chest or throat tightness or if you break out in hives. Do not take with aspirin.
Vitamin C	500 mg twice a day	Do not take high dosages if you are prone to kidney stones or gout.
Vitamin E	400 IU once a day	Take mixed tocopherols, the more active type of vitamin E. Consult healthcare provider first if you are taking a blood thinner.
Zinc	25 mg once a day	The best zinc supplements are zinc picolinate and zinc citrate. If you are taking zinc and iron supplements, take one in the morning and one in the evening. (Taking them together reduces the efficiency of both.)

SUN TANNER'S NUTRITION

Sunshine, although essential for health and well-being (particularly because it is our primary source of vitamin D), can also be hazardous to the body. Unprotected exposure to the sun's ultraviolet (UV) rays can cause eye damage, a weakened immune system, and certain cancers—skin cancer in particular. It is also implicated in skin damage, including age spots, wrinkles, and other signs of aging.

Antioxidants like vitamins C and E are important immune system protectors, guarding the body against the harmful effects of free radicals. These vitamins, however, are sensitive to the light—it takes just a few minutes in the sun to significantly reduce their presence in the skin. Along with the damage from UV rays, the lack of vitamins C and E leaves the skin vulnerable, accelerating the aging process. In addition to using a good broad-spectrum sunscreen, applying topical vitamin E to the skin helps fight wrinkles and other signs of aging. (Vitamin E is often contained in sunscreen.) Taken internally, supplemental vitamins C and E also help reduce some of the harmful effects of sun exposure.

If you are going to be in the sun for any length of time—whether relaxing at the beach, working in the garden, or playing an outdoor sport—be sure to apply protective sunscreen and topical vitamin E to your skin. Taking the following nutrients will provide you with further protection.

SUPPLEMENTS FOR SUN TANNERS		
Supplements	Dosage	Considerations
Coenzyme Q_{10}	30 to 100 mg once a day	May reduce the effects of blood thinners. Dosages over 100 mg may cause diarrhea.
N-acetylcysteine (NAC)	500 mg once a day	When taking NAC supplements, also take extra vitamin C, copper, and zinc.
Vitamin C	500 mg twice a day	Do not take high dosages if you are prone to kidney stones or gout.
Vitamin E	400 to 800 IU once a day	Take mixed tocopherols, the more active type of vitamin E. Consult healthcare provider first if you are taking a blood thinner.

SURGERY AND NUTRITION

Surgery of any kind, no matter how minor, requires a period of recovery. Implementing a good nutritional program both before and after the procedure will help support the body's healing process and pave a smooth road to recovery. People who are well nourished are more likely to heal better and more quickly than those who are not. Scientific studies have confirmed that patients who follow a healthy diet-supplement-exercise regimen are less prone to develop infections and other complications after surgery.

It is important to follow your surgeon's specific pre- and post-operative instructions during this time. As a general rule, however, you can help bolster your health by following the guidelines of the supplement program below. If possible, begin the program about two weeks before the surgery and continue it for four weeks after.

SUPPLEMENTS FOR BEFORE AND AFTER SURGERY

Supplements	Dosage	Considerations
Alpha-lipoic acid	200 to 300 mg once a day	Improves blood sugar levels so diabetics may be able to take less medication.
Arginine	1,000 to 5,000 mg once a day	If you have kidney disease, liver disease, or herpes, only take under a doctor's supervision.
Carnitine	1,500 mg once a day	
Coenzyme Q_{10}	30 mg once a day	May reduce the effects of blood thinners. Dosages over 100 mg may cause diarrhea.
EPA/DHA (fish oil)	1,000 mg once a day	Choose a source that contains vitamin E to prevent oxidation.
Glutamine	3,000 to 5,000 mg once a day	If you have a sensitivity to monosodium glutamate (MSG), use glutamine with caution. If you are taking medications for seizures, only take glutamine under the direction of your doctor.
Gota kola	1 to 3 capsules once a day	
Grape seed extract	200 mg once a day	
Magnesium	400 mg once a day	Consult healthcare provider for dosage if you have kidney disease. Discontinue use and see your doctor if you experience abdominal pain. Take a lower dose if it causes diarrhea.

Methylsulfonyl-methane (MSM)	3,000 to 10,000 mg once a day	When beginning supplementation, ingest with meals to avoid possible heartburn. May cause stomach upset in dosages larger than 6,000 mg.
N-acetylcysteine (NAC)	1,000 mg once a day	When taking NAC supplements, also take extra vitamin C, copper, and zinc.
Phosphatidylserine	300 mg once a day	
Probiotics	20 billion units once a day	If taking an antibiotic, wait three hours before taking probiotics.
Selenium	200 mcg once a day	
Taurine	1,000 to 3,000 mg once a day	Take between meals. Discontinue use if you suddenly have feelings of chest or throat tightness or if you break out in hives. Do not take with aspirin.
Vitamin A and mixed carotenoids	10,000 to 15,000 IU—vitamin A and half mixed carotenoids—once a day	Use caution when taking vitamin A supplements because they have the potential to be toxic. Do not take for extended periods of time. Do not take high dosages if you have liver disease, are a smoker, or are exposed to asbestos.
Vitamin C	500 to 1,000 mg twice a day	Do not take high dosages if you are prone to kidney stones or gout.
Zinc	25 to 50 mg once a day	The best zinc supplements are zinc picolinate and zinc citrate. If you are taking zinc and iron supplements, take one in the morning and one in the evening. (Taking them together reduces the efficiency of both.)

■ Supplements to Avoid for Two Weeks Before and One Week After Surgery

- Cayenne
- Garlic
- Ginkgo
- Large doses of eicosapentaenoic acid (EPA) or docosahexanoic acid (DHA)
- St. John's wort
- Vitamin E

WEIGHT LOSS

See Dieter's Nutrition.

WOMEN'S HEALTH

There are many steps women can take to maintain wellness. It is particularly important to realize that women's health is markedly different from men's health. For many years, most health considerations were determined by the results of studies on men. Unfortunately, these results are not necessarily applicable to women. For example, most people are aware that certain symptoms—such as chest discomfort, pain in the left arm, shortness of breath, nausea, vomiting, and general uneasiness—may indicate the occurrence of a heart attack. But while these signs are prevalent in men experiencing a heart attack, women usually have different signs. Women tend to have back or jaw pain, as well as a high incidence of weakness and fatigue. Time is critical when someone is having a heart attack, and mistaking the signs for a less serious problem can drastically alter a person's rate of recovery. Yet many women are unaware of these important differences.

Thankfully, medical studies have progressed with time and researchers have begun to acknowledge these differences. Yet there may be more conditions that have still not been properly examined. For this reason, all curious pains or abnormalities should be taken seriously and reported to a healthcare professional.

SUPPLEMENTS FOR HEALTHY WOMEN UNDER THE AGE OF FIFTY		
Supplements	Dosage	Considerations
B-complex vitamins	50 mg twice a day	I suggest taking a multi-vitamin.
Calcium	500 to 1,000 mg daily in 500 mg doses	Although most people are deficient in calcium, there is a danger in taking too much calcium. Do not ingest more than 1,000 to 1,200 mg of calcium a day.
Chromium	200 mcg once a day	Combining with the protein picolinate allows your body to absorb chromium more efficiently. However, some chromium picolinate supplements contain more chromium than necessary. Ask your healthcare provider for a recommendation.
Copper	1 to 2 mg once a day	Your copper-to-zinc ratio is very important for your health. Also, do not take copper supplement cupric oxide, which has a very low bioavailability.

EPA/DHA (fish oil)	1,000 mg once a day	Choose a source that contains vitamin E to prevent oxidation.
Magnesium	250 to 500 mg once a day	Consult healthcare provider for dosage if you have kidney disease. Discontinue use and see your doctor if you experience abdominal pain. Take a lower dose if it causes diarrhea.
Manganese	2 mg once a day	
Selenium	100 mcg once a day	
Vitamin A and mixed carotenoids	5,000 to 10,000 IU—half vitamin A and half mixed carotenoids—once a day	Use caution when taking vitamin A supplements because they have the potential to be toxic. Do not take for extended periods of time. Do not take more than 8,000 IU a day if you have liver disease, are a smoker, or are exposed to asbestos.
Vitamin C	500 to 1,000 mg twice a day	Do not take high dosages if you are prone to kidney stones or gout.
Vitamin D_3		Have your blood levels measured by your healthcare provider to determine proper dosage.
Vitamin E	400 IU once a day	Take mixed tocopherols, the more active type of vitamin E. Consult healthcare provider first if you are taking a blood thinner.
Zinc	15 mg once a day	The best zinc supplements are zinc picolinate and zinc citrate. If you are taking zinc and iron supplements, take one in the morning and one in the evening. (Taking them together reduces the efficiency of both.)

SUPPLEMENTS FOR HEALTHY WOMEN OVER THE AGE OF FIFTY

Supplements	Dosage	Considerations
Alpha-lipoic acid	100 mg once a day	Improves blood sugar levels so diabetics may be able to take less medication.
Bilberry	60 to 120 mg once a day	May cause low blood sugar levels.
B-complex vitamins	50 mg twice a day	I suggest taking a multi-vitamin.
Calcium	500 mg once or twice a day	Although most people are deficient in calcium, there is a danger in taking too much calcium. Do not ingest more than 1,000 to 1,200 mg of calcium a day.

Chromium	200 to 600 mcg once a day	Combining with the protein picolinate allows your body to absorb chromium more efficiently. However, some chromium picolinate supplements contain more chromium than necessary. Ask your healthcare provider for a recommendation.
Coenzyme Q_{10}	100 mg once a day	May reduce the effects of blood thinners. May cause diarrhea in dosages above 100 mg once a day.
Copper	2 to 3 mg once a day	Your copper-to-zinc ratio is very important for your health. Also, do not take copper supplement cupric oxide, which has a very low bioavailability.
EPA/DHA (fish oil)	2,000 mg once a day	Choose a source that contains vitamin E to prevent oxidation.
Gamma-linolenic acid (GLA)	240 to 480 mg once a day	It is important to maintain the proper ratio of omega-6 fatty acids to omega-3 fatty acids. (See page 110.)
Lutein	6 mg once a day	Do not take for extended periods of time. Do not take high dosages if you have liver disease, are a smoker, are exposed to asbestos, or are pregnant.
Magnesium	500 to 600 mg once a day	Consult healthcare provider for dosage if you have kidney disease. Discontinue use and see your doctor if you experience abdominal pain. Take a lower dose if it causes diarrhea.
Manganese	2 mg once a day	
Phosphatidylserine	300 mg once a day	
Selenium	100 to 200 mcg daily	
Vitamin A and mixed carotenoids	5,000 to 10,000 IU— half vitamin A and half mixed carotenoids— once a day	Use caution when taking vitamin A supplements because they have the potential to be toxic. Do not take for extended periods of time. Do not take more than 8,000 IU a day if you have liver disease, are a smoker, or are exposed to asbestos.
Vitamin B_9 (folate)	800 mcg once a day	High doses can deplete your body of other vitamins in the B complex.
Vitamin B_{12} (cobalamin)	500 to 1,000 mcg once a day	High doses can deplete your body of other vitamins in the B complex.

Vitamin C	1,000 to 2,000 mg twice a day	Do not take high dosages if you are prone to kidney stones or gout.
Vitamin D$_3$		Have your blood levels measured by your healthcare provider to determine proper dosage.
Vitamin E	400 to 800 IU once a day	Take mixed tocopherols, the more active type of vitamin E. Consult healthcare provider first if you are taking a blood thinner.
Vitamin K	100 mcg once a day	High dosages can cause toxicity. Consult your healthcare provider before taking if you are on an anticoagulant.
Zinc	25 mg once a day	The best zinc supplements are zinc picolinate and zinc citrate. If you are taking zinc and iron supplements, take one in the morning and one in the evening. (Taking them together reduces the efficiency of both.)

HORMONE REPLACEMENT THERAPY

When menopause occurs, the body has little use for the hormones that were responsible for menstruation. It therefore slows or stops their production, and progesterone and estrogen levels suddenly fall. This is the main cause of the uncomfortable and sometimes unpleasant feelings of menopause. The object of hormone replacement therapy (HRT) is to replenish the body with the hormones of which it is deficient, in order to improve the woman's well-being.

The most recommended therapy is bio-identical hormone replacement. It has the same chemical structure as your body, making it the best substitute. However, whether you take bio-identical or synthetic hormone replacement, the process can deplete your body of certain key nutrients. See page 372 for suggested nutritional supplements for women on hormone replacement therapy.

SUPPLEMENTS FOR WOMEN TAKING HORMONE REPLACEMENT THERAPY

Supplements	Dosage	Considerations
Alpha-lipoic acid	200 mg once a day	Improves blood sugar levels so diabetics may be able to take less medication.
B-complex vitamins	50 mg twice a day	I suggest taking a multi-vitamin.
Carnitine	1,000 mg once a day	
Gamma-linolenic acid (GLA)	240 mg once a day	It is important to maintain the proper ratio of omega-6 fatty acids to omega-3 fatty acids. (See page 110.)
Inositol	1,000 mg twice a day	May stimulate uterine contractions. Women who wish to become pregnant should consult their doctor regarding its use.
Magnesium	400 mg once a day	Consult healthcare provider for dosage if you have kidney disease. Discontinue use and see your doctor if you experience abdominal pain. Take a lower dose if it causes diarrhea.
Phosphatidylcholine (Lecithin)	2,000 mg once a day	Use with caution if you have malabsorption problems, as this could exacerbate them.
Vitamin B$_9$ (folate)	400 mcg twice a day	High doses can deplete your body of other vitamins in the B complex.
Vitamin B$_{12}$ (cobalamin)	500 mcg twice a day	High doses can deplete your body of other vitamins in the B complex.

Conclusion

Whether you wish to maintain your health or already have a certain disease process, you are now aware of many important and applicable nutrients. They can help in your effort to maintain good health and prevent disease by encouraging optimal biochemical activities in your body. A fellowship-trained anti-aging specialist can help you achieve your goals by encouraging the restoration of balance to your body.

Like the practices of anti-aging and functional medicines, the nutritional programs described in *What You Must Know About Vitamins, Minerals, Herbs, and More* are designed to treat the root cause of health problems, rather than mask the symptoms. These suggestions—which are based on an understanding of the physiological processes, environmental inputs, and role of genetic predisposition on well-being—can have a major and positive impact on your health.

Yet despite all its potentially helpful and effective information, *What You Must Know About Vitamins, Minerals, Herbs, and More* can only be as useful as you, the reader, make it. The key to good health is your taking responsibility for what you put into your body and how you live your life.

We are in a new age of medicine, one in which you, the patient, are an active participant in your own treatment. After all, your lifestyle choices—including food intake, exercise habits, spiritual practices, stress levels, and nutritional decisions—are very important to your overall health. Yet my job as a physician is not to blame your lifestyle choices. It is to assist you as you optimize your health and heal through education. It is my hope that this book has provided you with a reference that you and your healthcare provider can use as a framework to develop a nutritional program designed specifically for you.

Resources

FINDING A COMPOUNDING PHARMACY

Professional Compounding Centers of America
9901 South Wilcrest Drive
Houston, TX 77099
1-800-331-2498
www.pccarx.com

FINDING A FELLOWSHIP-TRAINED ANTI-AGING SPECIALIST

American Academy of Anti-Aging Physicians
1510 West Montana Street
Chicago, IL 60614
1-773-528-4333
www.worldhealth.net

Center for Health Living
30 locations nationwide
1-313-884-3288
www.cfhll.com

LABORATORY CONTACT INFORMATION

Age Diagnostic Laboratories
1341 West Fullerton Ave, Suite 123
Chicago, IL 60614
1-773-528-8500
www.adltests.com

Doctors Data Laboratory
3755 Illinois Avenue
St. Charles, IL 60174
1-800-323-2784
www.doctorsdata.com

Genova Diagnostics
63 Zillicoa Street
Asheville, NC 28801
1-800-522-4762
www.gdx.net

Metametrix Laboratory
3425 Corporate Way
Duluth, GA 30096
1-800-221-4640
www.metametrix.com

Spectracell
10401 Town Park Dr.
Houston, TX 77072
1-800-227-5227
www.spectracell.com

ZRT Laboratory
1815 NW 169th Place, Suite 5050
Beaverton, OR 97006
1-503-466-2445
www.zrtlab.com

PHARMACEUTICAL GRADE COMPANIES

You can find many good supplement brands at health food stores. Always make sure you buy pharmaceutical grade nutrients. The following pharmaceutical grade companies offer many quality nutritional supplements. Contact them for full product lists as well as for directions on ordering their products.

Designs for Health
2 North Road
East Windsor, CT 06088
1-800-847-8302
www.DesignsForHealth.com
Products include Policosanol + Gugulipid (for high cholesterol). New patient orders must be accompanied by the referral of a qualified healthcare professional.

Douglas Laboratories
600 Boyce Road
Pittsburgh, PA 15205
1-800-245-4440
www.douglaslabs.com

Life Extension Foundation
PO Box 407189
Fort Lauderdale, FL 33340
1-800-544-4440
www.lef.org

Metagenics
PO Box 1729
Gig Harbor, WA 98335
1-800-843-9660
www.metagenics.com

Products include CandiBactin (for yeast infections), Essential Defense (for colds), Insinase (for high levels of insulin), Kaprex AI (for immune disorders), Lipotain (for high cholesterol), Ultra Flora Plus (probiotics), and UltraInflamX (nutritional support for inflammation-related disorders).

Ortho Molecular Products
PO Box 1060
3017 Business Park Drive
Stevens Point, WI 54481
1-800-332-2351
www.orthomolecularproducts.
    com
Products include Candicid Forte (for yeast infections), Inflamma-bLOX (for gastointestinal problems), OrthoBiotics (probiotics), and Vessel Max (for varicose veins).

Pain and Stress Center
Billie Sahley, PhD
5282 Medical Drive, Suite 160
San Antonio, TX 78229
1-800-669-2256
www.painstresscenter.com

References

Fletcher, R, et al. "Vitamins for chronic disease prevention in adults." *JAMA* 2002; 287(23): 3116.

Hu, F, et al. "Diet, lifestyle, and the risk of type 2 diabetes mellitus in women." *NEJM* 2001; 345(11):790–797.

Murray, C, et al. "Alternative projections of mortality and disability by cause 1990–2020: global burden of disease study." *Lancet* 1997; 349:1498–1504.

Vita, Anthony, et al. "Aging, health risks, and cumulative disability." *NEJM* 1998; 338:1035–1041.

The Purpose of This Book

Bland, J. "Oxidants and antioxidants in clinical medicine: past, present, and future potential." *J. Nutr Environ Med* 1995; 5:255–280.

Challem, J. *Syndrome X.* New York, NY: John Wiley & Sons, Inc, 2000.

Colgan, M. *The New Nutrition.* Vancouver, BC: Apple Publishing, 1995.

Galland, L. "Person-centered diagnosis and chronic fatigue." *Metabolic Energy, Messenger Molecules, and Chronic Illness: The Functional Perspective.* Gig Harbor, WA: Institute for Functional Medicine, 2000.

Heller, L. "Healthy Women, Healthy Aging." Seminar, November 15–16, 2003.

Krebs-Smith, S, et al. "Fruits and vegetable intakes of children and adolescents in the United States." *Arch Ped Adolesc Med* 1996; 150(1):81–86.

Lieberman, S. *The Real Vitamin and Mineral Book.* New York, NY: Avery Publishing Group, 1997.

Pietrizk, K, et al. "Antioxidant, vitamins, cancer, and cardiovascular disease." *NEJM Letter to the Editor* 1996; 335(14):1065–1066.

Mixing Supplements, Drugs, and Food

Colgan, M. *The New Nutrition.* Vancouver, BC: Apple Publishing, 1995.

Fuhr, U, et al. "Drug interactions with grapefruit juice, extent, probable mechanism, and clinical relevance." *Drug Sci* 1998; 18:251–272.

Lieberman, S. *The Real Vitamin and Mineral Book.* New York, NY: Avery Publishing Group, 1997.

Meletis, C. *Interactions Between Drugs and Natural Medicines.* Sandy, OR: Electric Medical Publications, 1999.

Ulene, A. *Dr. Art Ulene's Complete Guide to Vitamins, Minerals, and Herbs.* New York, NY: Avery Publishing Group, 2000.

PART 1

CHAPTER 1: VITAMINS

Bateman, J. "Possible toxicity of herbal remedies." *Scottish Med J* 1998; 4:7–15.

Colgan, M. *The New Nutrition.* Vancouver, BC: Apple Publishing, 1995.

Hart, C. *The Insulin-Resistance Diet.* Chicago, IL: Contemporary Books, 2001.

Lieberman, S. *The Real Vitamin and Mineral*

377

Book. New York, NY: Avery Publishing Group, 1997.

Vitamin A

Bland, J. *Clinical Nutrition: A Functional Approach.* Gig Harbor, WA: Institute for Functional Medicine, 1999.

Brownstein, D. *The Miracle of Natural Hormones.* West Bloomfield, MI: Medical Alternatives Press, 1999.

Crook, T. *The Memory Cure.* New York, NY: Pocket Books, 1998.

Feskanich, D, et al. "Vitamin A intake and hip fracture among postmenopausal woman." *JAMA* 2002; 287(1):47–54.

Lark, S. *The Menopause Self Help Book.* Berkeley, CA: Celestial Arts, 1990.

Lieberman, S. *The Real Vitamin and Mineral Book.* New York, NY: Avery Publishing Group, 1997.

Paran, E, et al. "Effect of lycopene, an oral natural antioxidant, on blood pressure." *J Hypertens* 2001; 19:S74, Abstract P-1.204.

Paran, E, et al. "Effect of lycopene on blood pressure, serum lipoproteins, plasma homocysteine, and oxidative stress markers in grade I hypertensive patients." *Am J Hypertens* 2001; 140–141A, Abstract P-333.

Pietrizk, K, et al. "Antioxidant, vitamins, cancer, and cardiovascular disease." *NEJM Letter to the Editor* 1996; 335(14):1065–1066.

Semba, R, et al. "Vitamin A and immunity to viral, bacterial, and protozoan infections." *Proc Nutr Soc* 1999; 58(3):719–727.

Vitamin D

Al Farai, S, et al. "Vitamin D deficiency and chronic low back pain in Saudi Arabia." *Spine* 2003; 28(2):177–179.

Ali, F, et al. "Loss of seizure control due to anticonvulsant-induced hypocalcemia." *Amer Pharmacother* 2004; 38(6):1002–1005.

Borissova, A, et al. "The effect of vitamin D_3 on insulin secretion and peripheral insulin sensitivity in type 2 diabetic patients." *Int J Clin Pract* 2003; 57(4):258–261.

Bland, J. *Clinical Nutrition: A Functional Approach.* Gig Harbor, WA: Institute for Functional Medicine, 1999.

Chiu, K, et al. "Hypovitaminosis D is associated with insulin resistance and beta cell dysfunction." *Am J Clin Nutr* 2004; 79:820–825.

Christiansen, C, et al. "Anticonvulsant action of vitamin D in epileptic patients? A controlled pilot study." *Brit Med J* 1974; 2(913):258–259.

Collins, J. *What's Your Menopause Type?* Roseville, CA: Prima Publishing, 2000.

Dawson-Hughes, B, et al. "Effect of calcium and vitamin D supplementation on bone density in men and women 65 years of age or older." *NEJM* 1997; 337(10):670–676.

Dawson-Hughes, B, et al. "Effect of vitamin D supplementation on wintertime and overall bone loss in healthy postmenopausal women." *Ann Intern Med* 1991; 115(7):505–512.

Goldberg, P, et al. "Multiple sclerosis: decreased relapse rate through dietary supplementation with calcium, magnesium and vitamin D." *Med Hypotheses* 1986; 21(2):193–200.

Grant, W, et al. "An estimate of premature cancer mortality in the U.S. due to inadequate doses of solar ultraviolet-B radiation." *Cancer* 2002; 94(6):1867–1875.

Holick, M, et al. "Vitamin D and bone health." *J Nutr* 1996; 126:1159S–1164S.

Kini, S, et al. "A reversible form of cardiomyopathy." *J Postgrad Med* 2003; 49(1):85–87.

Krause, R, et al. "Ultraviolet D and blood pressure." *Lancet* 1998; 352(9129):709–710.

Lansdown, A, et al. "Vitamin D_3 enhances mood in healthy subjects during winter." *Psychopharm* 1998; 135(4):319–323.

McAlindon, T, et al. "Relation of dietary intake and serum levels of vitamin D to progression of osteoarthritis of the knee among participants in the Framingham study." *Ann Int Med* 1996; 125(5):353–359.

Plotnikoff, G, et al. "Prevalence of severe hypovitaminosis D in patients with persistent nonspecific musculoskeletal pain." *Mayo Clin Proc* 2003; 78(12):1463–1470.

Scragg, R, et al. "Myocardial infarction is inversely associated with plasma 25-hydroxyvitamin D_3 levels: a community-based study." *Int J Epidemiol* 1990; 19(3):559–563.

Thys-Jacob, S, et al. "Vitamin D and calcium dysregulation in the polycystic ovarian syndrome." *Steroids* 1999; 64(5):430–435.

Thys-Jacob, S. "Vitamin D and calcium in menstrual migraine." *Headache* 1994;34(9): 544–546.

Van de Berge, G, et al. "Bone turnover in prolonged critical illness: effect of vitamin D." *J Clin Endocrinol Metab* 2003; 88(10):4623–4632.

Vasquez, A, et al. "The clinical importance of vitamin D (cholecalciferol): a paradigm shift with implications for all healthcare providers." *Altern Therapies* 2004; 10(5):28–36.

Zittermann, A, et al. "Low vitamin D status: a contributing factor in the pathogenesis of congestive heart failure?" *J Am Coll Cardiol* 2003; 41:105–112.

Vitamin E

Behl, C, et al. "Vitamin E protects nerve cell from amyloid and protein toxicity." *Biochem Biophys J Res Communs* 1992; 186(2):944–950.

Bland, J. *Clinical Nutrition: A Functional Approach*. Gig Harbor, Washington: Institute for Functional Medicine, 1999.

Chan, A, et al. "Vitamin E and atherosclerosis." *J Nutr* 1998; 128(10):1593–1596.

Crook, T. *The Memory Cure*. New York, NY: Pocket Books, 1998.

Fillion, M. *Natural Prostate Healers*. Paramus, NJ: Prentice Hall Press, 1999.

Freedman, F, et al. "Alpha-tocopherol inhibits aggregation of human platelets by a protein kinase C-dependent mechanism." *Circulation* 1996; 94(10):2434–2440.

Gaby, A. *Nutritional Therapy in Medical Practice*. Carlisle, PA: Nutrition Seminars, 2003.

Lethem, R, et al. "Antioxidants and dementia." *Lancet* 1997; 348:1189.

Meydani, S, et al. "Vitamin E supplementation and in vivo immune response in healthy elderly subjects." *JAMA* 1997; 277:1380–1386.

Packer, L. *The Antioxidant Miracle*. New York, NY: John Wiley & Sons, Inc., 1999.

Paolisso, G, et al. "Vitamin E improves the action of insulin." *Diabetes Care* 1989; 12:265–269.

Qureshi, A, et al. "Lowering of serum cholesterol in hypercholesterolemic humans by tocotrienols (palmvite)." *Am J Clin Nutr* 1991; 53(4) Suppl:1021S–1026S.

Qureshi, A, et al. "Response of hypercholesterolemic subjects to administration of tocotrienols." *Lipids* 1995; 30(12):1171–1177.

Sano, M, et al. "A controlled trial of selegiline, alpha-tocopherol, or both as treatment for Alzheimer's disease. The Alzheimer's disease cooperative study." *NEJM* 1997: 336:1216–1222.

Tomeo, A, et al. "Antioxidant effects of tocotrienols in patients with hyperlipidemia and carotid stenosis." *Lipids* 1995; 30(12):1179–1183.

Vitamin K

Bland, J. *Clinical Nutrition: A Functional Approach*. Gig Harbor, WA: Institute for Functional Medicine, 1999.

Booth, S, et al. "Effects of a hydrogenated form of vitamin K on bone formation and resorption." *Amer Jour Clin Nutr* 2001; 74(6):783–790.

Booth, S, et al. "Skeletal functions of vitamin K-dependent proteins: not just for clotting anymore." *Nutr Rev* 1997; 55:282–284.

Booth, S, et al. "Warfarin use and fracture risk." *Nutr Rev* 2000; 58(1):20–22.

Collins, J. *What's Your Menopause Type?* Roseville, CA: Prima Publishing, 2000.

Davidson, R. "Conversion of K_1 to K_2." *Jour of Nutr* 1998; 128(2):220–223.

Demer, L, et al. "Novel mechanisms in accelerated vascular calcification in renal disease patients." *Curr Opin Nephrol Hypertens* 2002; 11(4):437–443.

Eguchi, T, et al. "Post-operative intracranial hemorrhage due to vitamin K deficiency: report of two cases." *No Shinkei Geka* 1992; 20(1): 73–77.

Feskanich, D, et al. "Vitamin K intake and hip fracture in women: a prospective study." *Am J Clin Nutr* 1999; 69:74–79.

Goepp, J. "Vitamin K's delicate balancing act." *Life Extension* April 2006; 59–67.

Graci, S. *The Bone-Building Solution*. Mississauga, Ontario, Canada: John Wiley & Sons Canada Ltd, 2006.

Hansen, L, et al. "Prevention and treatment of nonpostmenopausal osteoporosis." *Amer Jour Health Syst Pharm* 2004; 61(24):2637–2654.

Hidaka, T. "Treatment for patients with postmenopausal osteoporosis who have been placed on HRT and show a decrease in bone mineral density: Effects of concomitant administration of vitamin K_2." *J Bone Miner Metab* 2002; 20(4): 235–239.

Janein, B, et al. "Low vitamin K linked to coronary calcification risk: nutritional intervention might be possible." *Family Practice News* 2002; 32(1):1–2.

Philip, W, et al. "Decreased axial and peripheral bone density in patients taking long-term warfarin." *QJM* 1995; 88(9):635–640.

Plaza, S, et al. "Vitamin K_2 in bone metabolism and osteoporosis." *Altern Med Rev* 2005; 10(1): 24–35.

Reese, A, et al. "Low-dose vitamin K to augment anticoagulation control." *Pharmacotherapy* 2005; 25(12):1746–1751.

Vermeer, C, et al. "A comprehensive review of vitamin K and vitamin K antagonist." *Hematol Oncol Clin North Am* 2000; 14(2):339–353.

"Weak bones cause heart attacks and stoke." *Collector's Edition Life Extension*, 2003.

Witteman, J, et al. "Aortic calcified plaque and cardiovascular disease (the Framingham study)." *Am J Cardiol* 1990; 66:1060–1064.

Vitamin B Complex

Benjamin, J, et al. "Double-blind, placebo-controlled, crossover trial of inositol treatment for panic disorder." *Am J Psychiatry* 1995; 152: 1084–1086.

Berkson, B. *The Alpha Lipoic Acid Breakthrough.* Rocklin, CA: Prima Publishing, 1998.

Bland, J. *Clinical Nutrition: A Functional Approach.* Gig Harbor, WA: Institute for Functional Medicine, 1999.

Bland, J. "Nutrients as Biological Response Modifiers." *Applying Functional Medicine in Clinical Practice.* Gig Harbor, WA: Functional Medicine Institute, 2002.

Bland, K. "Disorders of the Brain: Emerging Therapies in Complex Neurologic and Psychiatric Conditions." Conference, 2002.

Boltiglieri, T, et al. "Folate, vitamin B_{12}, neuropsychiatric disorders." *Nutr Rev* 1996; 54(2):138–142.

Butterworth, C, et al. "Folate deficiency and cervical dysplasia." *JAMA* 1992; 267(4):528–533.

Chan, P, et al. "Randomized double-blind,

placebo-controlled study of the safety and efficacy of vitamin B complex in the treatment of nocturnal leg cramps in elderly patients with hypertension." *J Clin Pharm* 1998; 38(12):1151–1154.

Coggeshall, J, et al. "Biotin status and plasma glucose in diabetes." *Ann NY Acad Sci* 1985; 447:389.

Colgan, M. *The New Nutrition.* Vancouver, BC, Canada: Apple Publishing, 1995.

Collins, J. *What's Your Menopause Type?* Roseville, CA: Prima Publishing, 2000.

Crayhon, R. "Aging well in the 21st century." Seminar 2002.

Crook, T. *The Memory Cure.* New York, NY: Pocket Books, 1998.

DiPalma, J, et al. "Use of niacin as a drug." *Annu Rev Nutr* 1991; 11:169–187.

Gaby, A. *Nutritional Therapy in Medical Practice.* Carlisle, PA: Nutrition Seminars, 2003.

Gang, R, et al. "Niacin treatment increases plasma homocysteine levels." *Am Heart J* 1999; 138(6 Pt. 1):1082–1087.

Goldman, R. *Human Growth Factors.* Chicago, IL: American Academy of Anti-Aging Physicians, 2003.

Hochman, L, et al. "Brittle nails: response to daily biotin supplementation." *Cutis* 1993; 51 (4):303–305.

Koutsilos, D, et al. "Biotin for diabetic peripheral neuropathy." *Biomed Phamacother* 1990; 44(10):511–514.

Kwasniewska, A, et al. "Folate deficiency and cervical intraepithelial neoplasia." *Eur Jour Gynaecol Oncol* 1997; 18(6):526–530.

Lark, S. *The Menopause Self Help Book.* Berkeley, California: Celestial Arts, 1990.

Levine, J, et al. "Combination of inositol and serotonin reuptake inhibitors in the treatment of depression." *Biol Psychiatry* 1999; 45(3):270–273.

Maebashi, M, et al. "Therapeutic evaluation of the effect of biotin on hyperglycemia patients with non-insulin dependant diabetes mellitus." *Journ of Clin Biochem and Nutri* 1993; 14:211–218.

Miller, A, et al. "Homocysteine metabolism:

nutritional modulation and impact on health and disease." *Alt Med Rev* 1997; 2(4):234–254.

Perlmutter, D. "The brain on fire: the role of inflammation in neurodegenerative disorders." A4M Conference, 2003.

Polo, V, et al. "Nicotinamide improves insulin secretion and metabolic control in lean type 2 diabetic patients with secondary failure to sulphonylureas." *Acta Diabetol* 1998; 35(1):61–66.

Schaumberg, H, et al. "Sensory neuropathy from pyridoxine abuse: a new megavitamin syndrome." *NEJM* 1983; 309:445–448.

Schmidt, M. *Tired of Being Tired*. Berkeley, CA: Frog, Ltd., 1995.

Schulman, R. *Solve It With Supplements*. New York, NY: Rodale, Inc, 2007.

Schoenen, J, et al. "High-dose riboflavin as a prophylactic treatment of migraine: results of an open pilot study." *Cephalgia* 1994; 14(5): 328–329.

Schwaberdal, P, et al. "Pantothenic acid deficiency as a factor contributing to the development of hypertension." *Cardiology* 1985; 72(1) Suppl:187–189.

Shang, H, et al. "A high biotin diet improves the impaired glucose tolerance of long-term spontaneously hyperglycemic rats with non-insulin-dependent diabetes mellitus." *Jour Nutr Sci Vitamins* 1996; 42:517–526.

Sundkvist, G, et al. "Sorbitol and myo-inositol levels and morphology of neural nerve in relation to peripheral nerve function and clinical neuropathy in men with diabetic, impaired, and normal glucose tolerance." *Diabetic Med* 2000; 17:259–268.

Van Goor, L, et al. "Cobalamin deficiency and mental impairment in elderly people." *Age and Ageing* 1995; 24:536–542.

Weler, M, et al. "Periconceptional folic acid exposure and risk of occurrent neural tube defects." *JAMA* 1993; 269:1257–1261.

Vitamin C

Bland, J. *Clinical Nutrition: A Functional Approach*. Gig Harbor, WA: Institute for Functional Medicine, 1999.

Block, G, et al, "Ascorbic acid status and subsequent diastolic and systolic blood pressure." *Hypertension* 2001; 37:261–267.

Colgan, M. *The New Nutrition*. Vancouver, BC, Canada: Apple Publishing, 1995.

Collins, J. *What's Your Menopause Type?* Roseville, CA: Prima Publishing, 2000.

Debusk, R, et al. "Dietary supplements and cardiovascular disease." *Curr Atheroscler Rep* 2000; 2:508–514.

Feldman, E, et al. "The role of vitamin C and antioxidants in hypertension." *Nutrition and the MD* 1998; 24:1–4.

Fillion, M, *Natural Prostate Healers*. Paramus, NJ: Prentice Hall Press, 1999.

Fotherby, M, et al. "Effect of vitamin C on ambulatory blood pressure and plasma lipids in older persons." *J Hypertens* 2000; 18; 411–415.

Houston, M. *What Your Doctor May Not Tell You About Hypertension*. New York, NY: Warner Books, Inc., 2003.

Packer, L. *The Antioxidant Miracle*. New York, NY: John Wiley & Sons, Inc, 1999.

Perlmutter, D. *BrainRecovery.com*. Naples, FL: The Perlmutter Health Center, 2000.

Simon, J, et al. "Vitamin C and cardiovascular disease a review." *J Amer Coll Nutr* 1992; 11: 107–125.

Sinatra, S. "Alternative interventions for preventing and treating cardiovascular disease." A4M Conference, June 2003.

Trout, D, et al. "Vitamin C and cardiovascular risk factors." *Am J Clin Nutr* 1991; 53:322–325.

CHAPTER 2: MINERALS

Calcium

Bland, J. *Clinical Nutrition: A Functional Approach*. Gig Harbor, WA: Institute for Functional Medicine, 1999.

Colgan, M. *The New Nutrition*. Vancouver, BC, Canada: Apple Publishing, 1995.

Crook, T. *The Memory Cure*. New York, NY: Pocket Books, 1998.

Gaby, A. *Nutritional Therapy in Medical Practice*. Carlisle, PA: Nutrition Seminars, 2003.

Germano, R. *The Osteoporosis Solution*. New

York, NY: Kensington Publishing Corporation, 1999.

Nachtigall, L. *Estrogen: The Facts Can Change Your Life.* New York, NY: HarperCollins, 1995.

Nguyen, U, et al. "Aspartame ingestion increases urinary, calcium, but not oxalate excretion, in healthy subjects." *J Clin Endocrinol Metab* 1998; 83(1):165–168.

Smith, P. *HRT: The Answers.* Traverse City, MI: Healthy Living Books, 2003.

Chloride

LaValle, J. "Metabolic Consequences of Drug Induced Nutrient Depletion." Detroit, MI: Anti-Aging and Functional Medicine Fellowship, 2007.

Magnesium

Bland, J. *Clinical Nutrition: A Functional Approach.* Gig Harbor, WA: Institute for Functional Medicine, 1999.

Braverman, E. *Hypertension and Nutrition.* New Canaan, CT: Keats Publishing, Inc, 1996.

Crook, T. *The Memory Cure.* New York: Pocket Books, 1998.

Davis, W, et al. "Monotherapy with magnesium increases abnormally low HDL cholesterol: A clinical assay." *Curr Ther Res* 1984; 36:341–346.

Doghlan, H, et al. "Magnesium in mitral valve prolapse syndrome." *Magnesium Trace Elem* 1990; 9:319–320.

Faccinetti, F, et al. "Magnesium prohylaxis of menstrual migraine: effects on intracellular magnesium." *Headache* 1991; 31:298–304.

Gaby, A. *Magnesium.* New Canaan, CT: Keats Publishing, 1994.

Gaby, A. *Nutritional Therapy in Medical Practice.* Carlisle, PA: Nutrition Seminars, 2003.

Galland, L. "Magnesium and immune function: an overview." *Magnesium* 1988; 7:290–299.

Paolisso, G, et al. "Improved insulin response ad action by chronic magnesium administration in aged NIDDM subjects." *Diabetes Care* 1989; 12(4):265–272.

Ramadan, W, et al. "Low brain magnesium in migraine." *Headache* 1989; 29:590–593.

Simontacchi, C. *The Crazy Makers.* New York, NY: Jeremy P. Tarcher/Putnam, 2000.

Weaver, K, et al. "Magnesium and migraine." *Headache* 1990; 30:168.

Yang, C, et al. "Calcium and magnesium in drinking water and risk from cardiovascular disease." *Stroke* 1998; 29(2):411–414.

Phosphorus

Bland, J. *Clinical Nutrition: A Functional Approach.* Gig Harbor, WA: Institute for Functional Medicine, 1999.

Potassium

Bland, J. *Clinical Nutrition: A Functional Approach.* Gig Harbor, WA: Institute for Functional Medicine, 1999.

Gaby, A. *Nutritional Therapy in Medical Practice.* Carlisle, PA: Nutrition Seminars, 2003.

Sodium

Bland, J. *Clinical Nutrition: A Functional Approach.* Gig Harbor, WA: Institute for Functional Medicine, 1999.

Boron

Bland, J. *Clinical Nutrition: A Functional Approach.* Gig Harbor, WA: Institute for Functional Medicine, 1999.

Colgan, M. *The New Nutrition.* Vancouver, BC, Canada: Apple Publishing, 1995.

Hunt, C, et al. "Dietary boron as a physiological regulator of the normal inflammatory response: a review and current research progress." *J Trace Elem Med* 1999; 12:221–233.

Newnham, R, et al. "Essentiality of boron for healthy bones and joints." *Environ Health Perspect* 1994; 102 (Suppl) 7:83–85.

Penland, J, et al. "Dietary boron, brain function, and cognitive performance." *Environ Health Perspect* 1994; 102 (Suppl) 7:65–72.

Penland, J, et al. "The importance of boron nutrition for brain and psychological function." *Biol Trac Elem Res* 1998; 66:299–317.

Zhang, Z, et al. "Boron is associated with decreased risk of prostate cancer." *FASEB J* 2001; 1:394–397.

Chromium

Anderson, R, et al. "Effect of chromium supplementation on Cr excretion of human subjects and correlation of Cr excretion with selected clinical parameters." *J of Nutr* 1983; 113:276–281.

Bahadori, B, et al. "Treatment with chromium picolinate improves lean body mass in patients following weight reduction." *Inter Jour of Obesity* 1995; 19(Suppl)12:38.

Bland, J. *Clinical Nutrition: A Functional Approach.* Gig Harbor, WA: Institute for Functional Medicine, 1999.

Bland, J. "Nutrients as Biological Response Modifiers." *Applying Functional Medicine in Clinical Practice.* Gig Harbor, WA: Functional Medicine Institute, 2002.

Crayhon, R. *Robert Crayhon's Nutrition Made Simple.* New York, NY: M. Evans and Company, 1994.

Evans, G. *Chromium Picolinate.* New York, NY: Avery Publishing Group, 1996.

Lieberman, S. *The Real Vitamin and Mineral Book.* New York, NY: Avery Publishing Group, 1997.

Press, R, et al. "The effect of chromium picolinate on serum cholesterol and apoliporotein fractions in human subjects." *Western J of Med* 1990; 152:41–45.

Preuss, H, et al. "Chromium update: examining recent literature 1997–1998." *Curr Opin Clin Nutr Metab Care* 1998; 1:509–512.

Copper

Bland, J. *Clinical Nutrition: A Functional Approach.* Gig Harbor, WA: Institute for Functional Medicine, 1999.

Bland, J. "Nutrients as Biological Response Modifiers." *Applying Functional Medicine in Clinical Practice.* Gig Harbor, WA: Functional Medicine Institute, 2002.

Gaby, A. *Nutritional Therapy in Medical Practice.* Carlisle, PA: Nutrition Seminars, 2003.

Iodine

Bland, J. *Clinical Nutrition: A Functional Approach.* Gig Harbor, WA: Institute for Functional Medicine, 1999.

Brownstein, D. *Iodine: Why You Need It, Why You Can't Live Without It.* Bloomfield Hills, MI: Medical Alternatives Press, 2004.

Goldman, R. *Human Growth Factors.* Chicago, IL: American Academy of Anti-Aging Physicians, 2003.

Lark, S. *The Menopause Self Help Book.* Berkeley, CA: Celestial Arts, 1990.

Iron

Bland, J. *Clinical Nutrition: A Functional Approach.* Gig Harbor, WA: Institute for Functional Medicine, 1999.

Bland, J. "Nutrients as Biological Response Modifiers." *Applying Functional Medicine in Clinical Practice.* Gig Harbor, WA: Institute for Functional Medicine, 2002.

Gaby, A. *Nutritional Therapy in Medical Practice.* Carlisle, PA: Nutrition Seminars, 2003.

Schulman, R. *Solve It With Supplements.* New York, NY: Rodale, Inc., 2007.

Simontacchi, C. *The Crazy Makers.* New York, NY: Jeremy P. Tarcher/Putnam, 2000.

Manganese

Bland, J. *Clinical Nutrition: A Functional Approach.* Gig Harbor, Washington: Institute for Functional Medicine, 1999.

Bland, J. "Nutrients as Biological Response Modifiers." *Applying Functional Medicine in Clinical Practice.* Gig Harbor, WA: Institute for Functional Medicine, 2002.

Gaby, A. *Nutritional Therapy in Medical Practice.* Carlisle, PA: Nutrition Seminars, 2003.

Molybdenum

Bland, J. *Clinical Nutrition: A Functional Approach.* Gig Harbor, Washington: Institute for Functional Medicine, 1999.

Colgan, M. *The New Nutrition.* Vancouver, BC, Canada: Apple Publishing, 1995.

Gaby, A. *Nutritional Therapy in Medical Practice.* Carlisle, PA: Nutrition Seminars, 2003.

Selenium

Berkson, B. *The Alpha Lipoic Acid Breakthrough.* Rocklin, CA: Prima Publishing, 1998.

Bland, J. *Clinical Nutrition: A Functional Ap-*

proach. Gig Harbor, Washington: Institute for Functional Medicine, 1999.

Fillion, M. *Natural Prostate Healers.* Paramus, NJ: Prentice Hall Press, 1999.

Packer, L. *The Antioxidant Miracle.* New York, NY: John Wiley & Sons, Inc, 1999.

Vanadium

Bland, J, *Clinical Nutrition: A Functional Approach.* Gig Harbor, WA: Institute for Functional Medicine, 1999.

Goldfine, A, et al. "Vanadium improves insulin sensitivity." *Jour Clin Endocrinol Metabol* 1995; 80(11):3311–3319.

Zinc

Bland, J. *Clinical Nutrition: A Functional Approach.* Gig Harbor, WA: Institute for Functional Medicine, 1999.

Bland, J. "Nutrients as Biological Response Modifiers." *Applying Functional Medicine in Clinical Practice.* Gig Harbor, WA: Institute for Functional Medicine, 2002.

Fillion, M. *Natural Prostate Healers.* Paramus, NJ: Prentice Hall Press, 1999.

Gaby, A. *Nutritional Therapy in Medical Practice.* Carlisle, PA: Nutrition Seminars, 2003.

Goldman, R. *Human Growth Factors.* Chicago, IL: American Academy of Anti-Aging Physicians, 2003.

Schmidt, M. *Tired of Being Tired.* Berkeley, CA: Frog, Ltd, 1995.

Schulman, R. *Solve It With Supplements.* New York, NY: Rodale, Inc, 2007.

CHAPTER 3: FATTY ACIDS

Bates, D, et al. "A double-blind controlled trial of long-chain omega-3 polyunsaturated fatty acids in the treatment of multiple sclerosis." *J Neurol, Neurosurg Psych* 1989; 52: 18–22.

Belluzzi, A, et al. "Polyunsaturated fatty acids and inflammatory bowel disease." *Am J Clin Nutr* 2000; 71(1):339S–342S.

Belury, M, et al. "Conjugated dienoic linoleate: a polyunsaturated fatty acid with unique chemorotective properties." *Nut Res* 1995; 53(4Pt 1):83–89.

Bland, J. *Clinical Nutrition: A Functional Approach.* Gig Harbor, Washington: Institute for Functional Medicine, 1999.

Blankson, H, et al. "Conjugated linoleic acid reduces body fat mass in overweight and obese humans." *J Nutr* 2000; 130(12):2943–2348.

Bucher, H, et al. "N-3 polyunsaturated fatty acid in coronary heart disease: a meta-analysis of random-controlled trials." *Am J Med* 2002; 112(4)298–304.

Colgan, M. *The New Nutrition.* Vancouver, BC, Canada: Apple Publishing, 1995.

Connor, S, et al. "Are fish oils beneficial in the prevention and treatment of coronary artery disease?" *Am J Clin Nutr* 1997; 66(4 Suppl):1020S–1031S.

Doyle, L, et al. "Scientific forum explores CLA knowledge." *Inform* 1998; 9(1):69–72.

Epstein, F, et al. "Glucose transporters and insulin action: implication for insulin resistance and diabetes mellitus." *NEJM* 1999; 341(4):248–257.

Erasmus, Udo. *Fats that Heal, Fats that Kill.* Burnaby, BC, Canada: Alive Books, 1993.

Gaby, A. *Nutritional Therapy in Medical Practice.* Carlisle, PA: Nutrition Seminars, 2003.

Geusens, P, et al. "Long-term effect of omega-3 fatty acid supplementation in active rheumatoid arthritis (a 12-month, double-blind, controlled study." *Arthritis and Rheumatism* 1996; 37(6):824–829.

Goodman, J. *The Omega Solution.* Roseville, CA: Prima Publishing, 2001.

Harris, W, et al. "Omega-3 fatty acids and serum lipoproteins: human studies." *Am J Clin Nutr* 1997; 65:1645S–1654S.

Holman, R, et al. "The slow discovery of the importance of omega-3 essential fatty acids in human health." *J Nutr* 1998; 128:427S–433S.

Horrobin, D, et al. "The use of gamma-linolenic acid on human diabetic peripheral neuropathy." *Agents and Actions* 1992; 37S:120–144.

Hu, F, et al. "Fish and omega-3 fatty acid intake and risk of coronary heart disease in women." *JAMA* 2002; 287(14):1815–1821.

Kang, J, et al. "Prevention of fatal cardiac arrhythmias by polyunsaturated fatty acids." *Am J. Clin Nutr* 2000; 71(1Suppl):2025–2075.

Kremer, J, et al. "N-3 fatty acid supplements in rheumatoid arthritis." *Am J Clin Nutr* 2000; 71(1Suppl):349S–351S.

Kris-Etherton, P, et al. "American Heart Association Nutrition Committee: Fish consumption, fish oil, omega-3 fatty acids and cardiovascular disease." *Circulation* 2002; 106:2747–2757.

Lerman, R. "Nutrients as biological response modifiers: fatty acids and inflammation." *Applying Functional Medicine in Clinical Practice.* Gig Harbor, WA: Institute for Functional Medicine, 2002.

Lerman, R. "The essential fatty acids in psychiatric and neurological dysfunction." *Brain Biochemistry and Nutrition.* Gig Harbor Washington: Institute for Functional Medicine, 2002.

Lorenz, R, et al. "Supplementation with n-3 fatty acid from fish oil in chronic irritable bowel disease: A random, placebo-controlled, double-blind, cross-over trial." *J Intern Med Suppl* 1989; 225(731):225–232.

Marangell, L. "A double-blind, placebo-controlled study of the omega-3 fatty acid docosahexanoic acid in the treatment of major depression." *Am J Psychiatry* 2003; 160(3):996–998.

Mayser, P, et al. "Omega-3 fatty acid-based lipid infusion in patients with chronic plaque psoriasis: results of a double-blind, randomized, placebo-controlled, multicenter trial." *J Am Acad Of Derm* 1998; 38:539–547.

Mischoulon, D, et al. "Docosahexaenoic acid and omega-3 fatty acids in depression." Psychiatr Clin North Am 2000; 4:785–794.

Moya-Camarena, S, et al. "Conjugated linoleic acid is a potent naturally occurring ligand and activator of PPAR." *J Lipid Res* 1999; 40:1426–1433.

Nordvik, I, et al. "Effect of dietary advice and omega-3 supplementation in newly diagnosed MS patient." *Acta Neurol Scandia* 2000; 102(3):143–149.

Oliver, M, et al. "Diet and coronary disease." *Br Med Bull* 1981; 37:49–58.

Ornish, D, et al. "Intensive lifestyle changes for reversal of coronary heart disease." *JAMA* 1998; 280(23):2001–2007.

Pariza, M, et. al. "Conjugated dienoic derivatives of linolic acid: a new class of anticarcinogens." *Med Oncol Tumor Pharmacother* 1990; 7(2-3):169–171.

Riserus, U. "Conjugated linoleic acid (CLA) reduced abdominal adipose tissue in obese middle-aged men with signs of metabolic syndrome: a randomized controlled trial." *Int J Obes Relat Metab Disord* 2001; 25(8):1129–1135.

Ryder, J, et al. "Isomer-specific antidiabetic properties of conjugated linoleic acid. Improve glucose tolerance, skeletal muscle insulin action, and UCP-2 gene expression." *Diabetes* 2001; 50:1149–1157.

Schmidt, M. *Brain-Building Nutrition: The Healing Power of Fats and Oils.* Berkeley, CA: Frog, Ltd, 2001.

Siguel, E, et al. "Prevalence of essential fatty acid deficiency in patients with chronic gastrointestinal disorders." *Metabolism* 1996; 45(1):12–23.

Stevens, L, et al. "Essential fatty acid metabolism in boys with attention-deficit hyperactivity disorder." *Am J Clin Nutr* 1995; 62:762–768.

Tiemeier, H, et al. "Plasma fatty acid composition and depression are associated in the elderly: the Rotterdam study." *Am J Clin Nutr* 2003; 78(1):40–46.

Vognild, E, et al. "Effects of dietary marine oils and olive oil on fatty acid composition, platelet membrane fluidity, platelet responses, and serum lipids in healthy humans." *Lipids* 1998; 3(4):3427–3436.

Watanabe, T, et al. "The effect of a newly developed ointment containing eicosapentaenoic acid and docosahexaenoic acid in the treatment of atopic dermatitis." *J Med Inves* 1999; 46: 173–177.

CHAPTER 4: AMINO ACIDS

Sahley, B. *Control Hyperactivity ADD Naturally.* San Antonio, TX: Pain and Stress Publications, 1999.

Sahley, B. *Heal with Amino Acids and Nutrients.* San Antonio, TX: Pain and Stress Publications, 2000.

Alanine

Sahley, B. *Heal with Amino Acids and Nutrients.* San Antonio, TX: Pain and Stress Publications, 2000.

Arginine

Efron, D, et al. "Role of arginine in immunonutrition." *J Gastroenterol* 2000; 35(suppl 12):20–23.

Klatz, R. *The New Anti-Aging Revolution.* Laguna Beach, CA: Basic Health Publications, 2003.

Sahley, B. *Heal with Amino Acids and Nutrients.* San Antonio, TX: Pain and Stress Publications, 2000.

Siani, A, et al. "Blood pressure and metabolic changes during dietary L-arginine supplementation in human." *Am J Hypertens* 2000; 13(5, Pt.1):547–551.

Sinatra, S. *Heart Sense For Women.* Washington, DC: LifeLine Press, 2000.

Aspartic Acid

Sahley, B. *Heal with Amino Acids.* San Antonio, TX: Pain and Stress Publications, 2000.

Asparagine

Sahley, B. *Heal with Amino Acids and Nutrients.* San Antonio, TX: Pain and Stress Publications, 2000.

Carnitine

Arockia, R, et al. "Carnitine as a free radical scavenger in aging." *Exp Gerontol* 2001; 36:1713–1726.

Bland, J. *Clinical Nutrition: A Functional Approach.* Gig Harbor, WA: Institute for Functional Medicine, 1999.

Bland, J. "Nutrients as Biological Response Modifiers." *Applying Functional Medicine in Clinical Practice.* Gig Harbor, WA: Institute for Functional Medicine, 2002.

Brooks, J, et al. "Acetyl-L-Carnitine slows decline in younger patients with Alzheimer's disease: a reanalysis of a double-blind, placebo-controlled study using the trilinear approach." *Int Psychogeriatr* 1998; 10:192–203.

Crayhon, R. *The Carnitine Miracle.* New York, NY: M. Evans and Company, 1998.

De Angelis, C, et al. "Levocarnitine acetyl stimulates peripheral nerve regeneration and neuromuscular junction remodeling following sciatic nerve injury." *Int J Clin Pharmacol Re* 1992; 12:269–279.

Gaby, A. *Nutritional Therapy in Medical Practice.* Carlisle, PA: Nutrition Seminars, 2003.

Garzya, G, et al. "Evaluation of the effects of L-acetylcarnitine on senile patients suffering from depression." *Drugs Exp Clin Res* 1990; 16:101–106.

Klatz, R. *The New Anti-Aging Revolution.* Laguna Beach, CA: Basic Health Publications, 2003.

Retter, A, et al. "Carnitine and its role in cardiovascular disease." *Heart Disease* 1999; 1:108–113.

Sahley, B. *Heal with Amino Acids and Nutrients.* San Antonio, TX: Pain and Stress Publications, 2000.

Spoganoli, A, et al. "Long-term acetyl-L-carnitine treatment in Alzheimer's disease." *Neurology* 1991; 41:1726–1732.

Tanphaichitr, V, et al. "Carnitine metabolism and carnitine deficiency." *Nur* 1993; 9:246–254.

Carnosine

"The anti-aging effects of carnosine." *Life Extensions* 2003; January.

Boldyrev, A. "Biochemical and physiological evidence that carnosine is an endogenous neuroprotector against free radicals." *Cell Mol Neurobiol* 1997; 17(2):259–271.

Boldyrev, A, et al. "The antioxidative properties of carnosine, a natural histidine containing dipeptide." *Biochem Int* 1987; 15:1105–1113.

Gulyaeva, N, et al. "Superoxide-scavenging activity of carnosine in the presence of copper and zinc ions." *Biochemistry (Masc)* 1987; 52(7 Part 2):1051–1054.

Hipkiss, A, et al. "Carnosine protects proteins against methylglycoxal-mediated modifications." *Bochem Biophys Res Comm* 1998; 248(1): 28–32.

Horning, M, et al. "Endogenous mechanisms of neuro-protection: role of zinc, copper, and carnosine." *Brain Res* 2000; 852(1):56–61.

Price, D, et al. "Chelating activity of advanced glycation end-product inhibitors." *J Bio Chem* 2001; 276:48967–48672.

Quinn, P, et al. "Carnosine: its properties, functions, and potential therapeutic applications." *Mol Aspects Med* 1992; 13:379–444.

Ririe, D, et al. "Vasodilatory actions of the dietary peptide carnosine." *Nutrition* 2000; 16:168–172.

Roberts, OP, et al. "Dietary peptides improve wound healing following surgery." *Nutrition* 1998; 14:266–269.

Stvolinsky, S, et al. "Anti-ischemic activity of carnosine." *Biochemistry (Masc)* 2000; 65:849–855.

Stvolinsky, S, et al. "Carnosine: an endogenous neuroprotector in the ischemic brain." *Cell Mol Neurobiol* 1999; 19:4556.

Wang, A, et al. "Use of carnosine as a natural anti-senescence drug for human beings." *Biochemistry (Masc)* 2000; 65:869–871.

Cysteine

Gaby, A. *Nutritional Therapy in Medical Practice.* Carlisle, PA: Nutrition Seminars, 2003.

Klatz, R. *The New Anti-Aging Revolution.* Laguna Beach, CA: Basic Health Publications, 2003.

Sahley, B. *Heal with Amino Acids and Nutrients.* San Antonio, TX: Pain and Stress Publications, 2000.

Hydroxytryptophan (5-HTP)

Birdshell, T. "5-hydroxytryptophan: a clinically-effective serotonin precursor." *Alt Med Rev* 1998; 3:271–278.

den Boer, J, et al. "Behavior, neuroendocrine, and biochemical effects of 5-hydroxytryptophan administration in panic disorder." *Psychiatry Res* 1990; 31:267–278.

Ribeiro, C, et al. "5-hydroxytryptophan in the prophylaxis of chronic tension-type headache: a double-blind, random, placebo-controlled study for the Portuguese Head Society." *Headache* 2000; 40:451–456.

Sahley, B. *Heal with Amino Acids and Nutrients.* San Antonio, TX: Pain and Stress Publications, 2000.

Gamma-Aminobutyric Acid (GABA)

Klatz, R. *The New Anti-Aging Revolution.* Laguna Beach, CA: Basic Health Publications, 2003.

Sahley, B. *GABA: The Anxiety Amino Acid.* San Antonio, TX: Pain and Stress Publications, 1999.

Glutamine

Keast, D, et al. "Depression of plasma glutamine concentration after exercise stress and its possible influence on the immune system." *Med J Aust* 1995; 162(1):15–18.

Klatz, R. *The New Anti-Aging Revolution.* Laguna Beach, CA: Basic Health Publications, 2003.

Maskovitz, B, et al. "Glutamine metabolism and utilization: relevance to major problems in health care." *Pharmacol Res* 1994; 30(1):61–71.

Peck, L, et al. "Glutamine should be figured into inflammatory bowel disease formulations." *Family Practice News* June 1994.

Sahley, B. *Heal with Amino Acids and Nutrients.* San Antonio, TX: Pain and Stress Publications, 2000.

Shabert, J. *The Ultimate Nutrient Glutamine.* New York, NY: Avery Publishing Group, 1994.

Welbourne, T, et al. "Increased plasma bicarbonate and growth hormone after an oral glutamine load." *Am J Clin Nutr* 1995; 61(5): 1058–1061.

Glutathione

Klatz, R. *The New Anti-Aging Revolution.* Laguna Beach, CA: Basic Health Publications, 2003.

Perlmutter, D. *BrainRecovery.com.* Naples, Florida: The Perlmutter Health Center, 2000.

Glycine

Klatz, R. *The New Anti-Aging Revolution.* Laguna Beach, CA: Basic Health Publications, 2003.

Sahley, B. *Heal with Amino Acids and Nutrients.* San Antonio, TX: Pain and Stress Publications, 2000.

Histidine

Klatz, R. *The New Anti-Aging Revolution.* Laguna Beach, CA: Basic Health Publications, 2003.

Sahley, B. *Heal with Amino Acids and Nutrients.* San Antonio, TX: Pain and Stress Publications, 2000.

Lysine

Klatz, R. *The New Anti-Aging Revolution.* Laguna Beach, CA: Basic Health Publications, 2003.

Sahley, B. *Heal with Amino Acids and Nutrients.* San Antonio, TX: Pain and Stress Publications, 2000.

Methionine

Klatz, R. *The New Anti-Aging Revolution.* Laguna Beach, CA: Basic Health Publications, 2003.

Sahley, B. *Heal with Amino Acids and Nutrients.* San Antonio, TX: Pain and Stress Publications, 2000.

Phenylalanine

Klatz, R. *The New Anti-Aging Revolution.* Laguna Beach, CA: Basic Health Publications, 2003.

Sahley, B. *Heal with Amino Acids and Nutrients.* San Antonio, TX: Pain and Stress Publications, 2000.

Proline

Sahley, B. *Heal with Amino Acids and Nutrients.* San Antonio, TX: Pain and Stress Publications, 2000.

Serine

Klatz, R. *The New Anti-Aging Revolution.* Laguna Beach, CA: Basic Health Publications, 2003.

Sahley, B. *Heal with Amino Acids and Nutrients.* San Antonio, TX: Pain and Stress Publications, 2000.

Taurine

Birdsall, T, et al. "Therapeutic applications of taurine." *Altern-Med-Rev* 1998; 3:128–136.

Chapman, R, et al. "Taurine and the heart." *Cardiovasc Res* 1993; 27(3):358–363.

Collins, B. "Plasma and urinary taurine in epilepsy." *Clin Chem* 1988; 34(4):671–675.

Crayhon, R. "Aging well in the 21st century." Seminar, 2002.

Dawson, R. "An age-related decline in striatal taurine is correlated with a loss of dopaminergic markers." *Brain Res Bull* 1999; 48:319–324.

Desai, T, et al. "Taurine deficiency after intensive chemotherapy and/or radiation." *Am J Clin Nutr* 1992; 55(3):708–711.

Fujita, T. "Hypotensive effect of taurine. Possible involvement of the sympathetic nervous system and endogenous opiates." *J Clin Invest* 1988; 82(3):993–997.

Gaby, A. *Nutritional Therapy in Medical Practice.* Carlisle, PA: Nutrition Seminars, 2003.

Goldman, R. *Human Growth Factors.* Chicago, IL: American Academy of Anti-Aging Physicians, 2003.

Huxtable, R, et al. "Physiologic actions of taurine." *Physiol Rev* 1992; 72:101–163.

Kendler, B, et al. "Taurine: an overview of its role in preventive medicine." *Prev Med* 1989; 18(1):70–100.

Klatz, R. *The New Anti-Aging Revolution.* Laguna Beach, CA: Basic Health Publications, 2003.

Kumata, K, et al. "Restoration of endothelium-dependant relaxation in both hypercholesterolemic and diabetics by chronic taurine." *Eur J Pharmacol* 1996; 303:47–53.

Lombardini, J, et al. "Taurine: retinal function." *Brain Res Brain Res Rev* 1991; 16(2):151–169.

Nakagawa, M, et al. "Antihypertensive effect of taurine on the salt-induced hypertension." *Adv Exp Med Biol* 1994; 359:197–206.

Paauw, J, et al. "Taurine supplementation at three different dosages and its effect on trauma patients." *Am J Clin Nutr* 1994; 60(2):203–206.

Redmond, H, et al. "Immunonutrition: the role of taurine." *Nutrition* 1998; 14(7-8):599–604.

Sahley, B. *Heal with Amino Acids and Nutrients.* San Antonio, TX: Pain and Stress Publications, 2000.

Zackheim, H, et al. "Taurine and psoriasis." *J Invest Dermatol* 1968; 50(23):277–230.

Threonine

Great Smokies Interpretative Studies. Asheville, NC: Great Smokies Diagnostic Laboratory.

Klatz, R. *The New Anti-Aging Revolution.* Laguna Beach, CA: Basic Health Publications, 2003.

Tryptophan

Great Smokies Interpretative Studies. Asheville, NC: Great Smokies Diagnostic Laboratory.

Klatz, R. *The New Anti-Aging Revolution*. Laguna Beach, CA: Basic Health Publications, 2003.

Sahley, B. *Heal with Amino Acids and Nutrients*. San Antonio, TX: Pain and Stress Publications, 2000.

Tyrosine

Great Smokies Interpretative Studies. Asheville, NC: Great Smokies Diagnostic Laboratory.

Klatz, R. *The New Anti-Aging Revolution*. Laguna Beach, CA: Basic Health Publications, 2003.

CHAPTER 5: HERBS

Werbach, M. *Botanical Influences on Illness*. Tarzana, CA: Third Line Press, Inc, 2000.

Aloe Vera

Chalaprawat, M, et al. "The hypoglycemic effects of aloe vera in Thai diabetic patients." *Jour Clin Epidemiol* 1997; 50(1):3S–45S.

Heggers, J, et al. "Beneficial effects of Aloe in wound healing." *Phytoher Res* 1993, 7:S48–52.

Klatz, R. *The New Anti-Aging Revolution*. Laguna Beach, CA: Basic Health Publications, 2003.

Quillin, P. *Beating Cancer With Nutrition*. Tulsa, OK: Nutrition Times Press, Inc, 2000.

Shelton, R, et al. "Aloe vera, its chemical and therapeutic properties." *Int Jour Dermatol* 1991; 30:679–683.

Syed, T, et al. "Management of psoriasis with Aloe vera extract in a hydrophilic cream: a placebo-controlled, double-blind study." *Trop Med Int Health* 1996; 1(4):505–559.

Werbach, M. *Botanical Influences on Illness*. Tarzana, CA: Third Line Press, Inc, 2000.

Yongchaiyudha, S, et al. "Antidiabetic activity of Aloe vera L. juice. Int clinical trial in new cases of diabetes mellitus." *Phytomed* 1996; 3(3):241–243.

Ashwagandha Root

Collins, J. *What's Your Menopause Type?* Roseville, CA: Prima Publishing, 2000.

Heller, L. *Applying the Essentials of Herbal Care*. Gig Harbor, WA: Institute of Functional Medicine, 1999.

Bilberry

Klatz, R. *The New Anti-Aging Revolution*. Laguna Beach, CA: Basic Health Publications, 2003.

Black Cohosh

Lieberman, S. "A review of the effectiveness of Cimicifuga racemosa (Black cohosh) for the symptoms of menopause." *Jour of Women's Health* 1998; 7:525–529.

Liske, E. "Therapeutic efficacy and safety of Cimicifuga racemosa for gynecological disorders." *Adv Ther* 1998; 15:45–53.

Miksicek, R. "Commonly occurring plant flavonoids have estrogenic activity." *Molecular Pharmacology* 1993; 44:37–43.

Murray, M. *The Healing Power of Herbs*. Rocklin, CA: Prima Publications, 1995.

Ulene, A. *Art Ulene's Complete Guide To Vitamins, Minerals, and Herbs*. New York, NY: Avery Publishing Group, 2000.

Werbach, M. *Botanical Influences on Illness*. Tarzana, CA: Third Line Press, Inc, 2000.

Cat's Claw

Quillin, P. *Beating Cancer With Nutrition*. Tulsa, OK: Nutrition Times Press, Inc, 2000.

Cayenne

Klatz, R. *The New Anti-Aging Revolution*. Laguna Beach, CA: Basic Health Publications, 2003.

Yoshioka, M, et al. "Effects of red pepper added to high-fat and high-carbohydrate meals on energy metabolism and substrate utilization in Japanese women." *Brit Jour Nutr* 1998; 80(6):503–510.

Chamomile

Sinatra, S. *Optimum Health*. New York, NY: The Lincoln-Bradley Publishing Group, 1996.

Echinacea

Dorn, M, et al. "Placebo-controlled, double-blind study of Echinaceae pallidae radix in upper respiratory tract infections." *Comp Ther Med* 1997; 3:40–42.

Klatz, R. *The New Anti-Aging Revolution*. Laguna Beach, CA: Basic Health Publications, 2003.

Werbach, M. *Botanical Influences on Illness.* Tarzana, CA: Third Line Press, Inc, 2000.

Evening Primrose Oil

Khoo, S, et al. "Evening primrose oil and treatment of premenstrual syndrome." *Med Jour of Australia* 1990; 153:189–192.

Ulene, A. *Dr. Art Ulene's Complete Guide To Vitamins, Minerals And Herbs.* New York, NY: Avery Publishing Group, 2000.

Garlic

Ackermann, R, et al. "Garlic shows promise for improving some cardiovascular risk factors." *Arch Inter Med* 2001; 151:813–824.

Crayhon, R. *Robert Crayhon's Nutrition Made Simple.* New York, NY: M. Evans and Company, 1994.

Jarrell, S, et al. "Effects of wild garlic (allium ursinum) on blood pressure in systolic hypertension." *J Amer Coll Nur* 1996; 15:532.

Klatz, R. *The New Anti-Aging Revolution.* Laguna Beach, CA: Basic Health Publications, 2003.

Lieberman, S. *The Real Vitamin and Mineral Book.* New York, NY: Avery Publishing Group, 1997.

McMahon, F, et al. "Can garlic lower blood pressure? A pilot study." *Pharmacotherapy* 1993; 13:406–407.

Orckhov, A, et al. "Effects of garlic on atherosclerosis." *Nutrition* 1997; 13:656–663.

Pedraza-Chaverri, J, et al. "Garlic prevents hypertension induced by chronic inhibition of nitric oxide synthesis." *Life Sci* 1998; 62:71–77.

Rountree, R. *Immunotics.* New York, NY: Berkley Publishing Group, 2000.

Sendl, A, et al. "Inhibition of cholesterol synthesis in vitro by extracts and isolated compounds prepared from garlic and wild garlic." *Atherosclerosis* 1992:94:79–86.

Silagy, C, et al. "A meta-analysis of the effect of garlic on blood pressure." *J Hypertens* 1994; 12:463–468.

Ginkgo

Akiba, S, et al. "Inhibitory effect of the leaf extract of ginkgo biloba on oxidative stress-induced platelet aggregation." *Biochem Mol Bio Int* 1998; 46(6):1243–1248.

Chang, H, et al. "Ginkgo biloba extract increases ocular blood flow velocity." *J Ocul Pharmacol Therapy* 1999; 15(3):233–240.

Haramski, N, et al. "Effects of natural antioxidant ginkgo biloba extract (EGB 761) on myocardial ischemia-reperfusion injury." *Free Radic Biol Med* 1994; 16(6):789–794.

Kleijnen, J, et al. "Ginkgo biloba for cerebral insufficiency." *Br J Clin Pharmacol* 1992; 34(4): 352–358.

LeBars, P, et al. "A placebo-controlled, double-blind, random trial of an extract of ginkgo biloba for dementia." *JAMA* 1997; 278:1327–1332.

Lebars, P, et al. "Ginkgo biloba for dementia." *JAMA* 1997; 278:1327–1332.

Meyer, B, et al. "A multi-center, double-blind, drug vs. placebo study of gingko biloba extract in the treatment of tinnitus." *Prese Med* 1986; 5:1562–1564.

Packer, L. *The Antioxidant Miracle.* New York, NY: John Wiley & Sons, Inc, 1999.

Sikora, R., et al. "Ginkgo biloba extract in the therapy of erectile dysfunction." *J Urol* 1989; 141:188A.

Ginseng

Collins, J. *What's Your Menopause Type?* Roseville, CA: Prima Publishing, 2000.

Klatz, R. *The New Anti-Aging Revolution.* Laguna Beach, CA: Basic Health Publications, 2003.

Goldenseal

Klatz, R. *The New Anti-Aging Revolution.* Laguna Beach, CA: Basic Health Publications, 2003.

Werbach, M. *Botanical Influences on Illness.* Tarzana, CA: Third Line Press, Inc, 2000.

Green Tea

Hibasami, H, et al. "Induction of apoptosis in human stomach cancer cells by green tea catechins." *Oncol Rep* 1998; 5(2):527–529.

Imai, K, et al. "Cancer-preventive effects of drinking green tea among a Japanese population." *Prev Med* 1997; 26(6):769–775.

Klatz, R. *The New Anti-Aging Revolution.* Laguna Beach, CA: Basic Health Publications, 2003.

Luo, M, et al. "Inhibition of LDL oxidation by green tea extract." *Lancet* 1997; 349:360–361.

Quillin, P. *Beating Cancer With Nutrition*. Tulsa, OK: Nutrition Times Press, Inc, 2000.

Werbach, M. *Botanical Influences on Illness*. Tarzana, CA: Third Line Press, Inc, 2000.

Hawthorne

Klatz, R. *The New Anti-Aging Revolution*. Laguna Beach, CA: Basic Health Publications, 2003.

Milk Thistle

Bokemeyer, C, et al. "Silibinin protects against cisplatin-induced nephrotoxicity without compromising cisplatin or iposfamide anti-tumor activity." *Br J Cancer* 1996; 74:2036–2041.

Dehmlow, C, et al. "Inhibition of Kepffer cell functions as an explanation for the hepatoprotene properties of silibinin." *Hepatology* 1996; 23(4):749–754.

Dehmlow, C, et al. "Scavenging of reactive oxygen species and inhibition of arachidonic acid metabolism by silibinin in human cells." *Life Sci* 1996; 58:1591–1600.

Leng-Peschlow, E, et al. "Properties and medical use of flavonolignans (silymarin) from silybum marianum." *Phytother Res* 1996; 10(Suppl):S24–S26.

Skuttowa, M, et al. "Activity of silymarin and its flavonolignans upon low density lipoproteins oxidizability in vitro." *Phytother Res* 1999; 12:535–537.

Skottowa, N, et al. "Silymarin as a potential hypocholesterolemic drug." *Physiol Res* 1998; 47:1–7.

Velussi, M, et al. "Long-term treatment with antioxidant drug (silymarin) is effective on hyperinsulinemia, exogenous insulin need and malondialdehyde in cirrhotic diabetic patients." *J Hepatol* 1997; 26(4):871–879.

St. John's Wort

Bennett, D, et al. "Neuropharmacology of St. John's wort (Hyericum)." *Ann Pharmacother* 1998; 32(11):1201–1208.

Chatterjee, S, et al. "Hyperforin as a possible antidepressant component of hypericum extracts." *Life Sci* 1998; 63(6):499–510.

Cott, J, et al. "In vitro receptor binding and enzyme inhibition by Hypericum perforatum extract." *Pharmacopsychiatry* 1997; 30:108–112.

Harrer, G, et al. "Treatment of mild/moderate depression with Hypericum." *Phytomedicine* 1994; 1:3–8.

Linde, K, et al. "St. John's wort for depression—an overview and meta-analysis of randomised clinical trials." *Brit Med Jour* 1996; 313:253–258.

Neary, J, et al. "Hypericum, LI 160 inhibits uptake of serotonin and norephinephrine in astrocytes." *Brain Res* 1999; 816(2):358–363.

Werbach, M. *Botanical Influences on Illness*. Tarzana, CA: Third Line Press, Inc, 2000.

Saw Palmetto

Collins, J. *What's Your Menopause Type?* Roseville, CA: Prima Publishing, 2000.

Klatz, R. *The New Anti-Aging Revolution*. Laguna Beach, CA: Basic Health Publications, 2003.

Vinpocetine

Ley, B, et al. *Boost Your Brain Power with Periwinkle Extract*. Detroit Lakes, MN: BL Publications, 2000.

Miyazaki, M, et al. "The effect of a cerebral vasodilator vinpocetine, on cerebral vascular resistance evaluated by the Doppler ultrasonic technique in patients with cerebrovascular diseases." *Angiology* 1995; 46(1):53–58.

Taiji, H, et al. "Clinical study of vinpocetine in the treatment of vertigo." *JPN Pharmacol Ter* 1986; 14:577.

Inset: Medicinal Herbs

Astragalus

Chen, K. "Certain progress in the treatment of coronary heart disease with traditional medicinal plants." *Amer Jour Chinese Med* 1981; 9:193–196.

Hou, Y, et al. "Effect of Radix Astragali Seu Hedysari on the interferon system." *Chin Med Jour* 1981; 94:35–40.

Kou, W, et al. "Validity of Oriental Medicines. 2. Hypotensive principle of Astragalus and Hedysarum Roots." *Planta Medica* 1976; 30:297.

Bacopa

Stough, C, et al. "The chronic effects of an extract of Bacopa monniera (Brahmi) on cognitive function in healthy human subjects." *Psychopharmacology* (Berl) 2001; 156(4):481–484.

Baikal Skullcap

Awad, A, et al. "In vitro and in vivo (SCID mice) effects of phytosterols on the growth and dissemination of human prostate cancer PC-3 cells." *Eur Jour Cancer Prev* 2001; 10(6): 507–513.

Awad, A, et al. "Phytoserols reduce in vitro metastatic ability of MDA-MB-231 human breast cancer cells." *Nutr Cancer* 2001; 440(2): 157–164.

Guilliams, T, et al. "Managing chronic inflammation: natural solutions." *The Standard* 2006; 7(2):1–8.

Beta-Sitosterol

Berges, R, et al. "Treatment of symptomatic benign prostate hyperplasia with beta-sitosterol: an 18-month follow-up." *British Jour Urol Inter* 2000; 85(7):842–846.

Glynn, R, et al. "The development of benign prostatic hyperplasia among volunteers in the Normative Aging Study." *Amer Jour Epidemiol* 1985; 121(1):78–90.

Klippel, K, et al. "A multicentric, placebo-controlled, double-blind clinical trial of beta-sitosterol (phytosterol) for the treatment of benign prostatic hyperplasia." *Brit Jour Urol* 1997; 80(3):427–432.

Boswellia

Ammon, H, et al. "Inhibition of leukotriene B4 formation in rat peritoneal neutrophils by an ethanolic extract of gum resin exudate of Boswellia serrata." *Planta Med* 1991; 57(3): 203–207.

Etzel, R. "Special extract of Boswellia serrata (H15) in the treatment of rheumatoid arthritis." *Phytomed* 1996; 3:91–4.

Gupta, I, et al. "Effects of Boswellia serrata gum resin in patients with bronchial asthma: results of a double-blind, placebo-controlled, 6-week clinical study." *Eur Jour Med Res* 1998; 3(11):511–514.

Gupta, I, et al. "Effects of Boswellia serrata gum resin in patients with chronic colitis." *Planta Med* 2001; 67(5):391–395.

Guilliams, T, et al. "Managing chronic inflammation: natural solutions." *The Standard* 2006; 7(2):1–8.

Kimmakar, N, et al. "Efficacy and tolerability of Boswellia serrata extract in treatment of osteoarthritis of knee—a randomized double-blind placebo-controlled trial." *Phytomedicine* 2003; 10(1):3–7.

Roy, S, et al. "Regulation of vascular responses to inflammation: inducible matrix metalloproteinase-3 expression in human microvascular endotheial cells is sensitive to antiinflammatory boswellia." *Antioxid Redox Signal* 2006; 8(3-4):653–660.

Safahy, H, et al. "Inhibition by boswellic acids of human leukocyte elastase." *Jour Pharmacol Exp Ther* 1997; 281(1):460–463.

Chamomile

Avallone, R, et al. "Pharmacologic profile of apigenin, a flavonoid isolated from Matricaria chamomilla." *Biochem Pharmacol* 2000; 59: 1387–1394.

Klatz, R. *The New Anti-Aging Revolution.* Laguna Beach, CA: Basic Health Publications, 2003.

Curcumin

Aggarwal, B, et al. "Anti-cancer potential of curcumin: preclinical and clinical studies." *Anticancer Res* 2003; 23 (1A):363–398.

Bengmark, D. "Curcumin, a atoxic antioxidant and natural NFkappa B, cyclooxygenase-2, lipoxygenase, and inducible nitric oxide synthase inhibitor: a shield against acute and chronic diseases." *Jour Parenter Enteral Nutr* 2006; 30(1):45–51.

Bundy, R, et al. "Tumeric extract may improve irritable bowel syndrome symptomology in otherwise healthy adults: a pilot study." *Jour Altern Complement Med* 2004; 10(6):1015–1018.

Guilliams, T, et al. "Managing chronic inflammation: natural solutions." *The Standard* 2006; 7(2):1–8.

Holt, P, et al. "Curcumin therapy in inflammatory bowel disease: a pilot study." *Dig Dis Sci* 2005; 50(11):2191–2193.

Ng, T, et al. "Curry consumption and cognitive function in the elderly." *Amer Jour Epidemiol* 2006; 164(9):898–906.

Parodi, F, et al. "Oral administration of difenuloylmethane (curcumin) suppresses proinflammatory cytokines and destructive connective tissue remodeling in experimental abdominal aortic aneurysms." *Ann Vasc Sur* 2006; 20(3):360–368.

Prucksunand, C, et al. "Phase II clinical trial on effect of the long turmeric (Curcuma longa Linn) on healing of peptic ulcer." *Southeast Asian Jour Trop Med Pubic Health* 2001; 32(1): 208–215.

Tuttle, D. "Protecting your DNA from Lethal Mutations." *Life Extension* Sept 2005, 30–32.

Fenugreek

Bordia, A, et al. "Effect of ginger (Zingiber officinale Rosc.) and fenugreek (Trigonella foenum graecum L.) on blood lipids, blood sugar and platelet aggregation in patients with coronary artery disease." *Prost Leuko EFA* 1997; 56:379–384.

Haefele, C, et al. "Characterization of a dioxygenase from Trigonella foenum graecum involved in 4-hydroxyisoleucine biosynthesis." *Phytochem* 1997; 44:563–566.

Kaczmar, T. "Herbal support for diabetes management." *Clin Nutr Insights* 1998; 6(8):1–4.

Sharma, R. "Effect of fenugreek seeds and leaves on blood glucose and serum insulin responses in human subjects." *Nutr Re* 1986; 6:1353–1364.

Feverfew

Johnson, E, et al. "Efficacy of feverfew as prophylactic treatment of migraine." *Brit Med Jour* 1985; 291:569.

Murphy, J, et al. "Randomized double-blind trial of feverfew in migraine prevention." *Lancet* 1988; 2:189.

Weiner, M. *Weiner's Herbal*. Mill Valley, CA: Quantum Books, 1990.

Gotu Kola

Allegra, C. "Comparative capillaroscopic study of certain bioflavonoids and total triterpenic fraction of centella asiatica in venous insufficiency." *Clin Therap* 1984; 110:555–559.

Bonnett, G. "Treatment of localized cellulitis with Asiaticoside madecassol." *Progr Med* 1974; 102:109–110.

Murray, M. *Encyclopedia of Natural Medicine*. New York, NY: Three Rivers Press, 1998.

Pointel, J, et al. "Titrated extract of Centella asiatica (TECA) in the treatment of venous insufficiency of the lower limbs." *Angiology* 1987; 38:46–50.

Tenailleau, A. "On 80 cases of cellulitis treated with the standard extract of centella asiatica." *Quest Med* 1978; 31:919–924.

Guggulipid

Nityanand, S, et al. "Clinical trial with gugulipid, a new hypolipidemic agent." *Jour Assoc Phys India* 1989; 37:321–328.

Rose, J, et al. "Herbal support for a healthy cardiovascular system." *Clinical Nutriton Insights* 1999; 6(16):1–6.

Satayavanti, G. "Gugulipid: a promising hypolipidaemic agent from gum gugul." *Econ Med Plant Res* 1991; 5:47–82.

Urizar, N, et al. "A natural product that lowers cholesterol as an antagonist ligand for FXR." *Science* 2002; 296(5573):1703–1706.

Gymnema Sylvestre

Baskaran, K, et al. "Antidiabetic effect of a leaf extract from Gymnema sylvestre in non-insulin dependent diabetes mellitus patients." *Jour Ethnopharmacol* 1990; 30:295–305.

Shanmugasundaram, E, et al. "Use of Gymnema sylvestre leaf extract in the control of blood sugar in insulin-dependent diabetes mellitus." *Jour Ethnopharmacol* 1990; 30:281–294.

Jujube

Klatz, R. *The New Anti-Aging Revolution*. Laguna Beach, CA: Basic Health Publications, 2003.

Licorice

Klatz, R. *The New Anti-Aging Revolution*. Laguna Beach, CA: Basic Health Publications, 2003.

Modern Sage

Blumenthal, M, et al. Eds. *The Complete German Commission E Monographs: Therapeutic Guide to Herbal Medicines*. Austin, Texas: American Botanical Society, 1998.

Witchl, M. *Herbal Drugs and Phytopharmaceuticals*. Boca Raton, FL: CRC Press, 1993.

Olive Leaf Extract

Klatz, R. *The New Anti-Aging Revolution*. Laguna Beach, CA: Basic Health Publications, 2003.

Passion Flower

Klatz, R. *The New Anti-Aging Revolution.* Laguna Beach, CA: Basic Health Publications, 2003.

Weiner, M. *Weiner's Herbal.* Mill Valley, CA: Quantum Books, 1990.

Perilla Seed Extract

Hsu, H, et al. *Oriental Materia Medica: A Concise Guide.* Long Beach, CA: Oriental Healing Arts Institute, 1986.

Ishihara, T, et al. "Inhibition of antigen-specific T helper type 2 responses by Perilla Frutescens extract." *Arerugi* 1999; 48(4):443–450 (article in Japanese).

Kimata, M, et al. "Effects of luteolin and other flavonoids on IgE mediated allergic reactions." *Planta Med* 2000; 66(1):25–29.

Makino, T, et al. "Effect of oral treatment of Perilla frutescens and its constituents on type-1 allergy in mice." *Biol Pharm Bull* 2001; 24(10):1206–1209.

Osakabe, N, et al. "Rosmarinic acid, a major polyphenolic component of Perilla frutescens, reduces lipopolysaccharide (LPS)-induced liver injury in D-galactosamine (D-GalN)-sensitized mice." *Free Radic Biol Med* 2002; 33(6):798–806.

Robak, J, et al. "Screening of the influence of flavonoids on lipoxygenase and cyclooxygenase activity, as well as on nonenzymic lipid oxidation." *Pol Jour Pharmacol Pharm* 1988; 40(5):451–458.

Shimoi, K, et al. "Radioprotective effect of antioxidative flavonoids in gamma-ray irradiated mice." *Carcinogenesis* 1994; 15(11):2669–2672.

Shin, T, et al. "Inhibitory effect of mast cell-mediated immediated-type allergic reactions in rats by Perilla frutescens." *Immunopharmacol Immunotoxicol* 2000; 22(3):489–500.

Ueda, H, et al. "Anti-inflammatory and anti-allergic actions by oral administration of a perilla leaf extract in mice." *Biosci Biotechnol Biochem* 2001; 65(7):1673–1675.

Ueda, H, et al. "Luteolin as an anti-inflammatory and anti-allergic constituent of Perilla frutescens." *Biol Pharm Bull* 2002; 25(9):1197–1202.

Yamamoto, H. "Anti-allergic effects of perilla seed extract in patients with allergy." *Food & Dev* 1997; 32(9):41–43 (article in Japanese).

Yamamoto, H, et al. "Inhibitors of arachidonate lipoxygenase from defatted perilla seed." *Jour of Food Chem* 1998; 46:862–865.

Rhodiola Rosea

Abidov, M, et al. "Extract of rhodiola rosea radix reduces the level of C-reactive protein and creatinine kinase in the blood." *Bull Exp Biol Med* 2004; 138(1):63–64.

Anon. "Rhodiola rosea." *Monograph. Altern Med Rev* 2002; 7(5):421–423.

Kelly, G. "Rhodiola rosea: a possible plant adaptogen." *Altern Med Rev* 2001; 6(3):293–302.

Perricone, N. *Dr. Pericone's 7 Secrets to Beauty, Health, and Longevity: The Miracle of Cellular Rejuvenation.* New York, NY: Ballantine Books, 2006.

Shevtsov, V, et al. "A randomized trial of two different doses of a SHR-5 Rhodiola rosea extract versus placebo and control of capacity for mental work." *Phytomedicine* 2003; 10(2–3):95–105.

Theanine

Ayoub, S, et al. "Introduction of neutral endopeptidase (NEP) activity of SK-N-SH cells by natural compounds from green tea." *Jour Pharm Pharmacol* 2006; 58(4):495–501.

Cooper, R, et al. "Medicinal benefits of green tea: Part 1. Review of noncancer health benefits." *Jour Alter Complement* Med 2005; 11(3):521–528.

Johnson, T. "Quick relief from anxiety and stress without tranquilizer drugs." *Life Extension* Aug 2007; 31–36.

Yamada, T, et al. "Effect of theanine, r-glutamylethylamide, on neurotransmitter release and its relationship with glutamic acid neurotransmission." *Nutr Neurosci* 2005; 8(4):219–226.

Yokogoshi, H, et al. "Effect of theanine, r-glutamylethylamide, on brain monoamines and striatal dopamine release in conscious rats." *Neurochem Res* 1998; 23(5):667–673.

Yokogoshi, H, et al. "Reduction effect of theanine on blood pressure and brain 5-hydroxyindoles in spontaneously hypertensive rats." *Biosci Biotechnol Biochem* 1995; 59(4):615–618.

Zheng, G, et al. "Anti-obesity effects of three

major components of green tea, catechins, caffeine and theanine in mice." *In Vivo* 2004; 18(1):55–62.

Valerian

Klatz, R. *The New Anti-Aging Revolution*. Laguna Beach, CA: Basic Health Publications, 2003.

CHAPTER 6: OTHER NUTRIENTS

Alpha-Glyceryl Phosphoryl Choline

De Jesus Moreno, M. "Cognitive improvement in mild to moderate Alzheimer's dementia after treatment with acetylcholine precursor choline alfoscerate: a multicenter, double-blind, randomized, placebo-controlled trial." *Clin Ther* 2003; 25(1):178–193.

Drago, F, et al. "Behavioral effects of L-alpha glycerylphosphorylcholeine: influence on cognitive mechanisms in the rat." *Pharmacol Biochem Behav* 1992; 41(2):445–448.

Mandat, T, et al. "Preliminary evaluation of risk and effectiveness of early choline alphoscerate treatment in craniocerebral injury." *Neurol Neurochir Pol* 2003; 37(6):1231–1238.

Alpha-Lipoic Acid

Berkson, B. *The Alpha Lipoic Acid Breakthrough*. Rocklin, CA: Prima Publishing, 1998.

Estrada, D, et al. "Stimulation of glucose uptake by the natural coenzyme alpha-lipoic acid/thiotic acid: participation of elements of the insulin signaling pathway." *Diabetes* 1996; 45(12):1798–1804.

Jacob, S, et al. "Enhancement of glucose disposal in patients with type 2 diabetes by alpha lipoic acid." *Arzneimittel-Forshung/Drug Research* 1995; 45:872–874.

Nagamatsu, M, et al. "Lipoic acid improves nerve blood flow, reduces oxidative stress and improves distal nerve conduction in experimental diabetic neuropathy." *Diabetes Care* 1995; 18:1160–1167.

Packer, L, et al. "Alpha-lipoic acid: a metabolic antioxidant which regulates NF-kappaB signal transduction and protects against oxidative injury." *Drug Metab Rev* 1998; 30(2):245–275.

Packer, L, et al. "Neuroprotection by the metabolic antioxidant alpha lipoic acid." *Free-radical Biology and Medicine* 1997; 22:359–378.

Packer, L. *The Antioxidant Miracle*. New York, NY: John Wiley & Sons, Inc, 1999.

Coenzyme Q$_{10}$

Burke, B, et al. "Randomized double-blind, placebo-controlled trial of coenzyme Q$_{10}$ in isolated systolic hypertension." *Southern Med J* 2001; 94(11):1112–1117.

Digiesi, V, et. al. "Effect of coenzyme Q$_{10}$ on essential hypertension." *Curr Ther Res* 1990; 47:841–845.

Hoffman-Bang, C, et al. "Coenzyme Q$_{10}$ as an adjunctive treatment of congestive heart failure." *Am J Cardiol* 1992; Supp 19(3):216A.

Langsjoen, P, et al. "Overview of the use of coenzyme Q$_{10}$ in cardiovascular disease." *Bio Factors* 1999; 9:273–284.

Mortensen, S, et al. "Dose-related decrease of serum coenzyme Q$_{10}$ during treatment with HMG-COA reductase inhibitors." *Mol Aspects of Med* 1997; 18(suppl):S137–144.

Morisco, C. "Effect of coenzyme Q$_{10}$ therapy in patients with congestive heart failure: a long-term multicenter, randomized trial." *Clin Investig* 1993; 71:S134–S136.

Perlmutter, D. "The Basic Science of Neurodegenerative Disease." *Brain Biochemistry and Nutrition*. Gig Harbor, WA: Institute of Functional Medicine, 2002.

Perlmutter, D. "The brain on fire: the role of inflammation in neurodegenerative disorders." A4M Conference, 2003.

Peruman, S, et al. "Combined efficacy of tamoxifen and coenzyme Q$_{10}$ on the status of lipid peroxidation and antioxidants in DMBA induced breast cancer." *Mol Cell Biochem* 2005; 273(1-2):151–160.

Richardson, M, et al. "Complementary/alternative medicine use in a comprehensive cancer cener and the implications for oncology." *Jour Clin Oncol* 2000; 18(13):2505–2514.

Rozen, T, et al. "Open trial of coenzyme Q$_{10}$ as a migraine preventive." *Cephalalgia* 2002; 22(2):137–141.

Sinatra, S. *The Coenzyme Q$_{10}$ Phenomenon*. New Canaan, CT: Keats Publishing Inc, 1998.

Sinatra, S. "Cutting edge technology in the prevention and treatment of cardiovascular disease: alternative interventions in treating cardiovascular disease." A4M Conference, Dec 2003.

Singh, R, et al. "Coenzyme Q$_{10}$ and its role in heart disease." *J Clin Biochem Nutr* 1999; 26: 109–118.

Singh, R, et al. "Effect of hydrosoluble coenzyme Q$_{10}$ on blood pressures and insulin resistance in hypertensive patients with coronary artery disease." *J Human Hypertension* 1999; 13(3):203–208.

Enzymes

Valerio, D, et al. "Clinical effectiveness of a pancreatic enzyme supplement." *Jour Parenter Enternal Nutr* 1981; 5:110–14.

Wright, J. *Why Stomach Acid Is Good For You.* New York, NY: M. Evans and Company, 2001.

Fiber

Burke, V, et al. "Dietary protein and soluble fiber reduce ambulatory blood pressure in treatment of hypertensives." *Hypertension* 2001; 38(4):821–826.

Houston, M. *What Your Doctor May Not Tell You About Hypertension.* New York, NY: Warner Books, Inc, 2003.

Rountree, R. *Immunotics.* New York, NY: Berkley Publishing Group, 2000.

Indole-3-Carbinol

Bradlow, H, et al. "Indole-3-carbinol. A novel approach to breast cancer prevention." *Ann NY Acad Sci* 1995; 768:180–200.

Chinni, S, et al. "Indole-3-carbinol (I3C) induced cell growth inhibition, GI cell cycle arrest and apoptosis in prostate cancer cells." *Oncogene* 20:2927–2936.

Michnovicz, J, et al. "Changes in levels of urinary metabolites after oral indole-3-carbinol in humans." *J Nat Cancer Inst* 1997; 89(10):718–723.

Michnovicz, J, et al. "Induction of estradiol metabolism by dietary indole-3-carbinol in humans." *J Nat Cancer Inst* 1990; 82:9470–9489.

Melatonin

Collins, J. *What's Your Menopause Type?* Roseville, CA: Prima Publishing, 2000.

Cos, S, et al. "Influence of melatonin on invasive and metastic properties of MCF-7 human breast cancer cells." *Cancer Res* 1998; 58(19): 4383–4390.

Poeggeler, B, et al. "Melatonin: A highly potent endogenous radical scavenger and e-donor: new aspects of the oxidation chemistry of this indole-accessed in vitro." *Ann NY Acad Sci* 1994; 738:419–421.

Ram, P, et al. "Estrogen receptor transactivation in MCF-7 breast cancer cells by melatonin and growth factors." *Mol Cell Endocrinol* 1998; 141(1-2):53–64.

Sharkey, K, et al. "Melatonin phase shifts human circadian rhythms in a placebo-controlled simulated night-work study." *Am J Physiol Regul Integr Comp Physiol* 2002; 282(2):R454–463.

Methylsulfonylmethane

Jacob, S. *The Miracle of MSM.* New York, NY: Penguin Putnam, 1999.

Oligomeric Proanthocyanidins

Halpern, M, et al. "Red wine polyphenols an inhibition of platelet aggregation: possible mechanisms and potential use in health promotions and disease preventions." *J Int Med Res* 1998; 26(4):171–180.

Klatz, R. *The New Anti-Aging Revolution.* Laguna Beach, CA: Basic Health Publications, 2003.

Noir, N, et al. "Grape seed extract activates Th1 cells in vitro." *Clin Diagn Lab Immunol* 2002; 9(2):470–476.

Preuss, H, et al. "Effects of niacin bound chromium and grape seed proanthocyanidin extract on the lipid profile of hypercholesterolemic subjects: a pilot study." *J Med* 2000; 31(5-6):227–246.

Sinatra, S. *Heart Sense For Women.* Washington, DC: LifeLine Press, 2000.

Phosphatidylcholine

Barbagallo, S. "Alpha-GPC in the mental recovery of cerebral ischemic attacks, an Italian multicenter clinical trial." *Ann NY Acad Sc* 1994; 717:253–269.

Kidd, P, et al. "Phosphatidylcholine: a superior protectant against liver damage." *Alt Med Rev* 1996; 1(4):258–274.

Little, A, et al. "A double-blind, Placebo controlled trial of high-dose lecithin in Alzheimer's disease." *J Neurol Neurosurg* 1985; 4 8(8):736–742.

Olszewsik, A, et al. "Reduction of plasma lipid and homocysteine levels by pyridoxine, folate, cobalamin, choline, riboflavin, and troxerutin in atherosclerosis." *Atherosclerosis* 1989; 5(1):1–6.

Phosphatidylserine

Amaducci, L, et al. "Phosphatidylserine in the dosing of Alzheimer's disease: results of a multi-center study." *Psychopharmacology Bulletin* 24:130–134.

Cenacchi, T, et al. "Cognitive decline in the elderly: a double-blind, placebo-controlled multicenter study on efficacy of phosphatidylserine administration." *Aging: Clinical and Experiment Res* 1993; 5:123–133.

Crook, T, et al. "Effects of phosphatidylserine in age-associated memory impairment." *Neurology* 1991; 4:644–649.

Crook, T, et al. "Effects of phosphatidylserine in Alzheimer's disease." *Psychopharmacology Bulletin* 1992; 28:61–66.

Engel, R, et al. "Double-blind cross-over, study of phosphatidylserine vs. placebo in subjects with early cognitive deterioration of the Alzheimer's type." *Europen Neuropsychopharmacology* 1992; 2:149–155.

Heiss, W, et al. "Long-term effects of phosphatidylserine, pyritinol, and cognitive training in Alzheimer's disease." *Cognitive Deterioration* 1994; 5:88–98.

Kidd, P. *Phosphatidylserine.* New Canaan, CT: Keats Publishing, Inc, 1998.

Monteleone, P, et al. "Blunting of chronic phosphatidylserine administration of the stress-induced activation of the hypothalamo-pituitary adrenal axis in healthy men." *Eur J of Clin Pharm* 1992; 41:385–388.

Monteleone, P, et al. "Effects of phosphatidylserine on the neuroendocrine response to physical stress in humans." *Neuroendocrinology* 1990; 52:243–248.

Schmidt, M. *Brain-Building Nutrition: The Healing Power of Fats and Oils.*

Berkeley, CA: Frog, Ltd, 2001.

Probiotics

Friend, B, et al. "Nutritional and therapeutic aspects of lactobacilli." *Jour Appl Nutr* 1984; 36:125–52.

Perdigon, G. et al. "Probiotic bacteria for humans: clinical systems for evaluaton of effectiveness. Immune system stimulation by probiotics." *Jour Dairy Sci* 1995; 78:1597–1606.

Inset: Other Nutrients

Chlorella

Klatz, R. *The New Anti-Aging Revolution.* Laguna Beach, CA: Basic Health Publications, 2003.

Chondroitin Sulfate

Baici, A, et al. "Analysis of glycosaminoglycans in human sera after oral administration of chondroitin sulfate." *Rheumatol Inter* 1992; 12:81–88.

Murray, M. *Encyclopedia of Natural Medicine.* New York, NY: Three Rivers Press, 1998.

Colostrum

Klatz, R. *The New Anti-Aging Revolution.* Laguna Beach, CA: Basic Health Publications, 2003.

Cordyceps

Rouse, J. "Herbal support for adrenal function." *Clinical Nutrition Insights* 1998; 6(9):1–2.

Glucosamine

Drovanti, A, et al. "Therapeutic activity of oral glucosamine sulfate in osteoarthrosis: a placebo-controlled double-blind investigation." *Clin Ther* 1980; 3:260–272.

Matheson, A, et al. "Glucosamine: a review of its use in the management of osteoarthritis." *Drugs & Aging* 2003; 20(14):1041–1060.

Muller-Fassbender, H, et al. "Glucosamine sulfate compared to ibuprofen in osteoarthritis of the knee." *Osteoarthritis Cartilage* 1994; 2:61–69.

Murray, M. *Encyclopedia of Natural Medicine.* New York, NY: Three Rivers Press, 1998.

Noack, W, et al. "Glucosamine sulfate in osteoarthritis of the knee." *Osteoarthritis Cartilage* 1994; 2:51–59.

Glycerophosphocholine (GCP)

Barbagallo, S, et al. "Alpha-Glycerophospho-choline in the mental recovery of cerebral is-chemic attacks. An Italian multicenter clinical trial." *Ann NY Acad Sci* 1994; 717:253–269.

Barclay, L. "Nutritional strategies to preserve memory and cognition." *Life Extension* Feb 2007; 59–60.

De Jesus Moreno, M. "Cognitive improvement in mild to moderate Alzheimer's dementia after treatment with the acetylcholine precursors choline alfoscerate: a multicenter, double-blind, randomized, placebo-controlled trial." *Clin Ther* 2003 25(1):178–193.

Parnetti, L, et al. "Choline alphoscerate in cognitive decline and in acute cerebrovascular disease: an analysis of published clinical data." *Mech Ageing Dev* 2001; 122(16):2041–2055.

Parnetti, L, et al. "Multicentre study of l-alpha-glyceryl-phosphorylcholine vs ST200 among patients with probable senile dementia of Alzheimer's type." *Drugs Aging* 1993; 3(2):159–164.

Vega, J, et al. "Nerve growth factor receptor immunoreactivity in the cerebellar cortex of aged rats: effect of choline alfoscerate treatment." *Mech Ageing Dev* 1993; 69(1-1):119–127.

Malic Acid

Osiecki, H. *The Nutrient Bible.* Australia: Bio Concepts Publishing, 2004.

Ornithine Alpha-Ketoglutarate (OKG)

Klatz, R. *The New Anti-Aging Revolution.* Laguna Beach, CA: Basic Health Publications, 2003.

Policosanol

Gouni-Berthold, I, et al. "Policosanol: cllinical pharmacology and therapeutic significance of a new lipid-lowering agent." *Amer Heart Jour* 2002; 143(2):356–365.

Reiner, Z, et al. "Effects of rice policosanol on serum lipoproteins, homocysteine, fibrinogen and c-reactive protein in hypercholesterolaemic patients." *Clin Drug Invest* 2005; 25(11):701–707.

Quercetin

Guilliams, T, et al. "Managing chronic inflam-mation: natural solutions." *The Standard* 2006; 7(2):1–8.

Hertog, M, et al. "Dietary antioxidant flavo-noids and risk of coronary heart disease: the Zutphen Elderly Study." *Lancet* 1993; 342:1007–1011.

Kandere-Grzybowska, K, et al. "Regulation of IL-1 induced selective IL-6 release from human mast cells and inhibition by quercetin." *Brit Jour Pharmacol* 2006; 148(2):208–215.

Kell, S, et al. "Dietary flavonoids, antioxidant vitamins, and incidence of stroke: the Zutphen study." *Arch Inter Med* 1996; 156(6):6637–6642.

Pignatelli, P, et al. "The flavonoids quercetin and catechin synergistically inhibit platelet function by antagonizing the intracellular pro-duction of hydrogen peroxide." *Amer Jour Clin Nutr* 2000; 72:1150–1155.

Sanhueza, J, et al. "Changes in the xanthine dehydrogenase/xanthine oxidase ratio in the rat kidney subjected to ischemia-reprefusion stress: preventive effect of some flavonoids." *Res Commun Chem Pathol Pharmacol* 1992; 78(2):211–218.

Red Yeast Rice

Eisenstein, M. *Unlocking Nature's Pharmacy.* New Jersey: CMI Press, 2006.

Heber, D, et al. "Cholesterol-lowering effects of a proprietary Chinese red-yeast-rice dietary supplement." *Amer Jour of Clin Nutr* 1999; 69(2):231–236.

Kelly, L, et al. "Complementary and alterna-tive medicine in cardiovscular disease: a re-view of biologically based approaches." *Amer Heart Jour* 2004; 147(3).

Yang, H, et al. "Acute administration of red yeast rice (Monascus purpureus) depletes tis-sue coenzyme q(10) levels in ICR mice." *Brit Jour of Nutr* 2005; 93(1):131–135.

Tea Tree Oil

Klatz, R. *The New Anti-Aging Revolution.* Laguna Beach, CA: Basic Health Publications, 2003.

Pycnogenol

Packer, L. *The Antioxidant Miracle.* New York, NY: John Wiley & Sons, Inc, 1999.

Resveratrol

Cal., C, et al. "Resveratrol and cancer: chemoprevention, apoptosis, and chemoimmuno sensitizing activities." *Curr Med Chem Anti Cancer* Agents 2003; 3:77–93.

Chanvitayapongs, S, et al. "Amelioration of oxidative stress by antioxidants and resveratrol in PC12 cells." *Neuro Report* 1997; 8:1499–1502.

Heller, L. "Healthy Women, Healthy Aging." Seminar, November 15–16, 2003.

Hiroyuki, N, et al. "Resveratrol inhibits human breast cancer cell growth and may mitigate the effect of linoleic acid, a potent breast cancer cell stimulator." *J Cancer Res Clin Oncol* 2001; 127:258–264.

Jang, J, et al. "Protective effect of reservatrol on beta-amyloid-induced oxidative PC12 cell death." *Free Radic Biol Med* 2003; 34:1100–1110.

Lu, R. "Resveratrol, a natural product derived from grape, exhibits antiestrogenic activity and inhibits the growth of human breast cancer cells." *J Cell Physiol* 1999; 179:297–304.

Mitchell, S, et al. "Resveratrol inhibits the express and function of the androgen receptor in LNcaP prostate cancer cells." *Cancer Res* 1999; 59:5892–5895.

Mitchell, T. "Resveratrol: Cutting-Edge Technology Available Today." *Life Extensions December* 2003 (Suppl).

Zbikowska, H, et al. "Antioxidants with carcinostatic activity (reseveratrol, vitamin E, and selenium) in modulation of platelet adhesion." *J Physiol Pharmacol* 2000; 51:513–520.

PART 2

Acne

Block, W, et al. "Modulation of inflammation and cytokine production by dietary (n-3) fatty acids." *J Nutr* 1996; 126:1515–1533.

Crayhon, R. *Designs For Health Institute's Eating and Supplement Plans.* Boulder, CO: Designs for Health Institute, 2000.

Grattan, C, et al. "Essential-fatty-acid metabolites in plasma phospholipids in patients with ichthyosis vulgaris, acne vulgaris and psoriasis." *Clin Exp Dermatol* 1990; 15(3):174–176.

Wright, S, et al. "Oral evening primrose seed oil improves atopic eczema." *Lancet* 1982; 2:1120.

ADD/ADHD

Bekaroglu, M, et al. "Relationships between serum free fatty acids and zinc, and ADHD: A research note." *J Child Psychol Psychiatry* 1996; 37:225–227.

Breggin, P. *Talking Back to Ritalin.* Monroe, Maine: Common Conrage Press, 1998.

Brenner, A, et al. "The effects of megadoses of selected B complex vitamins on children with hyperkinesis: controlled studies with long term followup." *J Learning Dis* 1982; 15:258.

Colquhoun, V, et al. "A lack of essential fatty acids as a possible cause of hyperactivity in children." *Med Hypotheses* 1981; 7:681.

Crayhon, R. *Designs For Health Institute's Eating and Supplement Plans.* Boulder, CO: Designs for Health Institute, 2000.

Kozielec, T, et al. "Assessment of magnesium levels in children with ADHD." *Magnes Res* 1997; 10:143–148.

Lyon, M. *Healing the Hyperactive Brain.* Calgary AB: Focused Publishing, 2000.

Sahley, B. *Control Hyperactivity, ADD Naturally.* San Antonio, TX: Pain and Stress Publications, 1999.

Sahley, B. *Is Ritalin Necessary?* San Antonio, TX: Pain and Stress Publications, 1999.

Starobrat-Hermelin, B, et al. "The effects of magnesium physiological supplementation on hyperactivity in children with ADHD. Positive response to magnesium oral loading test." *Magnes Res* 1997; 10:149–156.

Stevens, L, et al. "Essential fatty acids metabolism in boys with attention-deficit hyperactivity disorder." *Am J Clin Nutr* 1995; 62:761–768.

Stordy, B. *The LCP Solution.* New York, NY: Balantine Books, 2000.

Van Oudheusden, L, et al. "Efficacy of carnitine in the treatment of children with attention-deficit hyperactivity disorder." *Prostaglandins Leukot Essent Fatty Acids* 2002; 67(1):33.

Adrenal Fatigue and Exhaustion

Bland, J. *Nutritional Endocrinology: Breakthrough*

Approaches for Improving Adrenal and Thyroid Function. Gig Harbor, WA: The Institute for Functional Medicine, 2002.

Collins, J. *What's Your Menopause Type?* Roseville, CA: Prima Publishing, 2000.

Crayhon, R. "Aging well in the 21st century." Seminar, 2002.

Darbinyan, V, et al. "Rhodiola rosea in stress induced fatigue(a double-blind crossover study of a standardized extract SHR-J with a repeated low dose regimen on the mental performance of healthy physicians during night duty." *Phytomed* 2000; 7(5):365–371.

Fulder, S, et al. "Ginseng and the hypothalamic pituitary control of stress." *Am J Chinese Med* IX (2):112–118.

Gaffney, B, et al. "Panax ginseng and Eleutherococcus senticosus (Siberian ginseng) may exaggerate an already existing biphasic response to stress via inhibition of enzymes which limit the binding of stress hormones to their receptors." *Med Hypothesis* 2001; 56(5): 567–572.

Grandi, A, et al. "A comparative pharmacological investigation of ashwagandha and ginseng." *J Ethnopharmacol* 1994; 44:131–135.

Kelly, G, et al. "Nutritional and botanical interventions to assist with the adaption to stress." *Altern Med Rev* 1999; 4(4):249–265.

Rege, N, et al. "Adaptogenic properties of six Rasuyana herbs used in ayurvedic medicine." *Phytotherapy Res* 1999; 13:275–292.

Schmidt, M. *Tired of Being Tired.* Berkeley, CA: Frog, Ltd., 1995.

Tully, D, et al. "Modulation of steroid receptor-mediated gene expression by vitamin B_6." *FASEB J* 1994; 8:343–349.

Zhu, U, et al. "The scientific rediscovery of an ancient Chinese herbal medicine: cordyceps sinensis." *J Alt Comple Med* 1998; 4(3):289–203.

Alzheimer's Disease

Aisen, P, et al. "Inflammatory mechanisms in Alzheimer's disease: implications for therapy." *Am J Psychiatr* 1995; 151:1105–1113.

Birkmayer, J, et al. "Coenzyme nicotinamide adenine dinucleotide: new therapeutic approach for improving dementia of the Alzheimer type." *Ann Clin & Lab Sci* 1996; 26(1): 1–9.

Breitner, J, et al. "Inflammatory processes and anti-inflammatory drugs in Alzheimer's disease: a current appraisal." *Neurobiol Aging* 1996; 17(5):789–794.

Christen, Y, et al. "Oxidative stress and Alzheimer's disease." *Am J Clin Nutr* 2000; 71 (Suppl):621S–629S.

Clarke, R, et al. "Folate, vitamin B_{12}, and serum total homocysteine levels in confirmed Alzheimer's disease." *Arch Neurol* 1998; 55:1449–1455.

Conquer, J, et al. "Fatty acid analysis of blood plasma of patients with Alzheimer's disease, other types of dementia, and cognitive impairment." *Lipids* 2000; 35:1305A–1312.

Crook, T, et al. "Effects of phosphatidylserine in aged-associated memory impairment." *Neurology* 1991; 41(5):644–649.

Gottfries, C, et al. "Therapy options in Alzheimer's disease." *BJCP* 1994; 48(6):327–330.

Kalmijn, S, et al. "Fatty acid intake and the risk of dementia and cognitive decline: a review of clinical and epidemiological studies." *J Nutr Health Aging* 2000; 4(4):202–207.

Kyle, D, et al. "Low serum docosahexaenoic acid is a significant risk factor for Alzheimer's dementia." *Lipids* 1999; 34:S245.

Laszy, J, et al. "Comparison of cognitive enhancer activity of acetylcholinesterase inhibitors and vinopcetine." *Neurobiol of Aging* 2002; 23(1)Suppl 1:357.

LeBars, P, et al. "A placebo-controlled double-blind randomized trial of an extract of ginkgo biloba for dementia." *JAMA* 1997; 2789(6): 1327–1332.

Morris, M, et al. "Homocysteine and Alzheimer's disease." *Lancet Neurol* 2003; 2(7):425A–428.

Newman, P, et al. "Could diet be used to reduce the risk of developing Alzheimer's disease?" *Med Hypothesis* 1998; 50:335–337.

Nichols, T, et al. "Alpha-lipoic acid: biological effects and clinical implications." *Alt Med Rev* 1997; 2(3):177–183.

Nourhashemi, F, et al. "Alzheimer's disease:

protective factors." *Am J Clin Nutr* 2000; 71(Suppl):643S–649S.

Pettegrew, J, et al. "Clinical and neuro-chemical effects of acetyl-L-carnitine in Alzheimer's disease." *Neurobiol Aging* 1995; 16(1):1–4.

Salvioli, G, et al. "L-acetylcarnitine treatment of mental decline in the elderly." *Drugs Exp Clin Res* 1994; 20:169A–176.

Sano, M, et al. "A controlled trial of selegeline, alpha-tocopherol, or both as treatment for Alzheimer's disease." *NEJM* 1997; 336:1216A–1222.

Seshadri, S, "Plasma homocystine as a risk factor for dementia and Alzheimer's disease." *NEJM* 2002; 346:476–483.

Tenissen, C, et al. "Homocysteine: a marker for cognitive performance? A longitudinal follow-up study." *J Nutr Health Aging* 2003; 7(3): 153–159.

Thal, L, et al. "A one-year multicenter placebo-controlled study of acetyl-L-carnitine in patients with Alzheimer's disease." *Neurology* 1996; 4793):705–711.

Villardita, C, et al. "Multicenter clinical trial of brain phosphatidyl serine in elderly patients with intellectual deterioration." *Clin Trials J* 1987; 24:84–93.

Wang, H, et al. "Vitamin B_{12} and folate in relation to the development of Alzheimer's disease." *Neurology* 1991; 56:1188–1194.

Anorexia Nervosa

Ward, N, et al. "Assessment of zinc status and oral supplementation in anorexia nervosa." *J Nutr Med* 1990; 1:171–177.

Anxiety

Sahley, B. *Anxiety Epidemic*. San Antonio, TX: Pain and Stress Publications, 1999.

Gaby, A. *Nutritional Therapy in Medical Practice*. Carlisle, PA: Nutrition Seminars, 2003.

Arteriosclerosis

Crayhon, R. *Designs For Health Institute's Eating and Supplement Plans*. Boulder, CO: Designs for Health Institute, 2000.

Langsjoen, P, et al. "Overview of the use of coenzyme Q_{10} in cardiovascular disease." *Bio Factors* 1999; 9:273–284.

Nuttall, S, et al. "Antioxidant therapy for the prevention of cardiovascular disease." *Q J Med* 1999; 92:239–244.

Plotnick, G, et al. "Effect of antioxidant vitamins on the transient impairment of endothelium-dependent brachial artery vasoactivity following a single high-fat meal." *JAMA* 1997; 276(20):1682–1686.

Price, J, et al. "Antioxidant vitamins in the prevention of cardiovascular disease." *Eur Heart Jour* 1997; 18:719–727.

Reaven, P, et al. "Effect of dietary antioxidant combinations in humans." *Arterioscler Throm* 1993; 13:590–600.

Rinnium, E, et al. "Vitamin E consumption and the risk of coronary disease in men." *NEJM* 1993; 328:1450–1456.

Simon, J, et al. "Vitamin C and cardiovascular disease: a review." *J Am Coll Nutr* 1992; 11: 107–125.

Stampfer, M, et al. "Vitamin E consumption and the risk of coronary disease in women." *NEJM* 1997; 328:144–149.

Asthma

Britton, J, et al. "Dietary magnesium, lung function, wheezing, and airway hyperactivity in a random adult population sample." *Lancet* 1994; 344(8919):357–362.

Crayhon, R. *Designs For Health Institute's Eating and Supplement Plans*. Boulder, CO: Designs for Health Institute, 2000.

Greene, L, et al. "Asthma and oxidant stress: nutritional, environmental, and genetic risk factors." *J Am Coll Nutr* 1995; 14(4):317–324.

Hatch, G, et al. "Asthma, inhaled oxidants, and dietary antioxidants." *Am J Clin Nutr* 1995; 61(3 Suppl):625S–630S.

Kadrabova, J, et al. "Selenium status is decreased in patients with intrinsic asthma." *Biol Trac Elem Res* 1996; 52(3):241–248.

Villani, F, et al. "Effect of dietary supplementation with polyunsaturated fatty acids on bronchial hyperreactivity in subjects with seasonal asthma." *Respiration* 1998; 65(4):265–269.

Weiss, S, et al. "Diet as a risk factor for asthma." *Ciba Found Symp* 1997; 206:244–257.

Cancer

Ames, B, et al. "Are vitamins and mineral deficiencies a major cancer risk?" *Nat Rev Center* 2002; 2:694.

Bradlow, H, et al. "Multifunctional aspects of the action of vitamin C as an antitumor agent." *Ann NY Acad Sci* 1999; 869:204–213.

Clark, L, et al. "Decreased incidence of prostate cancer with selenium supplementation: results of a double-blind cancer prevention trial." *Br J Urol* 1998; 81:730–734.

Clark, L, et al. "Effects of selenium supplementation for cancer prevention in patients with carcinoma of the skin." *JAMA* 1996; 276(24):1957–1963.

Colgan, M. *The New Nutrition.* Vancouver, BC, Canada: Apple Publishing, 1995.

Cram, E, et al. "Indole-3-carbinol inhibits CDK6 expression in human MCF-7 breast cancer cells by disruption 5p1 transcription factor interactions with a composite element in the CDK6 gener promotor." *J Biol Chem* 2001; 22:276(25):2332–2334.

Crayhon, R. *Designs For Health Institute's Eating and Supplement Plans.* Boulder, CO: Designs for Health Institute, 2000.

Giovannucci, E, et al. "Folate, methionine, and alcohol intake and risk of colorectal adenoma." *J Natl Cancer Inst* 1993; 85:875–884.

Giovannucci, E, et al. "Intake of carotenoids and retinal in relation to risk of prostate cancer." *J Natl Cancer Instit* 1995; 87:1767–1776.

Giovannucci, E, et al. "MVI use, folate and colon cancer in women." *Ann Int Med* 1998; 129:517–524.

Heinonen, O, et al. "Prostate cancer and supplementation with alpha-tocophenols and beta-carotene: incidence and mortality in a controlled trial." *J Natl Cancer Inst* 1998; 90(6):4400–4046.

Kucuk, O. "Phase II randomized clinical trial of lycopene supplementation before radical prostatectomy." *Cancer Epidemiol Biomarkers Prev* 2001; 10(8):861–868.

Mason, J, et al. "Folate and colonic carcino-

genesis: searching for a mechanistic understanding." *J Nutr Biochem* 1994; 5:170–175.

Olson, KB, et al. "Vitamins A and E: further clues for prostate cancer prevention." *J Natl Cancer Inst* 1998; 90(6):414–415.

Overad, K. "Coenzyme Q_{10} in health and disease." *European J of Clin Nutr* 1999; 53(10):764–770.

Prasad, K, et al. "Vitamin E and cancer prevention: recent advances and future potentials." *J Am Coll Nutr* 1992; 11:487–500.

Recommendations for Cancer Prevention. American Institute for Cancer Research. Sept 2007. <http://www.aicr.org/site/PageServer?pagename=dc_home_guides>.

WCRF UK's Recommendations for Cancer Prevention. World Cancer Research Fund. Sept 2007. <http://www.wcrf-uk.org/research_science/recommendations.lasso>.

White, E, et al. "Relationship between vitamin and calcium supplement use and colon cancer." *Cancer Epidemiol Biomarkers Prev* 1997; 6:769–774.

Willett, W, et al. "Nutrition and cancer: summary of the evidence." *Cancer Causes and Control* 1996; 7:178–180.

Wong, G, et al. "Dose-ranging study of indole-3-C for breast cancer prevention." *J Cell Biochem* 1997; 28-29:111–116.

Xing, N, et al. "Quercein inhibits the expression and function of the androgen receptor in LCCaP prostate cancer cells." *Carcinogenesis* 2002; 22(3):409–414.

Candidiasis

Crayhon, R. *Designs For Health Institute's Eating and Supplement Plans.* Boulder, CO: Designs for Health Institute, 2000.

Schmidt, M. *Tired of Being Tired.* Berkeley, CA: Frog, Ltd, 1995.

Cataracts

Babizhayeo, M, et al. "Efficacy of n-acetyl carnosine in the treatment of cataracts." *Drugs Research and Development* 2002; 3(2):87–103.

Cumming, R, et al. "Diet and cataract: the blue

mountains eye study." *Opthal* 2000; 107(3): 4505–4506.

Giblin, F, et al. "Gluthione: a vital lens antioxidant." *J Ocul Pharmacol Ther* 2000; 16(2): 121–135.

Head, K, et al. "Natural therapies for ocular disorders part two: cataracts and glaucoma." *Alt Med Rev* 2001; 6:141–166.

Jacques, P, et al. "Long-term nutrient intake and early age-related nuclear lens opacities." *Arch Opath* 2001; 119(7):1009–1019.

Jacques, P, et al. "Long-term vitamin C supplement use: prevalence of early age-related lens opacities." *Am J Clin Nutr* 1997; 66: 911–916.

Mares-Perlman, J, et al. "Vitamin supplement use and incident cataracts in a population-based study." *Arc Opthal* 2000; 118(11):1556–1563.

Olmedila, B, et al. "Serum status of carotenoids and tocopherols in patients with age-related cataracts: a case-control study." *J Nutr Health Aging* 2002; 6(1):66–68.

"Preserving Clear Vision." *Life Extension* Feb 2003.

Quinn, P, et al. "Carosine: its properties, functions and potential therapeutic applications." *Mol Aspects Med* 1992; 13(5):379–444.

Robertson, J, et al. "A possible role for vitamins C and E in cataract prevention." *Am J Clin Nutr* 1991; 53:346S–351S.

Robertson, J, et al. "Vitamin E intake and risk of cataract in humans." *Ann NY Acad Sci* 1993; 372–382.

Taylor, A, et al. "Long-term intake of vitamins and carotenoids and odds of early age-related cortical posterior subcapsular lens opacities." *Am J Clin Nutr* 2002; 75(3):540–549.

Varma, S, et al. "Scientific basis for medial therapy of cataracts by antioxidants." *Am J Clin Nutr* 1991; 53:335S–345S.

Wang, A, et al. "Use of carnosine as a natural anti-senescence drug from human beings." *Biochem* 2000; 65(7)869–871.

Cervical Dysplasia

Werbach, M. "Cervical dysplasia." *Townsend Letter,* Nov 2006; 143–44.

Chronic Fatigue Syndrome

Abraham, G, et al. "Management of fibromyalgia: rationale for the use of magnesium and maleic acid." *J Nutr Med* 1991; 3:49–59.

Behan, P, et al. "Effect of high doses of essential fatty acids on the post viral fatigue syndrome." *ACTA Neurologic Scand* 1990; 87(3): 209–216.

Bralley, J, et al. "Treatment of chronic fatigue syndrome with specific amino acid supplementation." *J App Nutr* 1994; 46(3):74–78.

Crayhon, R. *Designs For Health Institute's Eating and Supplement Plans.* Boulder, CO: Designs for Health Institute, 2000.

Dalakas, M, et al. "Zidovadine-induced mitochondrial myopathy is associated with muscle carnitine deficiency and lipid storage." *Ann Neurol* 1994; 35(4):482–487.

Forsyth, L, et al. "Therapeutic effect of oral NADH on the symptoms of patients with chronic fatigue syndrome." *Ann Allergy Asthma Immunol* 1999; 82:185–191.

Hawkes, K. *Breakthroughs in Managing Chronic Pain & Fibromyalgia.* Gig Harbor, WA: Metagenics Educational Programs, 2002.

Juhl, J, et al. "Fibromyalgia and the serotonin pathway." *Altern Med Rev* 1998; 3:367–375.

Land, L, et al. "Antioxidative effective effective of ubiquinines on mitochondrial membranes." *Biochem J* 1984; 222:463–466.

Maddock, J, et al. "Biological properties of acetyl cysteine: assay development and pharmacokinetic studies." *Eur J Respir Dis* 1980; 61(Suppl 111):52–58.

Nies, K, et al. "Treatment of the fibromyalgia syndrome." *J Musculoskel Med* 1992; 9(5):20–26.

Packer, L, et al. "Alpha-lipoic acid as a biological antioxidant." *Free Rad Biol Med* 1995; 19(2):227–250.

Plioplys, A, et al. "Electron-microscopic investigation of muscle mitochondria in chronic fatigue syndrome." *Neuropsycholbiol* 1995; 32: 175–181.

Plioplys, A, et al. "Serum levels of carnitine in chronic fatigue syndrome: clinical correlates." *Neuropsycholbiol* 1995; 32:132–138

Rigden, S, et al. "Evaluation of the effect of a

modified entero-hepatic resuscitation program in chronic fatigue syndrome patients." *J Adv Med* 1998; 11(4):247–262.

Romano, T, et al. "Magnesium deficiency in fibromyalgia syndrome." *J Nutr Med* 1994; 4:165-67.

Closed Head Injury

Crayhon, R. "Nutritional Medicine Update." Seminar, 2003.

Congestive Heart Failure

Azuma, J, et al. "Double-blind randomized cross-over trial of taurine in congestive heart failure." *Curr Ther Res* 1983; 34(4):543–557.

Azuma, J, et al. "Therapeutic effect of taurine in congestive heart failure: A double-blind crossover trial." *Clin Cardiol* 1985; 8:276–282.

Cohen, N, et al. "Metabolic and clinical effects of oral magnesium supplementation in furosemide-treated patients with severe congestive heart failure." *Clin Cardiol* 2000; 23(6):433–436.

Dzugan, S. "Natural Approaches in the treatment of congestive heart failure." *Life Extension* 2003.

Fugh-Berman, A, et al. "Herbs and dietary supplements in the prevention and treatment of cardiovascular disease." *Prev Cardiol* 2000; 3(1):24–32.

Gaby, A. *Nutritional Therapy in Medical Practice.* Carlisle, PA: Nutrition Seminars, 2003.

Gavagan, T, et al. "Cardiovascular disease." *Prim Care* 2002; 29(2):323–338.

Langsjoen, P, et al. "Long-term efficacy and effects of coenzyme Q$_{10}$ therapy for idiopathic dilated cardomyopathy." *Am J Cardiol* 1990; 65:521–523.

Langsjoen, P, et al. "Pronounced increase of survival of patients with cardiomyopathy when treated with coenzyme Q$_{10}$ and conventional therapy." *Int J Tissu Reac* 1990; 12: 163–168.

Morelli, V, et al. "Alternative therapies: part II, congestive heart failure and hypercholesterolemia." *Am Fam Physician* 2000; 62(6):1325–1330.

Morisco, C, et al. "Effect of coenzyme Q$_{10}$ ther-apy in patients with congestive heart failure: a long-term multicenter randomized study." *Clin Invest* 1993; 71(8 Suppl):S134–S136.

Puccjarelli, G, et al. "The clinical and hemodynamic effects of propionyl-l-carnitine in the treatment of congestive heart failure." *Clin Ther* 1992; 141(11):379–384.

Schaffer, S, et al. "Interaction between the actions of taurine and angiotension II." *Amino Acids* 2000; 18(4):305–318.

Schmidt, U, et al. "Efficacy of the hawthorn (crataegus) preparation, LI 132 in 78 patients with chronic congestive heart failure defined as NYHA functional class II." *Phytomedicine* 1994; 1:17–24.

Sole, M, et al. "Conditioned nutritional requirements and the pathogenesis and treatment of myocardial failure." *Curr Opin Clin Nutr Metabolic Care* 2000; 3(6):417–424.

Tran, M, et al. "Role of coenzyme Q$_{10}$ in clinical heart failure, angina, systolic hypertension." *Pharmacotherapy* 2001; 7:797–806.

Crohn's Disease

Belluzzi, A, et al. "Effect of an enteric coated fish-oil preparation or relapses in Crohn's disease." *NEJM* 1996; 334(24):1557–1560.

Calder, P, et al. "N-3 polyunsaturated fatty acids and cytokine production in health and disease." *Ann Nutr Metab* 1997; 41(4):203–234.

Crayhon, R. *Designs For Health Institute's Eating and Supplement Plans.* Boulder, CO: Designs for Health Institute, 2000.

Fernandes, G, et al. "Dietary lipids and risk of autoimmune disease." *Clin Immunopathol* 1994; 72(2):193–197.

Goldin, B, et al. "Health benefits of probiotics." *Br J Nutr* 1998; 80(4):S203–S207.

Lukaczer, D. "Gastroenterology, part II: gastrointestinal disorders: clinical applications using the functional medicine perspective." *Applying Functional Medicine in Clinical Practice.* Gig Harbor, WA: Institute for Functional Medicine, 2002.

Robinson, D, et al. "Suppression of autoimmune disease by dietary n-3 fatty acids." *J Lipd Res* 1993; 34(8):1435–1444.

Souba, W, et al. "The role of glutamine in

maintaining a healthy gut and supporting the metabolic response to injury and infection." *J Surgical Res* 1990; 48:383–391.

Shoda, R, et al. "Therapeutic efficacy of n-3 polyunsaturated fatty acid in experimental Crohn's disease." *J Gastroenter* 1995; 30 (Suppl 8):98–101.

Depression

Birdsall, T, et al. "5-hydroxytrytophan: a clinically-effective serotonin precursor." *Alter Med Rev* 1998; 3(4):271–280.

Bottiglieri, T, et al. "Folate, vitamin B_{12}, and neuropsychiatric disorders." *Nut Rev* 1996; 54(12):383–390.

Copper, A, et al. "Enhancement of the antidepressant action of fluoxetine by folic acid: a randomized placebo controlled trial." *J Affective Dis* 2000; 60:121–130.

Crayhon, R. *Designs For Health Institute's Eating and Supplement Plans.* Boulder, CO: Designs for Health Institute, 2000.

Edwards, R, et al. "Omega-3 polyunsaturated fatty acids levels in the diet and RBC membranes of depressed patients." *J Affective Dis* 1998; 48:149–155.

Ernst, E, et al. "Adverse effects profile of the herbal antidepressant St. John's wort (Hypercium perforatum L)." *Eur J Clin Pharmacol* 1998; 54:589–594.

Galland, L. "Neuroendocrine imbalance in patient care." *Functional Medicine Approaches to Endocrine Disturbances of Aging.* Gig Harbor, WA: Institute of Functional Medicine, 2001.

Garzya, G, et al. "Evaluation of the effects of L-acetyl carnitine on senile patients suffering from depression." *Drugs Exp Clin Res* 1990; 16:101–106.

Hays, B. "Estrogen and depression." *Disorders of the Brain: Emerging Therapies in Complex Neurologic and Psychiatric Conditions.* Gig Harbor, WA: The Institute for Functional Medicine, 2002.

Hedaya, R. *The Antidepressant Survival Guide.* New York, NY: Three Rivers Press, 2000.

Linde, K, et al. "St John's wort for depression-an overview and meta-analysis of randomized clinical trials." *Br Med J* 1996; 313:253–258.

Maes, M, et al. "Lowered omega-3 polyunsaturated fatty acids in serum phospholipids and cholestreyl esters of depressed patients." *Psychiatry Res* 1999; 85:275–291.

Mehta, A, et al. "Pharmacologic effects of Withania somnifera root extract on GABA receptor complex." *Indian J Med Res* 1991; 94: 213–215.

Penninx, B, et al. "Vitamin B_{12} deficiency and depression in physically disabled older women: epidemiological evidence from the women's health and aging study." *Am J Psy* 2000; 157:715–721.

Sahley, B. *Anxiety Epidemic.* San Antonio, TX: Pain and Stress Publications, 1999.

Sakina, M, et al. "A psycho-neuropharmacological profile of centella asiatica extract." *Fitoterrpin* 1990; LXI(4):291–296.

Tempesta, E, et al. "L-acetylcarnitine in depressed elderly subjects. A cross-over study vs. placebo." *Drugs Exp Clin Res* 1987; 13:417–423.

Werbach, M. *Nutritional Influences on Mental Illness: A Sourcebook of Clinical Research.* Tarzana, CA: Third Line Press, Inc, 1991.

Diabetes Mellitus

Anderson, R, et al. "Beneficial effects of chromium for people with type II diabetes." *Diabetes* 1996; 45:124A.

Anderson, R, et al. "Elevated intakes of supplemental chromium improve glucose and insulin variables in individuals with type 2 diabetes." *Diabetes* 1997; 46(11):1786–1791.

Boden, G, et al. "Effects of vanadyl sulfate on carbohydrate and lipid metabolism in patients with non-insulin-dependent diabetes mellitus." *Metabol* 1996; 45(9):1130–1135.

Bustamante, J, et al. "Alpha-lipoic acid in liver metabolism and disease." *Free Rad Biol Med* 1998; 24(6):1023–1039.

Chausmer, A, et al. "Zinc, insulin and diabetes." *J Amer Coll Nutr* 1998; 17(2):109–115.

Crayhon, R. *Designs For Health Institute's Eating and Supplement Plans.* Boulder, CO: Designs for Health Institute, 2000.

Cunningham, J, et al. "Micronutrients as nutriceutical interventions in diabetes mellitus." *J Am Coll Nutr* 1998; 17(1):7–10.

Cunningham, J, et al. "The glucose/insulin system and vitamin C: implications in IDDM." *J Amer Coll Nutr* 1998; 17(2):105–108.

Demattia, G, et al. "Reduction of oxidative stress by oral n-acetyl-L-cysteine treatment decreases plasma soluble vascular cell adhesion molecule-1 concentrations in non-obese, non-diplipidaemic, normotensive patients with non-insulin dependent diabetes." *Diabetologia* 1998; 41:1392–1396.

Del Toma, E, et al. "Soluble and insoluble dietary fiber in diabetic diets." *Eur J Clin Nutr* 1988; 42:313–319.

Dominguy, L, et al. "Magnesium responsiveness to insulin and insulin-like growth factor I in erythrocytes from normotensive and hypertensive subjects." *J Clin Endocrinol Metab* 1998; 83:4402–4407.

Elamin, A, et al. "Magnesium and insulin-dependent diabetes mellitus." *Diab Res Clin Pract* 1990; 10:203–209.

Fantus, I, et al. "Multifunctional actions of vanadium compounds on insulin signaling pathways: evidence for preferential enhancement of metabolic versus mitogenic effects." *Mol Cell Biochem* 1998; 182(1-2):109–119.

French, R, et al. "Role of vanadium in nutrition: metabolism essentiality and dietary considerations." *Life Sciences* 1992; 52:339–346.

Galvan, A, et al. "Insulin decrease circulating vitamin E levels in humans." *Metabolism* 1996; 45(8):998–1003.

Gerbi, A, et al. "Neuroprotective effect of fish oil in diabetic neuropathy." *Lipids* 1999; 34(Suppl):93–94.

Horrobin, D, et al. "Essential fatty acids in the management of impaired nerve function in diabetes." *Diabetes* 1997; 46(Suppl2):S90–S93.

Jacob, S, et al. "Oral administration of RAC-alpha-lipoic modulates insulin sensitivity in patients with type-2 diabetes mellitus: a placebo-controlled pilot trial." *Free Radic Biol Med* 1999; 27(3-4):309–314.

Keen, H, et al. "Treatment of diabetic neuropathy with gama-linolenic acid." *Diabetes Care* 1993; 16(1):8–15.

Konrad, T, et al. "Alpha-lipoic acid treatment decreases serum lactate and pyruvate cones and improves glucose effectiveness in lean and obese patients with type 2 diabetes." *Diabetes Care* 1999; 22(2):280–287.

Leclere, CJ, et al. "Viscous guar gums lower glycemic responses after a solid meal: mode of action." *Am J Clin Nutr* 1994; 59(Supp):776S.

Lefebure, P, et al. "Improving the action of insulin." *Clin Invest Med* 1995; 18(4):340–347.

Linday, L, et al. "Trivalent chromium and the diabetes prevention program." *Med Hypothesis* 1997; 49:47–49.

Lukaczer, D. "Applied Endocrinology: Insulin Resistance and Chronic Disease." *Applying Functional Medicine in Clinical Practice*. Gig Harbor, WA: Institute for Functional Medicine, 2002.

Lukaczer, D. "Nutritional support for insulin resistance." *App Nutrit Sci Rep* 2001.

Luo, J, et al. "Dietary polyunsaturated (n-3) fatty acids improve adipocyte insulin action and glucose metabolism in insulin resistant rats: relation to membrane fatty acids." *J Nutr* 1996; 126:1951–1958.

Macbash, M, et al. "Therapeutic evaluation of the effect of biotin on hyperglycemia in patients with non-insulin dependent diabetes mellitus." *J Clin Biochem Nutr* 1993; 14:211–218.

MacDonald, H, et al. "Conjugated linolenic acid and disease prevention: a review of current knowledge." *J Am Col Nutr* 2000; 19(2):111S–118S.

Malone, J, et al. "Diabetic cardiomyopathy and carnitine deficiency." *J Diabetes Complications* 1999; 13(2):86–90.

McCarty, M, et al. "Complementary measures for promoting insulin sensitivity in skeletal muscle." *Med Hyotheses* 1998; 51:451–464.

Morcos, M, et al. "Effect of alpha-lipoic acid on the progress of endothelial cell damage and albuminura in patients with diabetes mellitus: an exploratory study." *Diabet Res Clin Pract* 2001; 52:175–183.

Okuda, Y, et al. "Long-term effects of eicosapentsenoic acid on diabetic peripheral neuropathy and serum lipids in patients with type II diabetes mellitus." *J Diab Comp* 1996; 10:280–287.

Pacifici, L, et al. "Counter action on experimentally induced diabetic neuropathy by levocarnitine acetyl." *Int J Clin Pharmacol Res* 1992; 12:231–236.

Packer, L. *The Antioxidant Miracle.* New York, NY: John Wiley & Sons, Inc, 1999.

Paolisso, G, et al. "Daily magnesium supplements improve glucose handling in elderly subjects." *Am J Clin Nutr* 1992; 55:1161–1167.

Paolisso, G, et al. "Pharmacologic doses of vitamin E improve insulin action in healthy subjects and non-insulin-dependent diabetic patients." *Am J Clin Nutr* 1993; 57:650–656.

Philipson, H, et al. "Dietary fiber in the diabetic diet." *ACTA Med Scand.* 1983; 671(Suppl):91–93.

Pieper, G, et al. "Oral administration of the antioxidant, n-acetyl cysteine, abrogates diabetes-induced endothelial dysfunction." *J Cardiovascular Pharmacol* 1998; 32:101–105.

Preuss, H, et al. "The insulin system: influence of antioxidants." *J Am Coll Nutr* 1998; 17(2): 101–102.

Quatraro, A, et al. "Acetyl-L-carnitine for symptomatic diabetic neuropathy." *Diabetologia* 1993; 38:123.

Reaven, P, et al. "Dietary and pharmacologic regimens to reduce lipid peroxidation in non-insulin-dependent diabetes mellitus." *Am Clin Nutr* 1995; 62:1483S–1489S.

Reaven, G, et al. "Pathophysiology of insulin resistance in human disease." *Physiological Reviews* 1995; 75(3):473–485.

Ripa, S, et al. "Zinc and diabetes mellitus." *Minerva Med* 1995; 86(10):415–421.

Saltiel, A, et al. "Thiazolidinediones in the treatment of insulin resistance and type II diabetes." *Diabetes* 1996; 45:1661–1669.

Salway, J, et al. "Effect of myo-onositol on peripheral-nerve function in diabetes." *Lancet* 1978; 282–1284.

Samiec, P, et al. "Glutathione in human plasma: decline in association with aging, age-related macular degeneration, and diabetes." *Free Rad Biol Med* 1998; 24(5):699–704.

Seelig, M, et al. "Consequences of magnesium deficiency on the enhancement of stress reactions: preventive and therapeutic implications: a review." *J Am Coll Nutr* 1994; 13(5):429–446.

Shamberger, R, et al. "The insulin-like effects of vanadium." *J Adv Med* 1996; 9(2):121–131.

Takahashi, R, et al. "Evening primrose oil and fish oil in non-insulin-dependant diabetes." *Prostaglandins Leulcot Essent Fatty Acids* 1993; 49(2):569–571.

Tatuncu, B, et al. "Reversal of defective nerve conduction with vitamin E supplementation in type II diabetics; a preliminary study." *Diabetes Care* 1998; 21:1915–1918.

Thompson, D, et al. "Micronutrients and antioxidants in the progression of diabetes." *Nutr Res* 1995; 15(9):1377–1410.

Verma, S, et al. "Nutritional factors that can favorably influence the glucose/insulin system: vanadium." *J Am Coll Nutr* 1998; 17(1):11–18.

Wascher, T, et al. "Effects of low-dose L-arginine in non-insulin diabetes mellitus: a potential role for nitric oxide." *Med Sci Res* 1993; 21:669–770.

Welinhinda, J, et al. "Effect of Momordica charantia on the glucose tolerance in maturity onset diabetes." *J Ethnopharmacol* 1986; 17:277–282.

Ziegler, D, et al. "Treatment of symptomatic diabetic peripheral neuropathy with the antioxidant alpha-lipoic acid. A 3-week multicenter randomized controlled trial (ALADIN study)." *Diabetologia* 1995; 38:1425–1433.

Dry Eyes

Rose, M, et al. *Save Your Sight.* New York, NY: Warner Books, 1998.

Eczema

Block, W, et al. "Modulation of inflammation and cytokine production by dietary (n-3) fatty acids." *Nutr* 1996; 126:1515–1533.

Crayhon, R. *Designs For Health Institute's Eating and Supplement Plans.* Boulder, CO: Designs for Health Institute, 2000.

Grattan, C, et al. "Essential-fatty-acid metabolites in plasma phospholipids in patients with ichthyosis vulgaris, acne vulgaris and psoriasis." *Clin Exp Dermatol* 1990; 15(3):174–176.

Wright, S, et al. "Oral evening primrose seed

oil improves atopic eczema." *Lancet* 1982; 2:1120.

Food Allergies

Chan, M, et al. "Effects of three dietary phytochemicals from tea, rosemary and turmeric on inflammation-induced nitrite production." *Cancer Lett* 1995; 96(1):23–29.

Crayhon, R. *Designs for Health Institute's Level II Eating and Supplement Plans.* Boulder CO: Designs for Health Institute, Inc, 1999.

Jakazawa, T, et al. "Metabolites of orally administered perilla frutescens extract in rats and humans." *Biol Pharm Bul* 2000; 23(1): 122–127.

Kodama, M, et al. "Autoimmune disease and allergy are controlled by vitamin C treatment." *In Vivio* 1994; 8(2):251–257.

Musonda, C, et al. "Quercetin inhibits hydrogen peroxide (H2O2)-induced NF-KappaB DNA binding activity and DNA damage in Hep G2 cells." *Carcinogensis* 1998; 19(9):1583–1589.

Packer, L, et al. "Alpha-lipoic acid as a biological antioxidant." *Free Rad Biol Med* 1995; 19(2): 227–250.

Sahley, B. *Anxiety Epidemic.* San Antonio, TX: Pain and Stress Publications, 1999.

Sahley, B. *Control Hyperactivity ADD Naturally.* San Antonio, TX: Pain and Stress Publications, 1999.

Sult, T, et al. "Th1/Th2 balances: a natural therapeutic approach to Th2 polarization in allergy." *Applied Nutritional Science Reports* 2003.

Tate, G, et al. "Suppression of acute and chronic inflammation by dietary gamma linolenic acid." *J Rheumatol* 1989; 16(6):729–734.

Gall Bladder Disorders

"Understanding Fatigue: Addressing the Molecular Basis of Chronic Metabolic Disorders." ACE Seminar, 2001.

Gout

Shen, F, et al. "Inhibition of xanthine oxidase by purpurogallin and silymarin group." *Anticancer Res* 1998; 18(1A):263–267.

Hair Loss

Kobren, S. *The Truth About Women's Hair Loss.* Chicago, IL: Contemporary Books, 2000.

Hashimoto's Thyroiditis

Calder, P, et al. "N-3 polyunsaturated fatty acids and cytokine production in health and disease." *Ann Nutr Metab* 1997; 41(4):203–234.

Crayhon, R. *Designs For Health Institute's Eating and Supplement Plans.* Boulder, CO: Designs for Health Institute, 2000.

Fernandes, G, et al. "Dietary lipids and risk of autoimmune disease." *Clin Immunopathol* 1994; 72(2):193–197.

Robinson, D, et al. "Suppression of autoimmune disease by dietary n-3 fatty acids." *J Lipd Res* 1993; 34(8):1435–1444.

Hepatitis C

Crayhon, R. *Designs for Health Institute's Level II Eating and Supplement Plans.* Boulder CO: Designs for Health Institute, Inc, 1999.

Luper, S, et al. "A review of plants used in the treatment of liver disease: part I." *Alt Med Rev* 1998; 3(6):410–421.

Niederau, C, et al. "Polyunsaturated phosphatidyl choline and interferon alpha for treatment of chronic hepatitis B and C: a multicenter, randomized, double-blind, placebo-controlled trial, Leich Study Group." *Hepatogastroenterology* 1998; 45(21):797–804

Packer, L. *The Antioxidant Miracle.* New York, NY: John Wiley & Sons, Inc, 1999.

Stern, E, et al. "Two cases of hepatitis C treated with herbs and supplements." *J Alt Complemet Med* 1997; 3(1):77–82.

High Blood Pressure (Hypertension)

Appel, L, et al. "Does supplementation with fish oil reduce blood pressure? A meta-analysis of controlled clinical trials." *Arch Int Med* 1993; 153:1429–1438.

Borrello, G, et al. "The effects of magnesium oxide on mild essential hypertension and quality of life." *Curr Ther Res* 1996; 57:767–774.

Braverman, E. *Hypertension and Nutrition.* New Canaan, CT: Keats Publishing, Inc, 1996.

Colin, P, et al. "Effect of dietary patterns on

blood pressure control in hypertensive patients: results from the dietary approaches to stop hypertension (DASH) trial." *Am J Hypertens* 2000; 13:949–955.

Digiesi, V, et al. "Coenzyme Q$_{10}$ in essential hypertension." *Mol Aspects Med* 1994; 15(Suppl):S257–S263.

Duffy, S, et al. "Treatment of hypertension with ascorbic acid." *Lancet* 1999; 356:2048–2050.

Houston, M. "The role of vascular biology, nutrition and nutraceuticals in the prevention and treatment of hypertension." *The Heart on Fire: Modifiable Factors Beyond Cholesterol.* Gig Harbor, WA: Institute of Functional Medicine, 2003.

Houston, M. *What Your Doctor May Not Tell You About Hypertension.* New York, NY: Warner Books, Inc., 2003.

Levison, P, et al. "Effects of n-3 fatty acids in essential hypertension." *Am J Hypertens* 1990; 3:754–760.

Ortiz, M, et al. "Antioxidants block angiotensin II-induced increase in blood pressure and endothelin." *Hyptertension* 2001; 38(3 pt. 2):655–659.

Sacks, F, et al. "Effects on blood pressure of reduced dietary sodium and the dietary approaches to stop hypertension (DASH) diet." *NEJM* 2001; 344(1):3–9.

Sigh, R, et al. "Effects of hydrosoluble coenzyme Q$_{10}$ on blood pressures and insulin resistance in hypertensive patients with coronary artery disease." *J Human Hyper* 1999; 13:203–208.

Silagy, C, et al. "A meta-analysis of the effect of garlic on blood pressure." *J Hyperten* 1994; 12:463–468.

Sinatra, S. "Cutting edge technology in the prevention and treatment of cardiovascular disease: alternative interventions in treating cardiovascular disease." A4M Conference, 2003.

Sinatra, S. *Lower Your Blood Pressure in Eight Weeks.* New York, NY: Ballantine Books, 2003.

Stevens, V, et al. "Long-term weight loss and change in blood pressure results of the trials of hypertension prevention, phase II." *Ann Int Med* 2001; 34:1–11.

Vollmer, V, et al. "Effects of diet and sodium intake on blood pressure: subgroup analysis of the DASH-sodium trial." *Ann Int Med* 2001; 135:1019–1028.

Witteman, J, et al. "Reduction of blood pressure with oral magnesium supplementation in woman with mild to moderate hypertension." *Am J Clin Nutr* 1994; 60:129–135.

High Cholesterol

Adler, A, et al. "Effect of garlic and fish oil supplementation on serum lipid and lipoprotein concentration in hypercholesterolemic men." *Ann J Clin Nutr* 1997; 65:445–450.

Alcocer, L, et al. "A comparative study of policosanol versus acipimox in patients with type II hypercholesterolemia." *Int J Tissue React* 1999; XX(3):85–92.

Anderson, J, et al. "High-fiber diets for diabetic and hypertriglyceridemic patients." *Can Med Assoc J* 1980; 123:975.

Anderson, J, et al. "Oat-bran cereal lowers serum total and LDL cholesterol in hypercholesterolemic men." *Am J Clin Nutr* 1990; 52:495–499.

Arruzazabala, M, et al. "Comparative study of policosanol, aspirin, and the combination therapy of policosanol-aspirin on platelet aggregation in healthy volunteers." *Pharmacological Res* 1997; 36(4):293–297.

Avogaro, P, et al. "Effect of pantethine on lipids, lipoproteins and apolipoproteins in man." *Curr Ther Res* 1983; 33:488.

Braverman, E. *Hypertension and Nutrition* New Canaan, CT: Keats Publishing, Inc. 1996.

Castano, G, et al. "A long-term study of policosanol in the treatment of intermittent claudication." *Angiology* 2001; 52:115–125.

Castano, G, et al. "Comparisons of the efficacy and tolerability of policosanol with atorvastatin in elderly patients with type II hypercholesterolemia." *Drugs Aging* 2003; 20(2): 153–163.

Castano, G, et al. "Effects of policosanol and pravastatin in lipid profile, platelet aggregation and endothelemia in older hypercholesterolemic patients." *Int J Clin Pharm Res* 1999; 19:105–116.

Castano, G, et al. "Effects of policosanol on

older patients with hypertension and type II hypercholesterolemia." *Drugs in R&D* 2002; 3(3):402–408.

Castano, G, et al. "Effects of policosanol on postmenopausal women with type II hypercholesterolemia." *Gynecol Endocrinol* 2000; 14(3): 187–195.

Castano, G, et al. "Effects of policosanol treatment on the susceptibility of low density lipoprotein (LDL) isolated from healthy volunteers to oxidative modification in vitro." *Br J Clin Pharmacol* 2000; 50(3):255–262.

Colgan, M. *The New Nutrition.* Vancouver, BC, Canada: Apple Publishing, 1995.

Crayhon, R. "Aging well in the 21st century." Seminar, 2002.

Crespo, E, et al. "Comparative study of the efficacy and tolerability of policosanol and lovastatin in patients with hypercholesterolemia and noninsulin-dependent diabetes mellitus." *Int Jour Clin Pharm Res* 1999; 19:117–127.

Davis, W, et al. "Monotherapy with magnesium increases abnormally low high density lipoprotein cholesterol: a clinical assay." *Curr Ther Res* 1984; 36:341–346.

Gaby, A. *Nutritional Therapy in Medical Practice.* Carlisle, PA: Nutrition Seminars, 2003.

Gaddi, A, et al. "Controlled evaluation of pantethine, a natural hyplipidemic compound, in patients with different forms of hyperlipoproteinemia." *Atherosclerosis* 1984; 50:73.

Galeone, F, et al. "The lipid-lowering effect of panthethine in hyperlipidemic patients: a clinical investigation." *Curr Ther Res* 1983; 34:383.

Gittleman, A. *Super Nutrition for Menopause.* New York, NY: Avery Publishing Group, 1998.

Head, K, et al, "Inositol hexaniacinate a safer alternative to niacin." *Alt Med Rev* 1996; 1(3):176–184.

Heber, D, et al. "Cholesterol-lowering effects of a proprietary Chinese red-yeast-rice dietary supplement." *Am J Clin Nutr* 1999; 69:231–236.

Jain, S, et al. "Effect of modest vitamin E supplementation on blood glycated hemoglobin and triglyceride levels and red cell indices in Type I diabetic patients." *J Am Coll Nutr* 1996; 15(5):458–461.

Maebashi, M, et al. "Lipid-lowering effect of carnitine in patients with type IV hyperlipoproteinemia." *Lancet* 1978; 805–808.

Maggi, G, et al. "Pantethine: a physiological lipomodulating agent, in the treatment of hyperlipidemias." *Curr Ther Res* 1982; 32:380.

Maioli, M, et al. "Effect of pantethine on the subfractions of HDL in dyslipemic patients." *Curr Ther Res* 1984; 35:307.

Mas, R, et al. "Effects of policosanol in patients with type II hypercholesterolemia and additional coronary risk factors." *Clin Pharmacol Ther* 1999; 65:439–447.

Menendez, R, et al. "Policosanol modulates HMG-Co-A reducatase activity in cultured fibroblasts." *Archives Med Res* 2001; 32:8–12.

Nityanand, S, et al. "Clinical trials with gugulipid. A new hypolipidaemic agent." *Econ Med Plant Res* 1991; 5:47–82.

Ornish, D, et al. "Can lifestyle changes reverse coronary heart disease?" *Lancet* 1990; 336: 129–133.

Ortensi, E, et al. "A comparative study of policosanol versus simvastatin in elderly patients with hypercholesterolemia." *Curr Ther Res* 1997; 58:390–401.

Pola, P, et al. "Statistical evaluation of long-term L-carnitine therapy I hyperlipoproteinaemias." *Drugs Expti Clin Res* 1983; 9:925–934.

Press, R, et al. "The effect of chromium picolinate on serum cholesterol and apolipoprotein fractions in human subjects." *West J Med* 1990; 152:41–45.

Qureshi, A, et al. "Novel tocotrienols of rice bran modulate cardiovascular disease risk parameters of hypercholesterolemic humans." *Nutritional Biochem* 1997; 8:290–298.

Satyavati, G, et al. "Guggulipid: A promising hypolipidemic agent from gum guggul (Commiphora)." *Econ Med Plant Res* 1991; 5:47–80.

Singh, K, et al. "Guggulsterone, a potent hypolipidaemic, prevents oxidation of low density lipoprotein." *Phytother Res* 1997; 11: 291–294.

Singh, R, et al. "Hypolipidemic and antioxidant effects of Commiphora mukul as an adjunct to dietary therapy in patients with hypercholesterolemia." *Cardiovas Drugs Ther* 1994; 8(4):659–664.

Sprecher, D, et al. "Efficacy of psyllium in reducing serum cholesterol levels I hypercholesterolemic patients o high-or low-fat diets." *Ann Int Med* 1993; 119:545–554.

Tomeo, A, et al. "Antioxidant effects of tocotrienols in patients with hyperlipidemia and carotid stenosis." *Lipids* 1995; 12:1179–1183.

Urberg, M, et al. "Hypocholesterolemic effects of nicotinic acid and chromium supplementation." *J Family Pract* 1988; 27:603–606.

Verma, S, et al. "Effect of Commiphora mukul (gum guggulu) in patients with hyperlipidemia with special reference to HDL cholesterol." *Indian J Med Res* 1988; 87:356–360.

Warshafsky, E, et al. "Effect of garlic on total serum cholesterol." *Ann Int Med* 1993; 119: 599–605.

Wolever, T, et al. "Psyllium reduces blood lipids in men and women with hyperlipidemia." *Am J Med Sci* 1994; 307:269–273.

Hypothyroidism

Aihara, K, et al. "Zinc, copper, manganese, and selenium metabolism in thyroid disease." *Am J Clin Nutr* 1984:40(1):26–35.

Berry, M, et al. "The role of selenium in thyroid hormone action." *Endocrine Rev* 1992; 13:207–220.

Brownstein, D. *Overcoming Thyroid Disorders.* West Bloomfield, MI: Medical Alternatives Press, 2002.

Crayhon, R. *Designs For Health Institute's Eating and Supplement Plans.* Boulder, CO: Designs for Health Institute, 2000.

Divi, R, et al. "Anti-thyroid isoflavones from soybean: isolation, characterization, and mechanism of action." *Biochem Pharmacol* 1997; 54:10, 1087–1096.

Kohrle, J, et al. "The deiodinase family: selenoenzymes regulating thyroid hormone availability and action." *Cell Mol Life Sci* 2000; 57:1853–1863.

Maebashi, M, et al. "Urinary excretion of carnitine in patients with hyperthyroidism and hypothyroidism: augmentation by thyroid hormone." *Metabolism* 1977; 26(4):351–356.

Mano, T, et al. "Vitamin E and coenzyme Q_{10} concentrations in the thyroid tissues of patients with various thyroid disorders." *Am J Med Sci* 1998; 315(4):230–232.

Meinhold, H, et al. "Effects of selenium and iodine deficiency on iodothyronine diodinases in brain thyroid and peripheral tissue." *JAMA* 1992; 19:8–12.

Nishiyama, S, et al. "Zinc supplementation alters thyroid hormone metabolism in disabled patients with zinc deficiency." *J Am Coll Nutr* 1994; 13:62–67.

Pansini, F, et al. "Effect of the hormonal contraception on serum reverse triiodothyronine levels." *Gynecol Obstet Invest* 1987; 23:133.

Rachman, B. "Managing endocrine imbalance; autoimmune-induced thyroidopathy and chronic fatigue syndrome." *Functional Medicine Approaches to Endocrine Disturbances of Aging.* Gig Harbor, WA: Institute For Functional Medicine, 2001.

Rouzier, N. "Thyroid replacement therapy." Longevity and Preventive Medicine Symposium, 2002.

Shames, R. *Thyroid Power: 10 Steps to Total Health.* New York, NY: HarperResource, 2001.

Smith, P. *HRT: The Answers.* Traverse City, MI: Healthy Living Books, 2003.

Vliet, E. *Women, Weight and Hormones.* New York, NY: M. Evans and Company, 2001.

Inflammation

Rountree, R. "Immune Dysfunction and Inflammation, Part II." *Applying Functional Medicine I Clinical Practice.* Gig Harbor, WA: Institute for Functional Medicine, 2002.

Insomnia

Chesson, A, et al. "Current trends in the management of insomnia." *Emergency Med* April 2002.

Edling, C, et al. "Occupational exposure to organic solvents as a cause of sleep apnea." *Br J Indust Med* 1993; 50:276–279.

Garfinkel, D, et al. "Improvement of sleep quality in elderly people by controlled-release melatonin." *Lancet* 1995; 346(8974):541–544.

Goldman, R. *Sleep: Essential for Optimal Health.*

Chicago, IL: American Academy of Anti-Aging Physicians, 2003.

Haimov, I, et al. "Melatonin replacement therapy of elderly insomniacs." *Sleep* 1995; 18(7): 598–603.

Hornyak, M, et al. "Magnesium therapy for periodic leg movements-related insomnia and restless legs syndrome: an open pilot study." *Sleep* 1998; 21:501–505.

James, S, et al. "Melatonin administration in insomnia." *Neuropsychopharm* 1990; 3(1):19–23.

Pastora, J, et al. "Flavonoids from lemon balm (Melissa officinalis L, Lamiaceae)." *Acta Pol Pharm* 2002; 59(2):139–143.

Schmidt, M. *Tired of Being Tired*. Berkeley, CA: Frog, Ltd, 1995.

Speroni, E, et al. "Neuropharmacologicial activity of extracts from Passiflora incarnate." *Planta Med* 1988; 488–491.

Steiger, A, et al. "Effects of hormones on sleep." *Horm Res* 1998; 49(3-4):125–130.

Irritable Bowel Syndrome (IBS)

Belluzzi, A, et al. "Effect of an enteric coated fish-oil preparation or relapses in Crohn's disease." *NEJM* 1996; 334(24):1557–1560.

Crayhon, R. *Designs For Health Institute's Eating and Supplement Plans*. Boulder, CO: Designs for Health Institute, 2000.

Gupta, Il, et al. "Effects of Boswellia serrata gum resin in patients with ulcerative colitis." *Eur J Med Res* 1997; 2(1):37–43.

Liu, J, et al. "Enteric-coated peppermint-oil capsules in the treatment of irritable bowel syndrome: a prospective, randomized trial." *J Gastroenterol* 1997; 32(6):765–768.

Nobaek, S, et al. "Alteration of intestinal microflora is associated with reduction in abdominal bloating and pain in patients with IBS." *Am J Gastroenterol* 2000; 95(5):1231–1238.

Salomon, P, et al. "Treatment of ulcerative colitis with fish oil n-3-omega-fatty acid: an open trial." *J Clin Gastro* 1990; 12(2):157–161.

Schmidt, M. *Tired of Being Tired*. Berkeley, CA: Frog, Ltd, 1995.

Shoda, R, et al. "Therapeutic efficacy of n-3 polyunsaturated fatty acid in experimental Crohn's disease." *J Gastroenter* 1995; 30 (Suppl 8):98A–101.

Stenson, W, et al. "Dietary supplementation with fish oil in ulcerative colitis." *Ann Int Med* 1992; 116(8):607–614.

Leaky Gut Syndrome

Goldin, B, et al. "Health benefits of probiotics." *Br J Nutr* 1998; 80(4):S203–S207.

Lukaczer, D. "Gastroenterology, part II: gastrointestinal disorders: clinical applications using the functional medicine perspective." *Applying Functional Medicine in Clinical Practice*. Gig Harbor, WA: Institute for Functional Medicine, 2002.

Souba, W, et al. "The role of glutamine in maintaining a healthy gut and supporting the metabolic response to injury and infection." *J Surgical Res* 1990; 48:383–391.

Leg Cramps

Braverman, E. *Hypertension and Nutrition*. New Canaan, CT: Keats Publishing, Inc, 1996.

Lupus

Calder, P, et al. "N-3 polyunsaturated fatty acids and cytokine production in health and disease." *Ann Nutr Metab* 1997; 41(4):203–234.

Crayhon, R. *Designs For Health Institute's Eating and Supplement Plans*. Boulder, CO: Designs for Health Institute, 2000.

Fernandes, G, et al. "Dietary lipids and risk of autoimmune disease." *Clin Immunopathol* 1994; 72(2):193–197.

Robinson, D, et al. "Suppression of autoimmune disease by dietary n-3 fatty acids." *J Lipd Res* 1993; 34(8):1435–1444.

Macular Degeneration

Crayhon, R. "Aging well in the 21st century." Seminar, 2002.

Delcourt, C, et al. "Age-related macular degeneration and antioxidant status in the POLA study: POLA study Group, pathologies Oculaires Liees a l'Age." *Arch Opth* 1999; 117(10): 384–389.

Mares-Perlman, J, et al. "Association of zinc and antioxidants with age-related maculopathy." *Arch Ophth* 1996; 114:991–7.

Newsome, D, et al. "Zinc content of human retinal pigment epithelium decreases with age and macular degeneration, but superoxide dismutase activity increases." *Jour Trace Elem Environ Med* 1995; 193–9.

Seddon, J, et al. "Dietary carotenoids, vitamins A, C, and E, and advanced age-related macular degeneration; eye disease case-control study group." *JAMA* 1994; 272(18):1413–1420.

VandenLangenberg, G, et al. "Association between antioxidant and zinc intake and the 5-year incidence of early age-related maculopathy in the Beaver Dam Eye Study." *Amer Jour Epidemol* 1998; 148:204–14.

Winkler, B, et al. "Oxidative damage and age-related macular degeneration." *Mol Vis* 1999; 5:32.

Migraine Headaches

Crayhon, R. "Aging well in the 21st century." Seminar, 2002.

Crayhon, R. *Designs for Health Institute's Level II Eating and Supplement Plans.* Boulder, CO: Designs for Health Institute, Inc, 1999.

Gawel, M, et al. "The use of feverfew in the prophylaxis of migraine attacks." *Today's Ther Trends* 1995; 13(20):79–86.

McCaren, T, et al. "Amelioration of severe migraine by fish oil (n-3) fatty acids." *Am J Clin Nutr* 1985; 41:874.

Murphy, J, et al. "Randomized double-blind placebo-controlled trial of feverfew in migraine prevention." *Lancet* 1988; 2(8604): 189–192.

Rozen, T, et al. "Open-label trial of high-dose coenzyme Q-10 as a migraine preventive." *Cephalgia* 2001; 21:3880–3881. Abstract P2–130.

Schoenen, J, et al. "Effectiveness of high-dose riboflavin in migraine prophylaxis. A randomized controlled trial." *Neurol* 1998; 50(2):466–470.

Thomas, J, et al. "Serum and erythrocyte magnesium concentrations and migraine." *Magnes Res* 1992; 5(2):127–130.

Thys-Jacobs, S, et al. "Alleviation of migraines with therapeutic vitamin D and calcium." *Headache* 1994; 34(10):590–592.

Thys-Jacobs, S, et al. "Vitamin E and calcium in menstrual migraine." *Headache* 1994; 34(9):544–546.

Vogler, B, et al. "Feverfew as a preventive treatment for migraine: a systematic review." *Cephalalgia* 1998; 18(10):704–708.

Multiple Sclerosis

Delanty, N, et al. "Antioxidant therapy in neurologic disease." *Arch Neruol* 2000; 57:1265–1270.

Dworkin, R, et al. "Linoleic acid and multiple sclerosis: a reanalysis of three double-blind trials." *Neurology* 1984; 34:1441–1445.

Ghadrian, P, et al. "Nutritional factors in the aetiology of MS: A case-control study in Montreal Canada." *Int J Epidmiol* 1998; 27(5): 845–852.

Hayes, C, et al. "Vitamin D and multiple sclerosis." *Proc Soc Exp Biol Med* 1997; 216:121–127.

Laur, K, et al. "Diet and multiple sclerosis." *Neurology* 1997; 49(Suppl 2):S55–S61.

Lebrun, C, et al. "Levocarnitine administration in multiple sclerosis patients with immunosuppressive therapy-induced fatigue." *Mult Scler* 2006; 12:321–324.

Nieves, J, et al. "High prevalence of vitamin D deficiency and reduced bone mass in multiple sclerosis." *Neurol* 1994; 44(9):1687–1692.

Nordvik, I, et al. "Effect of dietary advice and n-3 supplementation in newly diagnosed multiple sclerosis patients." *Acta Neurol Scand* 2000; 102:143–149.

Perlmutter, D. *BrainRecovery.com.* Naples, FL: The Perlmutter Health Center, 2000.

Perlmutter, D. "Multiple Sclerosis functional approaches." *Townsend Letter For Doctors and Patients* Nov. 2003; 244.

Reynolds, E, et al. "Multiple sclerosis and vitamin B12 metabolism." *Jour Neuroimmun* 1992; 40:225–230.

Rudick, R, et al. "Management of multiple sclerosis." *NEJM* 1997; 337(22):1604–1667.

Swank, R, et al. "Effect of low saturated fat diet in early and late cases of MS." *Lancet* 1990; 336:37–39.

Swank, R, et al. "MS in rural Norway: its geographic and occupational incidence in relation to nutrition." *NEJM* 1952; 246:721–728.

Swank, R, et al. "MS: the lipid relationship." *Am J Clin Nutr* 1988; 48(6):1387–1339.

Swank, R, et al. "Multiple sclerosis: twenty years on a low fat diet." *Arch Neurol* 1970; 23:460–474.

Myasthenia Gravis

Calder, P, et al. "N-3 polyunsaturated fatty acids and cytokine production in health and disease." *Ann Nutr Metab* 1997; 41(4):203–234.

Crayhon, R. *Designs For Health Institute's Eating and Supplement Plans.* Boulder, CO: Designs for Health Institute, 2000.

Fernandes, G, et al. "Dietary lipids and risk of autoimmune disease." *Clin Immunopathol* 1994; 72(2):193–197.

Robinson, D, et al. "Suppression of autoimmune disease by dietary n-3 fatty acids." *J Lipd Res* 1993; 34(8):1435–1444.

Osteoarthritis

Drovanti, A, et al. "Therapeutic activity of oral glucosamine sulfate in osteoarthritis: a placebo-controlled, double-blind investigation." *Clin Ther* 1980; 3:260–272.

Flynn, D, et al. "Inhibition of human neutrophil-lipoxygenase activity by ginger dione shagaol, capsaicin, and related pungent compounds." *Prostaglandins Leukotr Med* 1986; 24:195–198.

McAlinton, T, et al. "Glucosamine and chondrotin for the treatment of ostoarthritis." *JAMA* 2002; 283:1469–1475.

Morreale, P, et al. "Comparison of the antiinflamatory efficacy of chondroitin sulfate and dicolfenac sodium in patients with knee osteoarthritis." *J Rheumatol* 1996; 23:1385–1391.

Reginster, J, et al. "Long-term effects of glucosamine sulfate on osteoarthritis progress, placebo-controlled trial." *Lancet* 2001; 357: 251–256.

Sato, M, et al. "Quercetin, a bioflavonoid, inhibits the induction of interleukin gamma and monocyte chemoattractant protein-expression by tumor necrosis factor-alpha in cultured human synovial cells." *J Rheumatol* 1997; 24(9): 1680–1694.

Srivastava, L, et al. "Ginger (Zingiber offici-nale) in rheumatism and musculoskeletal disorders." *Med Hypothesis* 1992; 39(4):342–348.

Travers, R, et al. "Boron and arthritis: the results of a double-blind pilot study." *J Nutr Med* 1990; 1:127–132.

Uebelhart, D, et al. "Effects of oral chondrotin sulfate on the progression of knee osteoarthritis: a pilot study." *Osteoarthritis Cartilage* 1998; 6(Suppl A): 39–46.

Vaz, A, et al. "Double-blind-clinical evaluation of the relative efficacy of ibuprofen and glucosamine sulfate in the management of the knee in out-patients." *Curr Med Resp Opin* 1982; 8:145–149.

Osteoporosis

Adami, S, et al. "Impriflavone prevents radical bone loss in postmenopausal woman with low bone mass over 2 years." *Osteoporosis Int* 1997; 7:119–126.

Agnusdei, D, et al. "Effects of ipriflavone on bone mass and calcium metabolism in postmenopausal osteoporosis." *Bone Mineral* 1992; 19(Suppl):S43–S48.

Coats, C, et al. "Negative effects of high protein diet." *Fam Prac Recert* 1990; 12(12):80–88.

Crayhon, R. *Designs For Health Institute's Eating and Supplement Plans.* Boulder, CO: Designs for Health Institute, 2000.

Dawson-Hughes, B, et al. "Effect of calcium and vitamin D supplementation in bone density in women and men 65 years of age or older." *NEJM* 1997; 337:670–676.

Dimai, H, et al. "Daily oral magnesium supplementation suppresses bone turnover in young adult males." *J Clin Endocrin Metab* 1998; 83(8):2742–2748.

Gaby, A. *Preventing and Reversing Osteoporosis.* Rocklin, CA: Prima Publishing, 1994.

Germano, R. *The Osteoporosis Solution.* New York, NY: Kensington Publishing Corp, 1999.

Gittleman, A. *Super Nutrition for Menopause.* New York, NY: Avery Publishing Group, 1998.

Head, K, et al. "Ipriflavone: an important bone-building isoflavone." *Altern Med Rev* 1999; 4(1):10–22.

Krall, E, et al. "Smoking increases bone loss

and decreases intestinal calcium absorption." *J Bone Miner Res* 1999; 14(2):215–220.

Kruger, M, et al. "Calcium, gamma-linolenic acid and eicosapentaenoic acid supplementation in senile osteoporosis." *Aging* 1998; 10(5): 385–394.

Lloyd, T, et al. "Dietary caffeine intake and bone status of postmenopausal women." *Am J Clin Nutr* 1997; 65(6):1826–1830.

Melhus, H, et al. "Smoking, antioxidant vitamins, and the risk of hip fracture." *J Bone Miner Res* 1999; 14(1):129–135.

Niewoehner, C, et al. "Steroid-induced osteoporosis. Are your asthmatic patients at risk?" *Postgrad Med* 1999; 105(3):79–83, 87–88, 91.

Ooms, M, et al. "Prevention of bone loss by vitamin D supplementation in elderly women." *J Clin Endocrinol Metabol* 1995; 80:1052–1058.

Peris, P, et al. "Etiology and presenting symptoms in male osteoporosis." *Br J Rheumatol* 1995; 34(10):935–941.

Reginster, Y, et al. "Ipriflavone: pharmacological properties and usefulness in postmenopausal osteoporosis." *Bone Mineral* 1993; 23:223–232.

Sojka, J, et al. "Magnesium supplementation and osteoporosis." *Nutr Rev* 1995; 53(3):71–74.

Tamatani, M, et al. "Decreased circulating levels of vitamin k and 25-OH vitamin D in osteopenic elderly men." *Metabol* 1999; 47(2): 195–199.

Vermeer, C, et al. "Effects of vitamin K on bone mass and bone metabolism." *J Nutr* 1996; 126(Supl 14):1187S–1191S.

Parkinson's Disease

Beal, M, et al. "Coenzyme Q_{10} as a possible treatment for neurodegenerative diseases." *Free Rad Res* 2002; 36(4):455–460.

DeRijk, M, et al. "Dietary antioxidants and Parkinson's disease: The Rotterdam study." *Arch Neurol* 1997; 54:762–765.

Fahn, S, et al. "A pilot trial of high-dose alpha-tocophero and ascorbate in early Parkinson's disease." *Ann Neurol* 1992; 32(Suppl):S128– S132.

Perlmutter, D. *BrainRecovery.com.* Naples, Florida: The Perlmutter Health Center, 2000.

Sato, Y, et al. "High prevalence of vitamin D deficiency and reduced bone mass in Parkinson's disease." *Neurol* 1997; 49(5):1273–1278.

Sechi, G, et al. "Reduced glutathione in the treatment of early Parkinson's disease." *Prog Neuropsychopharmacol Biol Psychi* 1996; 20(7): 1159–1170.

Shults, C, et al. "Effects of coenzyme Q_{10} in early Parkinson's disease: evidence of slowing of the functional decline." *Arch Neurol* 2002 59(10):1541–1550.

Shults, C, et al. "A possible role of coenzyme Q_{10} in the etiology and treatment of Parkinson's disease." *Biofactors* 1000; 9(2-4):267–272.

Periodontal Disease

Crayhon, R. *Designs for Health Institute's Level II Eating and Supplement Plans.* Boulder CO: Designs for Health Institute, Inc, 1999.

Hansen, I, et al. "Gingival and leukocytic deficiencies of coenzyme Q_{10} in patients with periodontal disease." *Res Commun Chem Pathol Pharmacol* 1976; 14(4):729–738.

Polycystic Ovarian Syndrome (PCOS)

Ahene, S, et al. "Polycystic ovary syndrome." *Nurs Stand* 2004; 18(26):40–4.

Boulman, M, et al. "Increased c-reactive protein levels in the polycystic ovary syndrome: a marker of cardiovascular disease." *J Clin Endocrinol Metabol* 2004; 89(5):2160–5.

Christian, R, et al. "Prevalence and predictors of coronary artery calcification in women with polycystic ovary syndrome." *J Clin Endocrinol Metab* 2003; 88(6):2562–8.

Danaif, A, et al. "Beta cell dysfunction independent of obesity and glucose intolerance in the polycystic ovary syndrome." *J Clin Endocrinol Metab* 1996; 81:942–7.

De Leo, V, et al. "Polycystic ovary syndrome and type 2 diabetes mellitus." *Minera Ginecol* 2004; 56(1):53–62.

Gambineri, A, et al. "Obesity and the polycystic ovary syndrome." *Int Jour Obes Relat Metab Disord* 2002; 26(7):883–96.

Gonzalez, C, et al. "Polycystic ovarian disease: clinical and biochemical expression." *Gynecol Obstet Mex* 2003; 71:253–8.

Harris, C. *The PCOS Protection Plan*. Carlsbad, CA: Hay House, Inc, 2006.

Kasim-Karakas, M, et al. "Metabolic and endocrine effects of a polyunsaturated fatty acid-rich diet in polycystic ovary syndrome." *J Clin Endocrinol Metabol* 2004; 89(2):615–20.

Lefebvre, P, et al. "Long-term risks of polycystic ovaries syndrome." *Gynecol Obstet Fertil* 2004; 32(3):193–8.

Legro, R, et al. "Prevalence and predictors of risk for Type 2 diabetes mellitus and impaired glucose tolerance in polycystic ovary syndrome: a prospective, controlled study in 254 affect women." *J Clin Endocrinol Metabol* 1999; 84(1):165–9.

Marantides, D, et al. "Management of polycystic ovary syndrome." *Nurse Pract* 1997; 22(12):34-8, 40-1.

Orio, F, et al. "The cardiovascular risk of young women with polycystic ovary syndrome: an observational analytical, prospective case-control study." *J Clin Endocrinol Metab* 2004; 89(8):3696–701.

Pelusi, B, et al. "Type 2 diabetes and the polycystic ovary syndrome." *Minerva Ginecol* 2004; 56(1):41–51.

Rai, R, et al. "Polycystic ovaries and recurrent miscarriage--a reappraisal." *Hum Repro* 2000; 15:612–5.

Rajkhowa, M., et al. "Polycystic ovary syndrome: a risk for cardiovascular disease." *Int Jour Obstet Gyn* 2000; 107(1):11–8.

Solomon, C, et al. "Long or irregular menstrual cycle as a marker for the risk of type 2 diabetes mellitus." *JAMA* 2001; 286(19):2421–6.

Talbott, E, et al. "Cardiovascular risk in women with polycystic ovary syndrome." *Obstet Gyn Clin North Amer* 2001; 28(1):111–33.

Wild, S, et al. "Cardiovascular disease in women with polycystic ovary syndrome at long-term follow-up: a retrospective cohort study." *Clin Endocril* 2000; 62(5):595–600.

Premenstrual Syndrome (PMS)

Hudson, T. "Menstrual cramps (dysmenorrhea): an alternative approach." *Townsend Letter*, Oct 2006; 130–34.

Murray, M. *The Healing Power of Herbs*. California: Prima Publications, 1995; 375.

Psoriasis

Block, W, et al. "Modulation of inflammation and cytokine production by dietary (n-3) fatty acids." *J Nutr* 1996; 126:1515–1533.

Crayhon, R. *Designs For Health Institute's Eating and Supplement Plans*. Boulder, CO: Designs for Health Institute, 2000.

Grattan, C, et al. "Essential-fatty-acid metabolites in plasma phospholipids in patients with ichthyosis vulgaris, acne vulgaris and psoriasis." *Clin Exp Dermatol* 1990; 15(3):174–176.

Wright, S, et al. "Oral evening primrose seed oil improves atopic eczema." *Lancet* 1982; 2:1120.

Rheumatoid Arthritis

Bland, J. "GALT: activation, inflammation, and premature aging." *Improving Genetic Expression in the Prevention of the Diseases of Aging*. Gig Harbor, WA: HealthComm International, Inc, 1998.

Brzeski, M, et al. "Evening primrose oil in patients with rheumatoid arthritis and side-effects of non-steroidal anti-inflammatory drugs." *Br J Rheumatol* 1991; 30:370–372.

Calder, P, et al. "N-3 polyunsaturated fatty acids and cytokine production in health and disease." *Ann Nutr Metab* 1997; 41(4):203–234.

Crayhon, R. *Designs For Health Institute's Eating and Supplement Plans*. Boulder, CO: Designs for Health Institute, 2000.

Deretz, A, et al. "Adjuvant treatment of recent onset of rheumatoid arthritis by selenium supplementation: preliminary observations." *Br J Rheumatol* 1992; 31:281–286.

Di Silvestro, R, et al. "Effects of copper supplementation on ceruloplasmin and copper-zinc superoxide dismutase in free-living rheumatoid arthritis patients." *Am J Clin Nutr* 1992; 11(2):177–180.

Fernandes, G, et al. "Dietary lipids and risk of autoimmune disease." *Clin Immunopathol* 1994; 72(2):193–197.

Kremer, J, et al. "Effects of high-dose fish oil on rheumatoid arthritis after stopping NSAID. Clinical and immune correlates." *Arthritis Rheum* 1995; 38:1107–1114.

Leventhal, L, et al. "Treatment of rheumatoid arthritis with black currant seed oil." *Br J Rheumatol* 1994; 33:847–852.

Robinson, D, et al. "Suppression of autoimmune disease by dietary n-3 fatty acids." *J Lipd Res* 1993; 34(8):1435–1444.

Tarp, U, et al. "Low selenium level in rheumatoid arthritis." *Scan J Rheumatol* 1985; 14:97–101.

Zurier, R, et al. "Gamma-linolenic acid treatment of rheumatoid arthritis: a randomized, placebo-controlled trial." *Arthritis Rheum* 1996; 39:1808–1817.

Scleroderma (Systemic Sclerosis)

Crayhon, R. *Designs for Health Institute's Level II Eating and Supplement Plans.* Boulder, CO: Designs for Health Institute, Inc, 1999.

Famularo, G, et al. "Carnitine deficiency in scleroderma." (letter) *Immunol Today* 1999; 20(5):246.

Herrick, A, et al. "Dietary intake of micronutrient antioxidants in relation to blood levels in patients with systemic sclerosis." *J Rheumatol* 1996; 23(4):650–653.

Sjögren's Syndrome

Calder, P, et al. "N-3 polyunsturated fatty acids and cytokine production in health and disease." *Ann Nutr Metab* 1997; 41(4):203–234.

Crayhon, R. *Designs For Health Institute's Eating and Supplement Plans.* Boulder, CO: Designs for Health Institute, 2000.

Fernandes, G, et al. "Dietary lipids and risk of autoimmune disease." *Clin Immunopathol* 1994; 72(2):193–197.

Robinson, D, et al. "Suppression of autoimmune disease by dietary n-3 fatty acids." *J Lipd Res* 1993; 34(8):1435–1444.

Stroke

Crayhon, R. "Aging well in the 21st century." Seminar, 2002.

Perlmutter, D. *BrainRecovery.com.* Naples, FL: The Perlmutter Health Center, 2000.

Ulcerative Colitis

Goldin, B, et al. "Health benefits of probiotics." *Br J Nutr* 1998; 80(4):S203–S207.

Gupta, Il, et al. "Effects of Boswellia serrata gum resin in patients with ulcerative colitis." *Eur J Med Res* 1997; 2(1):37-43.

Lukaczer, D. "Gastroenterology, part II: gastrointestinal disorders: clinical applications using the functional medicine perspective." *Applying Functional Medicine in Clinical Practice.* Gig Harbor, WA: Institute for Functional Medicine, 2002.

Salomon, P, et al. "Treatment of ulcerative colitis with fish oil n-3-omega-fatty acid: an open trial." *J Clin Gastro* 1990; 12(2):157–161.

Souba, W, et al. "The role of glutamine in maintaining a healthy gut and supporting the metabolic response to injury and infection." *J Surgical Res* 1990; 48:383–391.

Stenson, W, et al. "Dietary supplementation with fish oil in ulcerative colitis." *Ann Int Med* 1992; 116(8):607–614.

Varicose Veins

Crayhon, R. "Aging well in the 21st century." Seminar, 2002.

Diehmetal, C, et al. "Comparison of leg compression stocking and oral horse chestnut seed extract therapy in patients with chronic venous insufficiency." *Lancet* 1996; 292–294.

Facino, R, et al. "Anti-elastase and anti-hyluronidase activities of saponins and sapogenins from Hedera helix, Aesculus hippocastanum, and Ruscus aculeatus: factors contributing to their efficacy in the treatment of venous insufficiency." *Arch Pharm* 1995; 328(10):720–724.

Pittler, M, et al. "Horse-chestnut seed extract for chronic venous insufficiency. A criteria-based systemic review." *Arch Dermatol* 1998; 134:1356–1360.

Pointel, J, et al. "Titrated extract of Centella asiatica (TECA) in the treatment of venous insufficiency of the lower limbs." *Angiology* 1987; 38(1Part 1):46–50.

Siebert, U, et al. "Efficacy, routine effectiveness, and safety of horse chestnut seed extract in the treatment of chronic venous insufficiency. A meta-analysis of randomized controlled trials and large observational studies." *Ant Angiol* 2002; 21(4):305–315.

Wound Healing

Quinn, P, et al. "Carnosine: its properties, functions and potential therapeutic application." *Mol Aspects Med* 1992; 13:379–444.

Roberts, P, et al. "Dietary peptides improve wound healing following surgery." *Nutrition* 1998; 14:266–269.

Vaxman, F, et al. "Can the wound healing process be improved by vitamin supplementation? Experimental study on humans." *Eur Surg Res* 1996; 28:306–314.

Vaxman, F, et al. "Effect of pantothenic acid and ascorbic acid supplementation on human skin wound healing process; A double-blind, prospective and randomized trial." *Eur Surg Res* 1995; 27:158–166.

PART 3

Birth Control Pills and Nutrition

Yanick, P. *Prohormone Nutriton*. Montaclair, NJ: Longevity Institute International, 1998.

Dieter's Nutrition

Anderson, R, et al. "Effects of chromium on body composition and weight loss." *Nutr Rev* 1998; 56(9):266–270.

Blankson, H, et al. "Conjugated linoleic acid reduces body fat mass in overweight and obese humans." *J Nutr* 2000; 130:2943–2948.

Crayhon, R. "Aging well in the 21st century." Seminar, 2002.

Crayhon, R. *Designs For Health Institute's Eating and Supplement Plans*. Boulder, CO: Designs for Health Institute, 2000.

Smith, P. *Demystifying Weight Loss*. Traverse City, MI: Healthy Living Books, 2007.

Enhancing Detoxification

The Importance of Detoxificaion. Advanced Nutritional Publications, Inc, 2002.

"Understanding Fatigue: Addressing the Molecular Basis of Chronic Metabolic Disorders." ACE Seminar, 2001.

Enhancing Energy

Crayhon, R. *The Carnitine Miracle*. New York, NY: M. Evans and Company, 1998.

Johns, D, et al. "Mitochondrial DNA and disease." *NEJM* 1995; 333:638–644.

Enhancing Immunity

Barringer, T, et al. "Effect of a multivitamin and mineral supplement on infection and quality of life. A randomized, double-blind, placebo-controlled trial." *Ann Int Med* 2003; 138(5):365–371.

Burger, R, et al. "Echinacea-induced cytokine production by human macrophages." *Int J Immunopharmacol* 1997; 19(7):371–379.

Chandra, R, et al. "Nutrition and the immune system: an introduction." *Am J Clin Nutr* 1997; 66(2):460S–463S.

Crayhon, R. *Designs For Health Institute's Eating and Supplement Plans*. Boulder, CO: Designs for Health Institute, 2000.

Cunningham-Rundles, S, et al. "Nutrition and the immune system of the gut." *Nutrition* 1998; 14(7-8):573–579.

DeSimone, C, et al. "The role of probiotics in modulation of the immune system in man and in animals." *In J Immunother* 1993; IX(1):23–28.

Folkers, K, et al. "The activites of coenzyme Q_{10} and vitamin B_6 for immune responses." *Biochem Biophys Res Comm* 1993; 193(1):88–92.

Harbige, L, et al. "Dietary n-6 and n-3 fatty acids in imunity and autoimmune disease." *Pro Nutr Soc* 1998; 57(4):555–562.

Meydani, S, et al. "Vitamin E enhacement of T-cell-mediated function in healthy elderly: mechanism of action." Nutr Rev 1995; 53:552–558.

Meydani, S, et al. "Vitamin E supplementation and in vivo immune response in healthy elderly subjects." *JAMA* 1997; 277:1380–1386.

Rountree, R. *Immunotics*. New York, NY: Berkley Publishing Group, 2000.

Thurnham, D, et al. "Micronutrients and immune function: some recent developments." *J Clin Pathol* 1997; 50(11):887–891.

Liver Health

Albrecht, M, et al. "Therapies of toxic liver

pathology with legalon." *J Clin Med* 1992; 47:87–92a.

Crayhon, R. *Designs For Health Institute's Eating and Supplement Plans.* Boulder, CO: Designs for Health Institute, 2000.

Flora, K, et al. "Milk thistle (silybum marianum) for the therapy of liver disease." *Am J Gastroenterol* 1998; 93(2):139–143.

Goldin, B, et al. "Health benefits of probiotics." *Br J Nutr* 1998; 80(4):S203–207.

Luper, S, et al. "A review of plants used in the treatment of liver disease: part I." *Altern Med Rev* 1998;3(6):410–421.

Rountree, R. "Immune Dysfunction and Inflammation, Part II." *Applying Functional Medicine I Clinical Practice.* Gig Harbor, WA: Institute for Functional Medicine, 2002.

Memory Enhancement

Crook, T, et al. "Effects of phosphatidylserine in age-associated memory impairment." *Neurology* 1991; 41(5):644–649.

Goldman, R. *Brain Fitness.* New York, NY: Doubleday, 1999.

Kidd, P, et al. "A review of nutrients and botanicals in the integrative management of cognitive dysfunction." *Alter Med Rev* 1999; 4(3):144–161.

Ley, B. *Marvelous Memory Boosters.* Temecula, CA: BL Publications, 2000.

Morris, M, et al. "Vitamin E and vitamin C supplement use and risk of incident Alzheimer's disease." *Alz Dis Assoc Disord* 1998; 12(3):121–126.

Muldoon, M, et al. *Amer Jour Med* 2000; 108:538–546.

Perlmutter, D. *BrainRecovery.com.* Naples, Florida: The Perlmutter Health Center, 2000.

Schmidt, M. *Brain-Building Nutrition: The Healing Power of Fats and Oils.* Berkeley, CA: Frog, Ltd, 2001.

Schreiber, S, et al. "An open trial of plant-source derived phosphatidylserine for treatment of age-related cognitive decline." *Isr J Psychiatry Relat Sci* 2000; 37(4):302–307.

Seshadri, S, et al. "Plasma homocysteine as risk factor for dementia and Alzheimer's disease." *NEMJ* 2002; 346:476–483.

Men's Health

Braeckman, J, et al. "The extract of serenoa repens in the treatment of BPH: a multicenter open study." *Ther Res* 1994; 55(7)776–785.

Fillion, M. *Natural Prostate Healers.* Paramus, NJ: Prentice Hall Press, 1999.

Fotsis, T, et al. "Genistein, and dietary ingested isoflavonoid, inhibits cell proliferation and in vitro angiogenesis." *J Nutr* 1995; 125:790S–797S.

Leake, A, et al. "The effect of zinc on the 5 alpha-reducion of testosterone by the hyperplastic human prostate gland." *J Steroid Biochem* 1984: 20(2):651–655.

Liang, T, et al. "Inhibition of steroid 5 alpha-reductase by specific aliphatic unsaturated fatty acids." *Biochem J* 1992; 285:557–562.

Niederprum, H. et al. "Testosterone 5 alpha-reductase inhibition by free fatty acids from sabal serrulata fruits." *Phytomedicine* 1994; 1:127–133.

Shippen, E. *The Testosterone Syndrome.* New York, NY: M. Evans and Company, 1998.

Thomas, J, et al. "Diet, micronutrients, and the prostate gland." *Nutr Rev* 1999; 57(4):95–103.

Weisser, J, et al. "Effects of the sabal serrulata extract IDS 89 and its subfractions on 5 alpha-reductase activity in human benign prostatic hyperplasia." *Prostate* 1996; 28:300–306.

Wilt, T, et al. "Saw palmetto extracts for treatment of BPH." *JAMA* 1998; 280(18):1604–1609.

Smoker's Nutrition

Ames, B. "Micronutrient deficiencies: a major cause of DNA damage." *Metabolic Energy, Messenger Molecules, and Chronic Illness: The Functional Perspective.* Gig Harbor, WA: The Institute for Functional Medicine, 2000.

Murata, A, et al. "Smoking and vitamin C." *World Rev Nutr Bio* 1999; 64:31–57.

Scheetman, G, et al. "Ascorbic acid requirements for smokers: analysis of a populations survey." *Am J Clin Nutr* 1991; 53:1466–1470.

Sports Nutrition

Antonio, J, et al. "Glutamine a potentially useful supplement for athletes." *Can J App Physiol* 1999; 24:1–14.

Applegate, E, et al. "Effective nutritional ergogemic aids." *Int J Sport Nutr* 1999; 9(2): 229–239.

Balakrishnan, S, et al. "Exercise, depletion of antioxidants and antioxidant manipulation." *Cell Biochem Funct* 1998; 1694):269–275.

Bertelli, A, et al. "Carnitine and coenzyme Q_{10}: biochemical properties and functions, synergism, and complementary action." *Int J Tissue React* 1990; 12(3):183–186.

Brilla, L, et al. "Effect of magnesium supplementation on strength training in humans." *J Am Coll Nutr* 1992; 11(3):326–329.

Bucci L, et al. "Selected herbals and human exercise performance." *Am J Clin Nutr* 2000; 72(Suppl)624S–636S.

Campbell, W, et al. "Effects of resistance training and chromium picolinate on body composition and skeletal muscle in older men." *J Appl Physiol* 1999; 86(1):29–39.

Clancy, S, et al. "Effects of chromium picolinate supplementation on body composition, strength, and urinary chromium loss in football players." *Int J Sport Nutr* 1994; 4(2):142–153.

Colgan, M. *Optimum Sports Nutrition.* New York, NY: Advanced Research Press, 1993.

Cordova, A, et al. "Behavior of zinc in physical exercise: a special reference to immunity and fatigue." *Neurosci Bebehav Rev* 1995; 19(3):-439–445.

Couzy, F, et al. "Zinc metabolism in the athlete: influence of training, nutrition, and other factors." *Int J Sports Med* 1990; 263–266.

Crayhon, R. *Designs for Health Institute's Level II Eating and Supplement Plans.* Boulder, CO: Designs for Health Institute, Inc, 1999.

Elam, R, et al. "Effects of arginine and ornithine on strength, lean body mass and urinary hydroxyproline in adult males." *J Sports Med Phys Fitness* 1989; 29(1):52–56.

Heath, G, et al. "Exercise and the incidence of upper respiratory tract infections." *Med Sci Sports Ex* 1991; 23:152–157.

Huertas, R, et al. "Respiratory chain enzymes in muscle of endurance athletes: effect of L-arginine." *Biochem Biophys Res Commun* 1992; 188(1):102–107.

Kelly, G, et al. "Sports nutrition: A review of selected nutritional supplements for endurance athletes." *Alt Med Rev* 1997; 2:282–295.

Konig, D, et al. "Zinc, iron, and magnesium status in athletes-influence on the regulation of exercise-induced stress and immune function." *Exerc Immun Rev* 1998; 4:2–21.

Lancha, A, et al. "Effect of aspartate, asparagine, and carnitine supplementation in the diet on metabolism of skeletal muscle during a moderate exercise." *Physiol Behav* 1995; 5792: 367–371.

Mittleman, K, et al. "Branched-chain amino acids prolong exercise during heat stress in men and women." *Med Sci Sports Exerc* 1998; 30(1):83–91.

Pyke, S, et al. "Severe depletion in liver glutathione during physical exercise." *Biochem Biophys Res Com* 1986; 139:926–931.

Ryan, A, et al. "Over training in athletes: a roundtable." *Physician Sports Med* 1983; 11: 93–100.

Schmidt, M. *Tired of Being Tired.* Berkeley, CA: Frog, Ltd, 1995.

Sen, C, et al. "Exercise-induced oxidative stress: glutathione supplementation and deficiency." *J Appl Physiol* 1994; 77(5):2177–2187.

Shimomuray, M, et al. "Protective effects of coenzyme Q_{10} on exercise-induced muscle injury." *Biochem Biophys Res Com* 1991; 176: 349–355.

Sumida, S, et al. "Exercise-induced lipid peroxidation and leakage of enzymes before and after vitamin E supplementation." *Int J Biochem* 1989; 21:835.

Sun Tanner's Nutrition

Packer, L. *The Antioxidant Miracle.* New York, NY: John Wiley & Sons, Inc, 1999.

Surgery and Nutrition

Crayhon, R. "Aging well in the 21st century." Seminar, 2002.

Crayhon, R. *Designs for Health Institute's Level II Eating and Supplement Plans.* Boulder, CO: Designs for Health Institute, Inc, 1999.

Furukawa, K, et al. "Effects of soybean oil

emulsion and eicosapentaenoic acid on stress response and immune function after a severely stressful operation." *Ann Surg* 1999; 229(2):255–261.

Nezu, R, et al. "Role of zinc in surgical nutrition." *J Nutr Sci Vitaminol* 1992; Spec:530–533.

Okeda, A, et al. "Zinc in clinical surgery: a research review." *Jpn J Surg* 1990; 2096:635–644.

Snyderman, C, et al. "Reduced post-operative infections with an immune-enhancing nutritional supplement." *Laryngoscope* 1999; 109(6): 915-921.

Vegetarianism

Crayhon, R. *Designs for Health Institute's Level II Eating and Supplement Plans*. Boulder, CO: Designs for Health Institute, Inc, 1999.

Women's Health

Abrahm, G, et al. "Effect of vitamin B_6 on PMS symptomatology in women with PMS syndromes. A double-blind, crossover study." *Infertility* 1980; 3(2):155–165.

Abraham, G, et al. "Nutrition and the premenstrual tension syndromes." *J Appl Nutr* 1984; 36:103.

Barr, W, et al. "Pyridoxine supplements in the PMS." *Practioner* 1984; 228:425–427.

Bermond, P, et al. "Therapy of side effects of oral contraceptive agents with vitamin B_6." *Acta Vitaminol Enzymol* 1982; 4(102):45–54.

Bell, M, et al. "Place-controlled trial of indole-3-carbinol in the treatment of CIN." *Gynecol Oncol* 2000; 78:123–129.

Bendich, A, et al. "The potential for dietary supplements to reduce premenstrual syndrome (PMS) symptoms." *J Am Col Nutr* 2000; 19(1); 3–12.

Butterworth, C, et al. "Folate deficiency and cervical dysplasia." *JAMA* 1992; 267:528–533.

Crayhon, R. "Aging well in the 21st century." Seminar, 2002.

Crayhon, R. *Designs For Health Institute's Eating and Supplement Plans*. Boulder, CO: Designs for Health Institute, 2000.

Deutch, B, et al. "Menstrual discomfort in Danish women reduced by dietary supplements of omega-3-PUFA and B12 (fish oil or seal oil capsules)." *Nutr Res* 2000; 20:621–631.

Facchinetti, F, et al. "Oral magnesium successfully relieves PMS mood changes." *Obstet Gynecol* 1991; 78:177–181.

Franks, S, et al. "Nutrition, insulin, and polycystic ovary syndrome." *Rev Reprod* 1996; 1(1):47–53.

Harel, Z, et al. "Supplementation with omega-3 polyunsaturated fatty acids in the management of dysmenorrhea in adolescents." *Am J Obstet Gynecol* 1996; 174:1335–1338.

Hays, B. "Applied endocrinology: women's hormones and women's health." *Applying Functional Medicine in Clinical Practice*. Gig Harbor, WA: Institute of Functional Medicine, 2002.

Heller, L. *Applying the Essentials of Herbal Care*. Gig Harbor, WA: Institute of Functional Medicine, 1999.

Holte, J, et al. "Polycystic ovarian syndrome and insulin resistance: thrifty genes struggling with over-feeding and sedentary lifestyle?" *J Endocrinol Invest* 1998; 21(9):589–601.

Horrobin, D, et al. "The role of essential fatty acids and prostaglandins in the premenstrual syndrome." *J Reprod Med* 1983:28(7):465–468.

Kleijnen, J, et al. "Vitamin B_6 in the treatment of the premenstrual syndrome: a review." *Br J Obstetrics Gynaecol* 1990; 94:847–852.

Lauritzen, C, et al. "Treatment of PMS with vitex agnus-castus controlled double-blind study vs. pyridoxine." *Photomedicine* 1997; 4(3):183–189.

London, R, et al. "Effect of nutritional supplement on premenstrual symptomatology in women with pre-menstrual syndrome: a double-blind longitudinal study." *J Am Coll Nutr* 1991; 10(5):494–499.

Murray, M. *The Healing Power of Herbs*. Rocklin: Prima Publications, 1995.

Nestler, J, et al. "Ovulatory and metabolic syndrome and the effect of D-chiro-inositol in the PCOS." *NEJM* 1999; 340:1314–1320.

Penland, J, et al. "Dietary calcium and manganese effects on menstrual cycle symptoms." *Am J Obstet Gynecol* 1993; 168(5):1417–1423.

Pizzorno, J. "Natural hormone balance: assessing and forming treatment programs."

Index

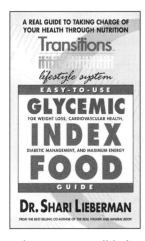

GLYCEMIC INDEX FOOD GUIDE

For Weight Loss, Cardiovascular Health, Diabetic Management, and Maximum Energy

Dr. Shari Lieberman

The glycemic index (GI) is an important nutritional tool. By indicating how quickly a given food triggers a rise in blood sugar, the GI enables you to choose foods that can help you manage a variety of conditions, as well as improve your overall health.

Whether you are interested in controlling your glucose levels to manage your diabetes, lose weight, increase your heart health, boost your energy level, or simply enhance your well-being, *Transitions Lifestyle System Glycemic Index Food Guide* is the best place to start.

$7.95 U.S. • 160 pages • 4 x 7-inch mass paperback • ISBN 978-0-7570-0245-8

THE ACID ALKALINE FOOD GUIDE

A Quick Reference to Foods & Their Effect on pH Levels

Dr. Susan E. Brown and Larry Trivieri, Jr.

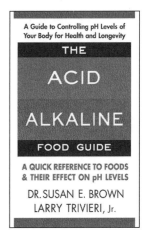

In the last few years, researchers around the world have reported the importance of acid-alkaline balance to good health. While thousands of people are trying to balance their body's pH level, until now, they have had to rely on guides containing only a small number of foods. *The Acid-Alkaline Food Guide* is a complete resource for people who want to widen their food choices.

The book begins by explaining how the acid-alkaline environment of the body is influenced by foods. It then presents a list of thousands of foods—single foods, combination foods, and even fast foods—and their acid-alkaline effects. *The Acid-Alkaline Food Guide* will quickly become the resource you turn to at home, in restaurants, and whenever you want to select a food that can help you reach your health and dietary goals.

$7.95 U.S. • 208 pages • 4 x 7-inch mass paperback • ISBN 978-0-7570-0280-9

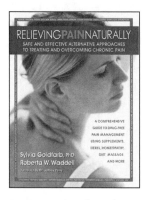

RELIEVING PAIN NATURALLY
Safe and Effective Alternative Approaches to Treating and Overcoming Chronic Pain
Sylvia Goldfarb, PhD and Roberta W. Waddell

For millions of Americans, severe pain is a fact of life. Standard drug therapies may offer relief, but come with a host of side effects, and can become less effective over time. While many would prefer nondrug options, the available information on alternative treatment has long been scattered or incomplete—or it was, until now. *Relieving Pain Naturally* is a comprehensive guide to drug-free pain management. Written in nontechnical language, this up-to-date resource is designed for ease of use and quick accessibility.

Relieving Pain Naturally begins by examining thirty-seven of the most common chronic pain-related conditions, from arthritis to tendonitis. It then offers twenty-seven drug-free therapies, including both conventional and alternative treatments. A resource section guides you to professional organizations that can help you find an appropriate therapist in your area. With *Relieving Pain Naturally*, it's easy to take that first step toward side-effect-free pain relief.

$18.95 US • 296 pages • 8.5 x 11-inch paperback • ISBN 978-0-7570-0079-9

NEVER SMOKE AGAIN
The Top 10 Ways to Stop Smoking Now & Forever
Grant Cooper, MD

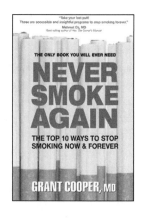

It isn't easy to stop smoking. Yet well over 45 million Americans have already quit. How? They found the method that worked for them and they stuck to it. This book can help you find the method that's right for you so that you never smoke again.

Never Smoke Again begins by explaining why you smoke cigarettes and how they keep you coming back for more. It then presents ten chapters, each of which focuses on one of the top ten techniques for quitting smoking: cold turkey; tapering off; nicotine patches, gum, lozenges, nasal spray, and inhalers; Zyban; Chantix; and hypnosis. For each method, you'll discover what it is, how it works, how you can best use it, what its risks and drawbacks are, and how effective it is compared with other techniques.

$12.95 US • 160 pages • 6 x 9-inch paperback • ISBN 978-0-7570-0235-9

NATURAL MEDICINE, OPTIMAL WELLNESS

The Patient's Guide to Health and Healing

Jonathan V. Wright, MD, and Alan R. Gaby, MD

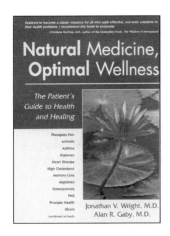

Imagine having holistic physicians at your fingertips to answer your medical questions. With *Natural Medicine, Optimal Wellness,* you do. For each condition, you'll sit in on a consultation between Dr. Jonathan Wright and a patient seeking advice. By the conclusion of each visit, you'll have a complete understanding of why Dr. Wright prescribes particular natural treatments. Then, Dr. Alan Gaby follows up with an analysis of the scientific evidence behind the treatments discussed, enabling you to make informed decisions about your health.

$21.95 • 400 pages • 8.5 x 11-inch paperback • ISBN 978-1-890612-50-4

THE YEAST CONNECTION HANDBOOK

How Yeasts Can Make You Feel "Sick All Over" and the Steps You Need to Take to Regain Your Health

William G. Crook, MD

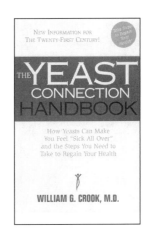

Most people don't realize how many health disorders can be caused by yeast. Fatigue, headache, depression, digestive problems, PMS, sexual dysfunction, asthma, ADHD, and autism can all be yeast-related. But once you recognize that yeast is the offender, what can you do to regain your health?

The Yeast Connection Handbook is a great resource for anyone who wants to learn about yeast-related problems. The book is comprehensive, not only discussing a wide range of health disorders, but also addressing a wide range of sufferers, including men, women, and children. Most important, this book provides a step-by-step program that effectively relieves health problems through dietary changes, nutritional supplements, medication, and simple lifestyle changes. If you've been looking for a solution to your yeast-related problem, *The Yeast Connection Handbook* provides the information you need to take charge of your health.

$15.95 • 288 pages • 6 x 9-inch paperback • ISBN 978-0-7570-0060-7

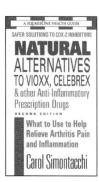

NATURAL ALTERNATIVES TO VIOXX, CELEBREX
& OTHER ANTI-INFLAMMATORY PRESCRIPTION DRUGS
Carol Simontacchi

Beyond today's headlines is an underlying truth—COX-2 inhibitors can be dangerous to your health. This guide points the way to far safer alternatives. It first examines the cause of arthritis pain, and then discusses the most effective supplements available for the treatment of this condition. Here is a vital resource for those looking for a better solution.

$5.95 • 128 pages • 4 x 7-inch mass paperback • ISBN 978-0-7570-0278-6

NATURAL ALTERNATIVES TO LIPITOR, ZOCOR
& OTHER STATIN DRUGS
Jay S. Cohen, MD

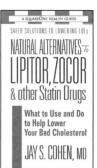

Elevated cholesterol and C-reactive proteins are markers linked to heart attack, stroke, and other cardiovascular disorders. While modern science has created a group of drugs known as statins to combat these problems, nearly 50 percent of the people who take them experience side effects. This guide explains the problems caused by statins and highlights the most effective natural alternatives.

$7.95 • 144 pages • 4 x 7-inch mass paperback • ISBN 978-0-7570-0286-1

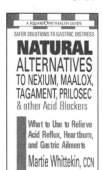

NATURAL ALTERNATIVES TO NEXIUM, MAALOX, TAGAMENT, PRILOSEC
& OTHER ACID BLOCKERS
Martie Whittekin, CCN

Natural Alternatives to Nexium, Maalox, Tagament, Prilosec & Other Acid Blockers begins by examining how acid blockers work, and discusses possible long-range side effects. It then explains those underlying causes of the problem that can be corrected. Finally, the author highlights the most important natural alternatives. If you suffer from the pain of recurrent gastric upset, or if you are currently using an acid blocker, *Natural Alternatives* can make a profound difference in the quality of your life.

$7.95 • 160 pages • 4 x 7-inch mass paperback • ISBN 978-0-7570-0210-6